Ethics and Human Values in Medical Sciences

A View from the Perspective of Indian Culture and Tradition

Niru Hazarika

CONCEPT PUBLISHING COMPANY PVT. LTD.
NEW DELHI-110059

ISBN-13: 978-93-5125-225-2

First Published 2016

Published and Printed by:

Concept Since 1974

Concept Publishing Company Pvt. Ltd.
A/15-16, Commercial Block, Mohan Garden,
New Delhi-110059 (INDIA)
Phones : 25351460, 25351794, *Fax* : 091-11-25357109
E-mail : publishing@conceptpub.com
Website: www.conceptpub.com

Editorial Office: H-13, Bali Nagar, New Delhi-110 015, India.

Cataloging in Publication Data—DK Courtesy: D.K. Agencies (P) Ltd. <docinfo@dkagencies.com>

Hazarika, Niru, 1947- **author.**

Ethics and human values in medical sciences : a view from the perspective of Indian culture and tradition / Niru Hazarika.

pages cm

Includes bibliographical references and index.

ISBN 9789351252252

1. Medical ethics—India. 2. Social values—India. 3. India—Civilization. I. Title.

R724.H39 2016 DDC 174.2 23

Dedicated to
all the physicians who are serving the
ailing people with due honour to
Human Rights and Ethical
principles of Medical Sciences

Acknowledgements

Being a student of Political Science with specialization in Public Administration I had to make an extra effort to understand the Indian Philosophy and ethical aspect of the major religions of the world while preparing the book. I depended heavily on the books authored by several eminent scholars on these subjects. I will be indebted to them throughout my life for enlightening me of insights of Indian culture and tradition.

I am extremely grateful to Dr. Sanjeev Bhoi, Additional Professor and In-charge, Department of Emergency Medicine, Additional Medical Superintendent, JPN APEX Trauma Centre, AIIMS, New Delhi for his valuable advice to proceed with my academic exercise in spite of his very busy schedule of work.

As regards the technical (medical) terms I had to depend upon Dr. Tej Prakash Sinha, Assistant Professor of the Department of Emergency Medicine, JPN APEX Centre, AIIMS, New Delhi for interpretation. I am extremely thankful to him for his kind cooperation by explaining the issues in a very clear and communicative way.

I am grateful to Dr. Dhruba Jyoti Bhowmick, Former Dean, School of Social Sciences, University of North Bengal for going through the manuscript and valuable suggestions for finalization of the book.

I must express my heartiest thanks to Dr. Himanta Biswa Sarma, Former Minister of Health and Education, Government of Assam for extending his kind cooperation to overcome the difficulties I faced to observe several formalities while undertaking the task.

My thanks are also due to Sri Jatindra Borah, IDOL, Gauhati University, Sri Dipu Kumar Das, Owner of a Computer Centre, Guwahati, Sri Joydeep Baruah, cricket player, Dr. Minu Hazarika, Jalukbari Higher Secondary School for extending cooperation in computerization, proof reading etc. whenever needed.

I am thankful to Sri Nagen Kalita and Sri Jyotish Talukdar, members of the Rukminigaon Housefed Apartment Family, Guwahati for helping me in various ways while preparing the book.

My thanks are also due to Concept Publishing Company (P) Ltd., New Delhi for undertaking the task of publication of the book.

Niru Hazarika

Preface

Rapid development of Information and Communication Technology (ICT) has brought radical changes in the administration-people interaction making it easy and fast. It has created the climate to conceive the ideas of 'Global Village' and 'e-governance.' It is no denying the fact that behind this progress of science and technology there remains the man's brain. Now, the task before us is to take the responsibility to transform the 'Global Village' into 'Global Human Village' for establishing peace and security in the world. It requires humanization of man's heart. In other words, integration of head, heart and hand of each individual in the modern democratic world is urgently needed. Mahatma Gandhi insisted on integration of word, work and thought of a man as a strong step towards this end. Since First World War efforts are being made by world leaders, especially through international organizations like League of Nations and United Nations of Organizations followed by various other organizations at the international and national levels towards peace and security of man. United Nations of Organizations is making serious efforts to sensitize the nations of the world about the significance of human rights in a democracy.

Health may be considered as a significant area to be taken care of for proving human security. Since 1970s, the responses of the UNO to health problems are noteworthy. Here mention may be made of 'Health for All' programme. It is a goal of the World Health Organization (WHO), which envisions securing the health and well-being of people around the world that has been popularized since then. It is the basis for the World Health Organization's primary health care strategy to promote health, human dignity, and enhanced quality of life.

Halfdan Mahler, Director General (1973-1983) of the WHO, defined 'Health For All' in 1981, as follows:

'Health For All' must be reachable to every individual within a country. "By 'Health' is meant a personal state of well-being not just the availability of health services—a state of health that enables a person to lead a socially and economically productive life. 'Health For All' implies the removal of the obstacles to health—that is to say, the elimination of malnutrition ignorance, contaminated drinking water and unhygienic housing – quite as much as it does the solution of purely medical problems such as lack of doctors, hospital beds, drugs and vaccines.

- Health For All means that health should be regarded as an objective of economic development.
- Health For All demands, ultimately, literacy for all. Until this becomes reality, it demands at least the beginning of an understanding of what health means for every individual.
- Health For All depends on continued progress in medical care and public health. The health services must be accessible to all through primary healthcare, in which basic medical help is available in every village, backed up by referral services to more specialized care. Immunization must similarly achieve universal coverage.
- Health For All is thus a holistic concept calling for efforts in agriculture, industry, education, housing and communications, just as much as in medicine and public health. Medical care alone is not enough to reach the hovels. Health for such people requires a whole new way of life and fresh opportunities to provide themselves with a higher standard of living." (en.wikipedia.org/wiki/Health_For_All)

In 1978, 134 health ministries signed the Alma Ata Declaration. The Declaration set a deadline of the year 2000 for achieving a level of health that would enable all of the world's people to lead a socially and economically productive life. The strategy to achieve this goal was focused on primary healthcare with the emphasis on community participation and tackling the underlying causes of disease such as poverty, illiteracy and poor sanitation.

In 1998, a new global health policy "Health for All in the 21st Century", incorporated additional elements not considered in Alma Ata. The importance of a gender perspective and the need to see health as central to sustainable human development are both emphasized. Also included the recognition of the growing importance of civil society in health governance. The new policy confirmed the goals of Health for All as:

- To attain health security for all.
- To achieve global health equity.
- To increase healthy life expectancy.
- To ensure access for all to essential health care of good quality.

More recently, and as a reflection of civil society's stronger influence on and participation in global health issues, the People's Health Assembly has produced a People's Health Charter. Based on an analysis of world health problems, as well as existing policies and porgramme, the Charter makes a set of recommendations to Governments as well as international organizations, the business sector, and non-governmental organizations. The Charter asserts that health is a human right and that "Health and human rights should prevail over economic and political concerns" and calls for the provision of "Universal and comprehensive primary health care, irrespective of people's ability to pay". (*http://www.who.int/trade/gloss ory03ary/st9/en*)

The above declarations and attempts of the World Health Organization underline importance of human right, civil society and human dignity in the mission to 'Health for All'. The healthcare service providers, especially the physicians in India are also concerned about human values and ethics. This had explicit expression in the International Conference on Health Policy : Ethics and Human Values held in New Delhi in 1986 under the auspices of Indian Council of Medical Research in collaboration with the Council of International Organization of Medical Sciences (Geneva). The physicians across the country participated in the conference and discussed various aspects of the problem and serious attempt was made to explore ways to safeguard human values.

WHO Director General Lee Jong-wook (2003-2006) reaffirmed the concept in the World Health Report 2003:

> "Health For All became the slogan for a movement. It was not just an ideal but an organizing principle everybody needs and is entitled to the highest possible standard of health. The principles remain indispensable for a coherent vision of global health. Turning that vision into reality calls for clarity both on the possibilities and on the obstacles that have slowed and in some cases reversed progress towards meeting the health needs of all

people. We have a real opportunity now to make progress that will mean longer, healthier lives for millions of people, turn despair into realistic hope, and lay the foundations for improved health for generations to come." (*http:/Wikipedia.org/wiki/Health_For_All*)

Recently, Narenda Modi, Prime Minister of India has indicated the effort of his Government to establish SMART Governance in the country. The SMART Governance is nothing but Simple, Moral, Accountable, Responsive and Transparent Governance. It is a strong step towards achievement of Global Human Village. No service to humanity which neglects the human aspect of it can be considered as a service in the true sense of the term.

Here reference may be made of the realization of the need of value-based administration in the United States mirrored in the books, 'Towards a New Public Administration : The Minnowbrook Perspective' and 'Public Administration in a Time of Turbulence' edited by Frank Marini and Dwight Waldo respectively which underline the values such as humanism, individual dignity, social justice etc. which engineered discussion on value-laden public administration under the leadership of Dwight Waldo and active participation of young scholars of the country in 1971. Further Osborne and Gaebler indicate some significant features of administration in the book, titled, 'Reinventing Government'. They emphasize on empowerment of the people to solve the problems rather than simply to deliver services, mission oriented service instead of rule-oriented service, investment on preventing problems rather than caring crises etc.

In India since ancient time the religious books, customs and tradition are giving priority to human values and dignity in administrative as well as social culture. The freedom struggle under the leadership of Mahatma Gandhi in India and the Constitution of India always remind us about the significance of human dignity and values. Today, it is the Prime Minister of India, Narendra Modi who is trying his best to strengthen the moral dimension of the governance in the country.

The most significant threshold in the path of human security is the United Nations declaration of 21st June as the International Yoga Day adopting the proposal of the Prime Minister of India Narendra Modi. It is really a great achievement for India to get the approval of the proposal by the 193-member UN General Assembly by consensus a resolution establishing a day to commemorate the ancient practice, which Modi called in September 2014 during his inaugural address to the world body.

UN Secretary General Ban Ki-moon said the International Day of Yoga would bring attention to Yoga's holistic benefits. "Yoga can contribute to resilience against non-communicable diseases. Yoga can bring communities together in an inclusive manner that generates respect." Ban said in a statement, " Yoga is a sport that can contribute development and peace. Yoga can even help people in emergency situations to find relief from stress." (*www.reuters-com/article/2014/12/11/us-un-yoga-iduskBNOJP20V20141211*)

Z.Bankowski, in his article, '*Ethics and Values in Health Policy*' (published in the World Health Forum, Volume 17, 1996) also said, "Mankind's most fundamental beliefs are those that concern life, suffering and death. They stem from what different societies hold and teach about the origin of man, the purpose of life, the significance of death. Health is influenced by beliefs. Hence, the understanding of beliefs can be of great help in formulating effective health policies which meet the requirements of ethical values and social justice."

Indian families till recently played a significant role inculcating the human values and dignity in the minds of the children. I have this experience in my own life. I had the privilege of spending more time with my grand parents during my childhood from whom I heard many stories with the very appealing messages to respect human beings in different ways – to elderly persons through service and obedience with utmost regards, to children through affection by offering some eatable things, because it is the simplest way to convey love and affection to them, to friends with interchange of opinion and exchange of ideas on day to day affairs. From the primary level to the University level, I had the opportunity of coming close to several teachers with strong personality and conviction that service to humanity is the service to God and for that one requires perseverance, and commitment to the cause of one's own profession and self-confidence. Thus, the values in human dignity are taught in the family itself in a most informal and convincing way in the day-to-day life itself through talk, control of behaviour of the children, guidance to maintain social relationships, narration of stories etc. On many occasions they used to control our behaviour by saying "should not do" or "should do" without explaining the reasons for it. In traditional societies generally ascriptive value system existed in the healthcare services also. The maintenance of secrecy was a common practice while giving advice to undertake certain activities or to behave in a particular manner while administering medicine for curing diseases and taking preventative measures for protection of health. Faith on the senior members of the family was the driving force to carry out our daily duties at home as well as at school.

Since ancient time, India is constructing the path on which people with different cultures can walk smoothly for rendering service to humanity through institutional devices as well as through customs and traditions which have been transmitted from generation to generation verbally. The achievements of the Takshashila University is very well known to all of us. The university was established more than 2700 years back where over 10,500 students from over the world came for higher studies in more than 64 different subjects. Chanakya, Panini, Charaka, Jivak etc. were the products of that University.

Next to Krishna and Shakuni, Chanakya occupies the position as an administrative consultant. Krishna is at the top in giving guidance to Pandavas in *Mahabharata* and then comes Shakuni for his guidance to Kauravas. Then comes Chanakya who guided Chandragupta Mauryan Empire. His *Niti-Shastra* focuses political ethics, addresses many problems of the administration and family and society.These have relevance even to-day. (*http://www.hibp.com/articles/history/takshashila-taxila-oldest-university*)

The customs, traditions, religions which are the important components of Indian social culture provide various ways to serve the human society effectively. The concept of administration and service can be understood with reference to human being only. Man is a social being and he is related to the society by some fundamental social needs as well as to realize his own self as human being. Every man has thinking faculty. The reasoning power of a man makes him supreme amongst all the beings in the world. So, the concept of man indicates not merely the physical organism, but also the inner and inherent qualities acquired by him through the mechanism of birth and the process of socialization or social environment. To move from 'being' to 'becoming' every person requires full development of personality. Then the personal qualities of a man must be activated or directed for the service to humanity as well as to retrain his own self to be away from all kinds of self-destructive acts. Because it will cause in the long run unrepairable damage to the society to which he belongs. Further, every organization or institution or society is judged on the basis of the qualities of the personnel associated with it. And it is the man not the machine who can inculcate moral and human values in the services. The deviation from the moral and human values by the service providers may cause serious constraints on the very survival of man. Because they are the role models for most common people.

The moral principles must be the driving force along with other devices provided by science and technology to achieve human security and peace in the world. Peace cannot be imposed from outside or by the laws of a country. It has to be generated by inner strength of a man. Laws can simply create an environment for it. But laws are essential and so is the case with society. The role of the family members and the immediate neighbours in creating congenial environment for enhancement of mental strength of a man can never be underestimated. Human culture flourishes in such situations. Every nation is in need of it and each nation is determining its goals considering good of its members based on these principles. In other words, the human society can be established only by human beings; just democracy can be made workable only by a democrat or by those who practice democratic principles with whole-hearted effort. Unless one is committed to the principles of democracy or unless a man realizes the significance of democracy he cannot apply his self with commitment in the process of democracy. Because to be committed to a particular ideals one must have understanding of it. The ethical principles induce a man to have clear and in-depth understanding of the concepts of human security, human dignity, peace of mind and their implications which go long way in the progress of a nation.

It is not the law nor the money nor the infrastructure nor the comfort provided by science and technology which can establish peace and security if there is ethical vacuity in the society. Unless the leaders realize the values of human dignity, develop love and affection for their countrymen, be sympathetic to weak and poor and take special care for the weak and hungry men they cannot help the nation to achieve its goals. The nation will certainly fail to be benefitted by their professional excellence only. The man who does not orient his professional excellence to the human goodness fails to grasp the philosophy of the laws of the country he is to serve. He misses the path to reach the nation's destiny. In contemporary India, we have to give a serious thought to the ability of the service providers who are not sensitive to the human values to take leading role in establishing good governance in the country and to what extent they can help India to contribute towards establishing a Global Human Village in the fast changing situation brought by the progress of science and technology.

The experience shows that the Insensitiveness of modern Indians to 'moral security' has become visible. They do not care to expose themselves to the 'moral risk'. The concept of service has changed to a great extent.

The elements like dedication, honesty, sense of mission to humanity etc. are thrown out of the concept of 'Service.'

The moral foundation of any public service organization in a democracy requires that administrators and public officials show a genuine care for their fellow citizens. Democratic values, such as equality, law, justice, right and freedom have moral connotations and demand an unwavering commitment from those who govern. Public servants are obliged to uphold these values. These values are enshrined in the Preamble to the Constitution of India itself. Democratic values warn us to view governmental efforts as moral endeavour.

The human values and ethical principles are rooted in the ancient society. Naturally with the progress of the society and modernization of way of life there emerges the ambiguity in the concept of morality. The co-existence of both tradition and modernity, the practice of modern way of living and at the same time valuing the age old tradition makes a man in modern India indecisive and creates confusing situation. (Presidential Address of O.P.Dwivedi :1988)

It is difficult to deny that the progress of science and technology cannot do away with the need of ethics in any society however modern it is. Democracy whether political or social must be based on ethical principles. It is true that the facilities and comfort provided by the modern technology expedites the development of a nation, helps solving very complicated problems caused by nature, relieves the suffering of the patients and provides scope to maintain good health, brings information from any part of the world within a moment to us.

Today a man is no longer satisfied with food, cloth and shelter only. His minimum needs have been increased with the changing situations. What is needed today is to explore the ways to safeguard the human aspect of the global society. It requires efforts to make modern man realize the dangerous consequences of ethical vacuity in our way of life. We must proceed in the escalator of progress of life but must carry with us the stick of humanism without which deviation from the path of progress is inevitable.

The Healthcare service is not only a great privilege, it is also a great responsibility. It is constrained by various limitations also. In many countries healthcare systems are facing enormous difficulties in meeting demands such as, distributing resources and providing adequate care due to the large number of patients in need. As these healthcare systems become larger and more bureaucratic, both practitioners and patients experience dehumanization. Healthcare practitioners often experience high levels of stress and burnout. The increase of the number of patients causes various kinds of hindrances in rendering service by the doctors and others effectively. The rising costs of medical services, technology and medication are becoming unaffordable for many patients preventing these individuals from receiving adequate healthcare. Experience also shows that poor doctor-patient relationship results in law suits against healthcare providers. The law suits have become a major burden to medical personnel and have risen in both number and cost (*en.wikipedia.org/wiki/ Humanistic medicine*).

Thus, the doctors often face a conflict between the professional commitment to the individual patient and social responsibility. Recently media has focused how the healthcare providers are exposed to conflicts or confrontations with the relatives and attendants of patients in India. It appears in *The Times of India*, a leading newspaper of the country that those who save lives are themselves at risk. More than 75 per cent of across the country have faced at least some form of violence as per initial findings of Indian Medical Association (IMA). (*timesofindia.indiatimes.com/india/ over-75%-of-doctors-have- faced-violence-at-work-study-finds/article show/147143806*)

At the same time allegations are also appearing in media on cases of medical errors and negligence, corrupt practices in the healthcare services due to which harm is done to the patients. While dealing with these issues, it has to be mentioned that the 55th World Health Assembly resolved in October 2005 at WHO headquarters on patient safety while Global Patient Safety Challenge as the core programme of the "World Alliance for patient Safety" launched in that year.

India, which was one of the eight prominent member countries to participate in the event, has committed to work towards the cause of promoting Patient Safety. A pledge to this effect was signed by the Ministry of Health and Family Welfare, Government of India, in the presence of the WHO representatives on 14th July, 2006 at New Delhi. Keeping the commitment in mind the Department of Hospital Administration, AIIMS in collaboration of WHO has taken the lead to launch the programme, 'National Initiative on Patient Safety' (NIPS) in 2009. Series of comprehensive workshops have been organized, involving multidisciplinary teams comprising of senior surgeons, physicians, microbiologists, medical superintendents and nursing officers from various medical colleges and hospitals across India under the leadership of Dr. Shakti Gupta as the Programme Director of NIPS and Head of the Department of Hospital Administration, AIIMS.

While taking care of the safeguard of the patients, it is difficult to ignore the safeguard of rights and health of the medical service providers in the face of conflicts, degradation of faith of the patients on them, experience of violent situations while in service to the patients, and various other constraints in the process.

Ethics deals with all aspects of human behaviour and decision-making. It is a very large and complex field of study with many branches and sub-divisions. The book is a modest effort to discuss ethics and human values in a limited way with the experience in India. As an academic discipline, medical ethics has developed its own vocabulary, including many terms that have been borrowed from philosophy. I depend heavily on the writings of several scholars in the field and the literature published by different organizations at international and national levels to express my ideas.

There is a close relationship between human rights and medical ethics. With growth and development of the concept of human rights emphasis is given on medical ethics. In recent years medical ethics has been greatly influenced by development of human rights. In a pluralistic and multi-cultural world, with many moral traditions, the major international human rights agreements can provide a foundation to medical ethics that is acceptable across national and cultural boundaries. Moreover, physicians frequently have to deal with problems resulting from violation of human rights. They are also greatly affected by the debate over whether healthcare is a human right.

Medical ethics is also closely related to law. In many countries there are laws that specify how physicians are required to deal with ethical issues in patient's care and research.

Gauhati **Niru Hazarika**
12.2.2016

Contents

ONE
Introduction

Humanism places a high value on human beings. To-day humanism in healthcare reminds us that illness and recovery, living and dying are an integral part of the life of a person. In the healthcare system like any other human system every person involves in it is human being. It also reminds us that we are all the members of a human society. The Health service is not only a great privilege to the service providers to enjoy it is also a great responsibility for them to be carried out at every moment with commitment to the profession.
(*www.arts.auckland.ac.nz/hoa/social-science-for-for-public health.*)

One must try to integrate head, heart and hand not only in the healthcare system, but in each and every system. Humanistic medicine or value-based medicine is an interdisciplinary field, in the practice of clinical care, aimed at addressing the problems of contemporary healthcare. The fundamental principles of humanistic medicine are open communication, mutual respect and emotional connection between physicians and their patients, relationship-centred or patient-centred care, in contrast to case-centred or disease-centred care.

In many countries with modern medical technology, healthcare systems are facing enormous difficulties in meeting demands such as, distributing resources and providing adequate care due to the large number of patients in need. As these healthcare systems become larger and more bureaucratic, both practitioners and patients experience dehumanization. Healthcare practitioners often experience high levels of stress and burnout. Doctors facing a large number of patients are not in a position to give the patients due attention they need. This situation is experienced specially in the public or government hospitals. The rising costs of medical services, technology and medication are becoming unaffordable for many patients preventing these individuals from receiving adequate healthcare.

Experience also shows that poor doctor-patient relationship results in law suits against healthcare providers. The law suits have become a major burden to medical personnel and have risen in both number and cost (*en.wikipedia.org/wiki/Humanistic medicine*).

A global and serious thought was given, after the global efforts during Second World War to safeguard human rights of the peoples, on the eve of the thirtieth anniversary of the Universal Declaration of Human Rights. UNESCO, with the close co-operation of the Government of the Federal Republic of Austria, convened the first International Congress on the Teaching of Human Rights. The Congress served dual purposes—first, it marked this anniversary with a stock-taking of the situation in the world concerning education for human rights, thirty years after the General Assembly proclaimed the Universal Declaration of Human Rights, "as a common standard of achievement for all peoples and all nations, to the end that every individual and every organ of society, keeping this Declaration constantly in mind, shall strive by teaching and education to promote respect for these rights and freedoms...." Secondly, it provided an opportunity for specialists in human rights teaching research, together with those responsible for education policies of UNESCO member states, to exchange their views and experience freely to adopt a series of conclusions and recommendations.

The sequence of events leading to the convening of the Congress began with the proposal for such a meeting made by Willibald Pahr, Federal Minister of Foreign Affairs of the Republic of Austria, to the Nineteenth General Conference of UNESCO, held in Nairobi, Kenya in November 1976. Ultimately, United Nations Commission on Human Rights, in Resolution No. 3 at its 33rd session (February-March 1977), recommended that education for human rights be chosen as an appropriate theme to mark the thirtieth anniversary year of the Universal Declaration of Human Rights.

The International Congress on the Teaching of Human Rights was set for 12-16 September, 1978 in the Kongresszentrum of the Hofburg Palace, Vienna. Experts from all regions of the world were invited by the Director-General to participate in their individual capacities. Representatives from organizations of the United Nations system and observers from non-governmental organizations in consultative status with UNESCO were invited to attend the Congress. The Congress was opened on 12th September by Amadou-Mahtar M' Bow, Director General of UNESCO.

The Congress along with other recommendations relating to teaching and research in human rights, suggested the following: "The concept of human rights should not be formulated in traditional or classical terms but should include the history and contributions of all peoples particularly in relation to the major contemporary problems, such as self-determination and all forms of discrimination and exploitation."

Human Rights education and teaching must aim at:

(i) Fostering the attitudes of tolerance, respect and solidarity inherent in human rights;
(ii) Providing knowledge about human rights, in both their national and international dimensions, and the institutions established for their implementation; and
(iii) Developing the individual's awareness of the ways and means by which human rights can be translated into social and political reality at both the national and international levels.

Further it was also suggested that human rights must be seen as an aspect of professional, ethical and social responsibility in all fields of research, study, teaching and work.

Referring to the teaching of human rights and professional ethics in the faculties or schools of medicine, it is found that a world survey on the subject was carried out, at UNESCO's request, by the International Institute of Human Rights in 1977-78. The Surveyors made it clear that without slackening the attention paid to law and political science, efforts were made to discover the importance attached to this question in the framework of the teaching of medicine and medical sciences in order that it may be possible to evaluate what needs to be done and what resources are required to develop medical ethics in the faculties of schools concerned. Further UN Commission on Human Rights has been regularly considering the topic of Human Rights and Scientific and Technological Developments. The relationship between human rights and medical ethics occupies a prominent place in the discussion at the international level and India cannot remain isolated from it as the progress of science and technology in the field of medicine and medical sciences is entering into the process of healthcare process of the country. (UNESCO: 1978)

The concept of health is no longer confined to the curing of diseases and absence of disease. The responsibility of medical professionals in taking care of public health must be shared by the public. The concept of health is too wide in scope and meaning. It embraces almost each and every aspect of individual as well as social life. Healthcare may be considered even as a social responsibility to be carried out at the moral and expert leadership of medical professionals in a country. It is more true in the case of a country like India because of its cultural uniqueness.

The evolving nature of the concept of 'health' is coming to surface very prominently since 1970s when the global community realized the importance of primary healthcare service at the grassroots level with the active cooperation of the people across the world through their day-to-day activities. The global effort to achieve health for all goal is a very strong threshold towards translating the idea of global village along with the effort of Information and Communication Technology (ICT). Further, healthcare service is a significant component of human security service.

Rapid development of ICT has brought radical changes in the administration-people interaction and make it easy and fast in the modern democracy. It has created the climate to conceive the ideas of 'Global Village' and 'e-governance.' Behind the progress of science and technology there remains the man's brain. The efforts of global community to achieve the aim of health for all embracing major issues of human society places before us the noble task of taking the responsibility to transform the 'Global Village' to 'Global Human Village' for establishing peace and security in the world. It requires humanization of man's heart. In other words, integration of head, heart and hand of each individual in the modern democratic world is urgently needed. Mahatma Gandhi insisted on integration of word, work and thought of a man as a strong step towards this end. Since First World War efforts are being made by world leaders, especially through international organizations like League of Nations and United Nations of Organizations followed by various other efforts at the international and national levels towards peace and security of man. United Nations of Organizations is making serious efforts to sensitize the members of the nations of the world about the significance of human rights in a democracy. Health may be considered as a significant area to be taken care of for providing human security, in its broader perspective. Growth of the concept of health of the people embracing the major issues of a human society is mirrored in the efforts of the United Nations of Organization since 1970s.

More recently, and as a reflection of civil society's stronger influence on and participation in global health issues, the People's Health Assembly has produced a People's Health Charter. Based on an analysis of world health problems, as well as existing policies and programmes, the Charter makes a set of recommendations to governments as well as international organizations, the business sector, and non-governmental organizations. The Charter asserts that health is a human right and that "Health and human rights should prevail over economic and political concerns" and calls for the provision of "Universal and comprehensive primary healthcare, irrespective of people's ability to pay". (*http://www.who.int/trade/gloss ory03ary/st9/en*)

Gradually, there has been vigorous global response to human security problems underlining the issues like human dignity, human rights and education and more significantly the health issues at the primary level of healthcare encompassing all communities and individuals living even in the remote areas of the world. In September 1978, an international conference was held in Alma-Ata, USSR (now Almaty, Kazakhstan) on Primary Healthcare issue. The conference expressed "the need for urgent action by all Governments, all health and development workers, and the world community to protect and promote the health of all people of the world." It is not only the first international declaration, but also a milestone in the global efforts for protection and promotion of the health of the people in the face of modern concepts of human security and human rights and duties of each one of us as human being in addition to other social responsibilities. It is reflected in the Declaration of Alma-Ata which states, "health is a state of complete physical, mental and social wellbeing, and not merely the absence of disease or infirmity, is a fundamental human right and that the attainment of the highest possible level of health is a most important worldwide social goal...." It goes on to call for all governments, regardless of politics and conflicts, to work together toward global health. (*http:/www.cliffsnotes.com/cliffsnotes/history/what-is-almaata-declaration, accessed on 6.5.2015*)

At the Alma-Ata Conference, Health Ministers from 134 countries, in association with the WHO and UNICEF set a goal of achieving "Health For All by the Year 2000" and identified primary healthcare as the device to achieve it. However, due to continued and deepened health inequalities on 8th December, 2000, 1453 delegates from 92 countries met at Savar, Bangladesh for the *First People's Health Assembly* which initiated the People's Health Movement (PHM) and the drafting of the People's Charter for Health. People's Health Movement is a global network of grassroots health activists, civil society organizations and academic institutions particularly from developing countries. Currently PHM has bases in more than 70 countries including both individuals and well established circles with their own governance structures. It has chapters in South Asia (India, Bangladesh, Sri Lanka), Africa (South Africa), Pacific (Australia), South America (Brazil, Ecuador), Central America (El Salvador, Nicaragua, Guatamala), North America (USA, Canada), Europe (Italy, Switzerland,

UK, Greece) and several other countries. The primary aim of PHM is to work for revitalization of Primary Healthcare as indicated in the Alma-Ata Declaration of 1978 with the following vision:

> "Equality, ecologically-sustainable development and peace are at the heart of our vision of a better world—a world in which a healthy life for all is a reality: a world that respects, appreciates and celebrates all life and diversity; a world that enables the flowering of people's talents and abilities to enrich each other; a world in which people' voices guide the decisions that shape our lives..."
>
> *http://en.wikipedia.org/wiki/people%27s_Health_Movement 6.5.2015*

The Alma-Ata Declaration of 1978 emerged as a major milestone of the twentieth century in the field of public health and it identified primary healthcare as the key to the attainment of the goal of Health for All. The following are excerpts from the declaration:

- The conference strongly reaffirms that health, which is a state of complete physical, mental and social wellbeing, and not merely the absence of diseases or infirmity, is a fundamental human right and that the attainment of the highest possible level of health is a most important worldwide social goal whose realization requires the action of many other social and economic sectors in addition to the health sector.
- The existing gross inequality in the health status of the people, particularly between developed and developing countries as well as within countries, is politically, socially and economically unacceptable and is, therefore of common concern to all countries.
- The people have a right and duty to participate individually and collectively in the planning and implementation of their healthcare.
- Primary healthcare is essential healthcare based on practical, scientifically sound, and socially acceptable methods and technology made universally accessible to individuals and families in the community through their full participation and at a cost that the community and the country can afford to maintain at every stage of their development in the spirit of self-reliance and self-determination. It forms an integral part of both of the

country's health system, of which it is the central function and main focus, and of the overall social and economic development of the community. It is the first level of contact of individuals, the family and community with national health system bringing healthcare as close as possible to where people live and work and constitutes the first elements of continuing healthcare process.

- An acceptable level of health for all the people of the world by the year 2000 can be attained through a fuller and better use of the world's resources, a considerable part of which is now spent in armaments and military conflicts. A genuine policy of independence, peace, détente and disarmament could and should release additional resources that could well be devoted to peaceful aims and in particular to the acceleration of social and economic development of which primary healthcare, as an essential part, should be allotted its proper share.

(http://www.who.int/social_determinants/tools/multimedia/alma_ata/en)

The People's Charter for Health echoes many of the principles of the Alma-Ata Declaration by recognizing health as "a social, economic and political issue and above all a fundamental human right". It identified inequality, poverty, exploitation, violence and injustice as the major drivers of all ill health and calls for "Health for All Now" through the involvement of people's organizations in health decision making.

Significantly, the PHM works to address the social determinants of health and pointed out that growing inequity within and between nations attributed to unfair economic structures which lock the people into poverty and poor health. The PHM helped to include the Social Determinants of Health on the global agenda through continued engagement with the World Health Organization. It became easy due to appointment of Professor Fran Baum from Australia, who was the chairman of PHM, as the Commissioner of the WHO Commission on Social Determinants of Health Steering Council. The engagement of PHM with the activities of the Commission resulted in the publication of a Civil Society Report on Social Determinants of Health in August 2008. In 2011, the PHM participated in the Conference on Social determinants of Health in Rio de Janeiro.

A significant contribution of the PHM is the formation of Global Health Watch as a searching device to answer the questions raised by the people across the globe. The question is, why is so little progress being made in promoting health of the people in the world in an increasingly integrated, globalized world with new cross bordered threats to health, widening disparities in both health and access to healthcare, and an unacceptable level of human suffering and premature mortality in developing countries ? The Global Health Watch aims to:

- Promote human rights as the basis for health policy.
- Counterbalance liberal and market-driven perspectives.
- Shift the health policy agenda to recognize the political, social and economic barriers to better health.
- Improve civil society's capacity to hold national and international governments, global international financial institutions and corporations to account (including WHO and the World Bank).
- Strengthen the links between civil society organizations around the world.
- Provide a forum for magnifying the voice of the poor and vulnerable.

(http://en.wikipedia.org/wiki/people%27s_Health_Movement 6.5.2015

Halfdan Mahler, Director General (1973-1983) of the WHO, defined "Health For All" in 1981, as follows:

"Health For All" must be reachable to every individual within a country. "By 'Health' is meant a personal state of wellbeing not just the availability of health services—a state of health that enables a person to lead a socially and economically productive life. "Health For All" implies the removal of the obstacles to health—that is to say, the elimination of malnutrition, ignorance, contaminated drinking water and unhygienic housing—quite as much as it does the solution of purely medical problems such as a lack of doctors, hospital beds, drugs and vaccines.

- "Health For All" means that health should be regarded as an objective of economic development and not merely as one of the means of attaining it.
- "Health For All" demands, ultimately, literacy for all. Until this becomes reality it demands at least the beginning of an understanding of what health means for every individual.
- "Health For All" depends on continued progress in medical care and public health. The health services must be accessible to all through primary healthcare, in which basic medical help is available in every village, backed up by referral services to more specialized care. Immunization must similarly achieve universal coverage.

"Health For All" is thus a holistic concept calling for efforts in agriculture, industry, education, housing and communications, just as much as in medicine and public health. Medical care alone cannot bring health to hovels. Health for such people requires a new way of life and fresh opportunities to provide themselves with a higher standard of living." (*en.wikipedia.org/wiki/Health_For_All*)

WHO Director General Lee Jong-wook (2003-2006) reaffirmed the concept in the World Health Report 2003:

"Health for All" became the slogan for a movement. It was not just an ideal, but an organizing principle everybody needs and is entitled to the highest possible standard of health. The principles remain indispensable for a coherent vision of global health. Turning that vision into reality calls for clarity both on the possibilities and on the obstacles that have slowed and in some cases reversed progress towards meeting the health needs of all people. We have a real opportunity now to make progress that will mean longer, healthier lives for millions of people, turn despair into realistic hope, and lay the foundations for improved health for generations to come." (*http:/Wikipedia.org/wiki/Health_For_All*)

The above declarations and attempts of the World Health Organization underline importance of human right, civil society and human dignity in the mission to "Health for All". The healthcare service providers, especially the physicians in India are also concerned about human values and ethics. This had explicit expression in the International Conference on Health Policy: Ethics and Human Values held in New Delhi in 1986 under the auspices of Indian Council of Medical Research in collaboration with the Council of International Organization of Medical Sciences (Geneva). The physicians across the country participated in conference and discussed various aspects of the problem and serious attempt was made to explore ways to safeguard human values.

India is also responding to health issues significantly since ancient time till date. With effect from 1st April, 1999, the Government of India restructured the Comprehensive Rural Sanitation Programme and launched the Total Sanitation Campaign (TSC) and later it was renamed as *Nirmal Bharat Abhiyan* (NBA). The Government of India under the leadership of Narendra Modi as the Prime Minister launched officially *Swachchh Bharat Abhiyan* (Clean India Mission) on 2nd October, 2014 at Rajghat, New Delhi where Prime Minister himself cleaned the road which is considered as the India's biggest ever cleanliness drive. (*en.wikipedia.org/wiki/Swachh_bharat_Abhiyan*)

The significant effort of the Prime Minister Narendra Modi towards maintenance of health is the recent declaration by United Nations Organizations on 11th December, 2014 of 21st June as an International Yoga Day. The declaration was made after the call by Narendra Modi, Prime Minister of India to the United Nations on 27th September, 2014 during his address to the UN General Assembly. He called the UN General Assembly for adopting 21st June as an International Yoga Day to get all the benefits of yoga for the people all around the world.

Modi has said in his address to the UN General Assembly, "Yoga is an invaluable gift of India's ancient tradition. It embodies unity of mind and body; thought and action; restraint and fulfillment; harmony between man and nature, a holistic approach to health and wellbeing. It is not about exercise but to discover the sense of oneness ...."

The celebration of the event International Yoga Day is supported by various global leaders. It is celebrated by the people of more than 170 countries including USA, China, Canada etc. It is celebrated at the international level by organizing activities like yoga training camps, yoga competitions and various other activities to enhance the awareness about the yoga benefits among common public all-over the world. It is celebrated to let people know that regular yoga practice lead to the better mental, physical and intellectual health. It positively changes the lifestyle of the people and increase the level of wellbeing.

The objectives of World Yoga Day are:

- To let people know amazing and natural benefits of yoga.
- To connect people to the nature by practicing yoga.
- To make people get used of meditation through yoga.
- To draw attention of people worldwide towards holistic benefits of yoga.
- To reduce the rate of health challenging diseases all-over the world.
- To bring communities much close together to spend a day for health from busy schedule.
- To enhance development and spread of peace all-through the world.
- To help people to get relief by themselves from stress through yoga.
- To strengthen the global coordination among people through yoga.

- To make people aware of physical and mental diseases and their solutions through yoga.
- To prevent unhealthy practices and promote and respect the good practices to make health better.
- To let people know their rights of good health and healthy life-style to enjoy the highest standard of physical and mental health.
- To link between protection of health and sustainable development
- To meet health challenges through regular yoga practice.
- To promote mental and physical health of the people.

(http://www.indiacelebrating.com/events/international-day-yoga/

In 1998, a New Global Health Policy "Health for All in the 21st Century", incorporated additional elements not considered in Alma-Ata. The importance of a gender perspective and the need to see health as central to sustainable human development are both emphasized. Also included the recognition of the growing importance of civil society in health governance. The new policy confirmed the goals of "Health for All" as:

- To attain health security for all.
- To achieve global health equity.
- To increase healthy life expectancy.
- To ensure access for all to essential healthcare of good quality.

More recently, and as a reflection of civil society's stronger influence on and participation in global health issues, the People's Health Assembly has produced a People's Health Charter. Based on an analysis of world health problems, as well as existing policies and programmes, the Charter makes a set of recommendations to Governments as well as international organizations, the business sector, and non-governmental organizations. The Charter asserts that health is a human right and that "Health and human rights should prevail over economic and political concerns" and calls for the provision of "Universal and comprehensive primary healthcare, irrespective of people's ability to pay". (*http://www.who.int/trade/gloss ory03ary/st9/en*)

The most significant threshold in the path of human security is the United Nations declaration of 21st June as the International Yoga Day adopting the proposal of the Prime Minister of India Narendra Modi. It is really a great achievement for India to get the approval of the proposal by the 193-memebr UN General Assembly by consensus a resolution establishing a day to commemorate the ancient practice, which Modi called in September 2014 during his inaugural address to the world body.

UN Secretary General Ban Ki-moon said the International Day of Yoga would bring attention to Yoga's holistic benefits. "Yoga can contribute to resilience against non-communicable diseases. Yoga can bring communities together in an inclusive manner that generates respect." Ban said in a statement, " Yoga is a sport that can contribute development and peace. Yoga can even help people in emergency situations to find relief from stress." (*www.reuters-com/article/2014/12/11/us-un-yoga-iduskBNOJP20V20141211*)

Z. Bankowski, in his article, '*Ethics and Values in Health Policy*' (published in the World Health Forum, Volume 17, 1996) also said, "Mankind's most fundamental beliefs are those that concern life, suffering and death. They stem from what different societies hold and teach about the origin of man, the purpose of life, the significance of death. Health is influenced by beliefs. Hence, the understanding of beliefs can be of great help in formulating effective health policies which meet the requirements of ethical values and social justice."

Narenda Modi, Prime Minister of India has also indicated the effort of his Government to establish SMART Governance in the country. The SMART Governance is nothing, but Simple, Moral, Accountable, Responsive and Transparent Governance. It is a strong step towards achievement of Global Human Village. No service to humanity which neglects the human aspect of it can be considered as a service in the true sense of the term. It has specific significance in the healthcare services. Wide application of modern scientific equipment demands more ethical accountability of the medical service providers. Further, modern technology has its own limitations. The expanded concept of 'Health' is humanity oriented and bended towards self-control or self-governance rooted in most cases in the social culture and tradition.

The normative concept of governance is a value laden concept. It may be termed as Good Governance. The norms of a society are ultimately an expression of its values—socially shared ideas about what is good, right, and desirable. The difference between values and norms is that values are abstract and general concepts, whereas norms are behavioural rules or guidelines for people in particular kinds of situations. In India to-day health of a person is valued most. It is reflected in self-healthcare, practice of Yoga, diet control and morning walk, periodic health check-up, taking care of food nutrition of the children, revival of the system of midday meal in school, taking advice periodically from the family doctors etc. are the indicators giving value in priority to the health. However, most rural areas have yet to be sensitized about healthcare.

Here reference may be made of the realization of the need of value-based administration in the United States mirrored in the books, "Towards a New Public Administration: The Minnow brook Perspective" and "Public Administration in a Time of Turbulence" edited by Frank Marini and Dwight Waldo respectively which underline the values such as, humanism, individual dignity, social justice etc. which engineered discussion on value-laden public administration under the leadership of Dwight Waldo and active participation of young scholars of the country in 1971. Further Osborne and Gaebler indicate some significant features of administration in the book, titled, "Reinventing Government". They emphasize on empowerment of the people to solve the problems rather than simply to deliver services, mission oriented service instead of rule-oriented service, investment on preventing problems rather than caring crises etc.

In India since ancient time the religious books, customs and tradition are giving priority to human values and dignity in administrative as well as social culture. The freedom struggle under the leadership of Mahatma Gandhi in India and the Constitution of India always remind us about the significance of human dignity and values. Today it is the Prime Minister of India, Narendra Modi who is trying to strengthen the moral dimension of the governance in the country.

Indian families till recently played a significant role in inculcating the human values and dignity in the minds of the children. The values in human dignity are taught in the family in a most informal and convincing way in the day to day life itself through conversation, clearing the queries of the young children in day to-day family affairs, control of behaviour of the children, guidance to maintain social relationships, narration of stories etc. On many occasions they used to control our behaviour by saying "should not do" or "should do" without explaining the reasons for it. In traditional societies generally ascriptive value system existed and the maintenance of secrecy was a common practice while giving advice to undertake certain activities or to behave in a particular manner or while administering medicine for curing diseases and taking preventative measures for protection of health. Faith on the senior members of the family was the driving force to carry out our daily duties at home as well as at school.

Healthcare service is a very strong tie to keep all people together irrespective of caste, creed, religion, sex, place of birth etc. Because it is nothing but a service to humanity. Since ancient time India is constructing the path on which people with different cultures can walk smoothly for rendering service to humanity through institutional devices as well as through customs and traditions which have been transmitted from generation to generation verbally. The achievements of the Takshashila University is very well known to all of us. The university was established more than 2700 years back where over 10,500 students from over the world came for higher studies in more than 64 different subjects. Chanakya, Panini, Charaka, Jivak etc. were the products of that University.

Next to Krishna and Shakuni, Chanakya occupies the position as an administrative consultant. Krishna is at the top in giving guidance to Pandavas in *Mahabharata* and then comes Shakuni for his guidance to Kauravas. Then comes Chanakya who guided Chandragupta Mauryan Empire. His *Niti-Shastra* focuses political ethics and addresses many problems of the administration and family and society. These have relevance even to-day. (*http://www.hibp.com/articles/history/takshashila-taxila-oldest-university*)

The customs, traditions, religions which are the important components of Indian social culture provide various ways to serve the human society effectively. The concept of administration and service can be understood with reference to human being only. Man is a social being and he is related to the society by some fundamental social needs as well as to realize his own self as human being. Every man has thinking faculty. The reasoning power of a man makes him supreme amongst all the beings in the world. So, the concept of man indicates not merely the physical organism, but also the inner and inherent qualities acquired by him through mechanism of birth and the process of socialization or social environment. To move from 'being' to 'becoming' every person requires full development of personality. Then the personal qualities of a man must be activated or directed for the service to humanity as well as to retrain his own self to be away from all kinds of self-destructive acts. Because it will cause in the long run unrepairable damage to the society to which he belongs. Further, every organization or institution or society is judged on the basis of the qualities of the personnel associated with it. And it is the man not the machine who can inculcate moral and human values in the services. The deviation from the moral and human values by the service providers may cause serious constraints on the very survival of it. Because they are the role models for most common people.

The moral principles must be the driving force along with other devices provided by science and technology to achieve human security and peace in the world. Healthcare service will contribute with certainty to human security widening the path of establishing peace in the mind of an individual as well as in the society.

Peace cannot be imposed from outside or by the laws of a country. It has to be generated by inner strength of a man. Laws can simply create an environment for it. But laws are essential and so is the case with society. The role of the family members and the immediate neighbours in creating congenial environment for enhancement of mental strength of a man can never be underestimated. Human culture flourishes in such situations. Every nation is in need of it and each nation is determining its goals considering good of its members based on these principles. In other words, the human society can be established only by human beings; just as democracy can be made workable only by a democrat or by those who practice democratic principles with whole-hearted effort. Unless one is committed to the principles of democracy or unless a man realizes the significance of democracy he cannot apply his self with commitment in the process of democracy. Because to be committed to a particular ideals one must have understanding of it. The ethical principles induce a man to have clear and in-depth understanding of the concepts of human security, human dignity, peace of mind and their implications which go long way in the progress of a nation.

It is not the law nor the money nor the infrastructure nor the comfort provided by science and technology which can establish peace and security if there is ethical vacuity in the society. Unless the leaders realize the values of human dignity, develop love and affection for their countrymen, be sympathetic to weak and poor and take special care for the weak and hungry men they cannot help the nation to achieve its goals. The nation will certainly fail to be benefitted by their professional excellence. The man who does not orient his professional excellence to the human goodness fails to grasp the philosophy of the laws of the country he is to serve. He misses the path to reach the nation's destiny. In contemporary India there we have to give a serious thought to the ability of the service providers who are not sensitive to the human values to take leading role in establishing good governance in the country and to what extent they can help India to contribute towards establishing a Global Human Village in the fast changing situation brought by the progress of science and technology.

O.P. Dwivedi has rightly pointed out that the insensitiveness of modern Indians to 'moral security' has become visible. They do not care to expose themselves to the 'moral risk'. The concept of service has changed to a great extent. The elements like dedication, honesty, sense of mission to humanity etc. are thrown out of the concept of 'Service.'

The moral foundation of any public service organization in a democracy requires that administrators and public officials show a genuine care for their fellow citizens. Democratic values, such as equality, law, justice, right and freedom have moral connotations and demand an unwavering commitment from those who govern. Public servants are obliged to uphold these values. These values are enshrined in the Preamble to the Constitution of India itself. Democratic values warn us to view governmental efforts as moral endeavour.

The human values and ethical principles are rooted in the ancient society. Naturally, with the progress of the society and modernization of way of life there emerges the ambiguity in the concept of morality. The co-existence of both tradition and modernity, the practice of modern way of living and at the same time valuing the age old tradition makes a man in modern India indecisive and creates confusing situation. (Presidential Address of O.P. Dwivedi: 1988)

It is difficult to deny that the progress of science and technology cannot do away with the need of ethics in any society however modern it is. Democracy whether political or social must be based on ethical principles. It is true that the facilities and comfort provided by the modern technology expedites the development of a nation, helps solving very complicated problems caused by nature, relieves the suffering of the patients and provides scope to maintain good health, brings information from any part of the world within a moment to us.

Today a man is no longer satisfied with food, cloth and shelter only. His minimum needs have been increased with the changing situations. What is needed today is to explore the ways to safeguard the human aspect of the global society. It requires efforts to make modern man realize the dangerous consequences of ethical vacuity in our way of life. We must proceed in the escalator of progress of life, but must carry with us the stick of humanism without which deviation from the path of progress is inevitable.

The doctors often face a conflict between the professional commitment to the individual patient and social responsibility. Recently, media has focused how the healthcare providers are exposed to conflicts or confrontations with the relatives and attendants of patients in India. It appears in *The Times of India*, a leading newspaper of the country that those who save lives are themselves at risk. More than 75 per cent of across the country have faced at least some form of violence as per initial findings of Indian Medical Association (IMA).

(timesofindia.indiatimes.com/india/over-75%-of-doctors-have-faced-violence-at-work-study-finds/articleshow/147143806)

At the same time allegations are also appearing in media on cases of medical errors and negligence, corrupt practices in the healthcare services due to which harm is done to the patients. While dealing with these issues, it has to be mentioned that the 55th World Health Assembly resolved in October 2005 at WHO headquarters on patient safety while Global Patient Safety Challenge as the core programme of the "World Alliance for patient Safety" launched in that year.

India, which was one of the eight prominent member countries to participate in the event, has committed to work towards the cause of promoting Patient Safety. A pledge to this effect was signed by the Ministry of Health and Family Welfare, Government of India, in the presence of the WHO representatives on 14th July, 2006 at New Delhi. Keeping the commitment in mind, the Department of Hospital Administration, AIIMS in collaboration of WHO has taken the lead to launch the programme, National Initiative on Patient Safety (NIPS) in 2009. Series of comprehensive workshops, involving multidisciplinary teams comprising of senior surgeons, physicians, microbiologists, medical superintendents and nursing officers from various medical colleges and hospitals across India under the leadership of Dr. Shakti Gupta as the Programme Director of NIPS and Head of the Department of Hospital Administration, AIIMS.

While taking care of the safeguard of the patients it is difficult to ignore the safeguard of rights and health of the medical service providers in the face of conflicts, degradation of faith of the patients on them, experience of violent situations while in service to the patients, and various other constraints in the process.

Ethics deals with all aspects of human behaviour and decision-making. It is a very large and complex field of study with many branches and sub-divisions. The book is a modest effort to discuss ethics and human values in a limited way with the experience in India. As an academic discipline, medical ethics has developed its own vocabulary, including many terms that have been borrowed from philosophy. I depend heavily on the writings of several scholars in the field and the literature published by different organizations at international and national levels to express my ideas.

There is a close relationship between human rights and medical ethics. With growth and development of the concept of human rights emphasis is given on medical ethics. In recent years medical ethics have been greatly influenced by development of human rights. In a pluralistic and multi-cultural world, with many moral traditions, the major international human rights agreements can provide a foundation to medical ethics that is acceptable across national and cultural boundaries. Moreover, physicians frequently have to deal with problems resulting from violation of human rights. They are also greatly affected by the debate over whether healthcare is a human right.

Having in mind all the abovementioned health related issues and emergence of new areas in the domain of healthcare inviting cooperation and self-help or self-rule of the individuals in different capacities and appreciating the human culture and tradition of India since ancient time I have the temptation to prepare the book titled, ***"Ethics and Human Values in Medical Sciences: A View from the Perspective of Indian Culture and Tradition"*** which is an attempt to understand the state of human culture in the medical services of India. Ethics is an intrinsic part of medical practice. The concept of medical ethics in its broader connotation and dynamic nature embraces the human values, behaviour, attitude and belief applicable to the individual as well as the society. It is not merely about avoidance of doing harm to the patient, rather it is all about norms, values and principles. These norms, values and principles are intended to govern medical conduct.

Ian Robertson in his book, '*Sociology*' has analyzed different aspects of culture comprehensively and in a simple way. The survival of society depends on the transmission of culture from one generation to other. The most fascinating feature of the process of cultural transmission is that it always adds new elements to the old culture. Culture does not grow, it develops at the deliberate efforts of the members of the society. Generally, in the traditional society elderly members used to transmit culture to the young generation. The process of education was informal. With the emergence of the formal educational institutions knowledge, skill, values etc. are transmitted in a formal and systematic way. Since in the traditional society members were not mobile and were not exposed to the outside world, the social changes were very slow. Naturally, the process of transmission of culture was not only very simple it was also free from ambiguities and controversy. But the modern society is influenced by the progress of science and technology, spread of education and various other facilities provided by the Governments of a democratic State. Under these circumstances cultural transmission has become a very complex affair.

Further socio-cultural changes take place due to changes in the physical environment, such as earthquake, floods, deforestation, erosion, migration, increase of population, technological innovation, new policies at the national and international levels etc. making the social changes very fast. All changes do not bring reforms of the society. Experience shows that these have both positive and negative impact on our society. In most cases we have given up our old well established traditions required for establishing healthy human relationship. The role of the family and school in inculcating human values in the younger generations has become fragile. Very often it is noticed that the concepts like 'modernity', 'standard of life', 'advance', 'backward' are misinterpreted or interpreted superficially. It is difficult to deny that our old culture and traditions were not created in vacuum, these were based on long experience of elderly members of the traditional society with moral or ethical implications of social life. We cannot throw them out in the plea of being modern.

Medical professionals occupy a unique position in the human society as they deal with the ailing members of it and their decisions and performance of duties have immediate impact on the right to life of the patients. In India the patient population is increasing day by day and at the same time the situation of medical services is gravitated by the problems like unaccounted medical errors, medical negligence and involvement in unethical activities including corrupt practices by the medical professionals. It is a serious threat to human rights of the Indians as well as to Indian economy. The process of dehumanization of the old well established Indian society based on human culture must be prevented and we expect a good beginning will be made by the medical professional of the country very soon through realization of the deep rooted harm caused by it to the nation. Efforts must be made for emergence of genuine commitment to the service to humanity.

The health of human being is one of the basic requirements for survival of the global society with peace and tranquility as well as for the progress of human civilization. The birth of United Nations of Organization on 24th October, 1945 in New York, the meeting of World Medical Association in London in 1946, the beginning of World Health Organization on 7th April, 1948 as the directing and coordinating authority for health as a significant part of the UN system underlines the sincere efforts of the world leaders to safeguard the human rights of men and women in the interest of peace and security of the world. It also focuses the place occupied by the health and human rights of individuals in the discussion of the world leaders during the Second World War for the formation of UNO and this was followed by another strong step by the adoption of the Universal Declaration of Human Rights on 10th December, 1948 by the UN General Assembly towards this end.

The concept of democracy, whether political or social centers round human beings and their dignity. The need for ethical guidelines exist as soon as people start living together. The concept of democracy cannot be divorced from the ethical or moral principles as the means and end of it. It demands development of human personality requiring environment in which mutual respect for each other, co-existence of difference of opinion, development of the feeling of brotherhood. Only in this environment full development of individual's personality is possible and then only political democracy can work effectively in the greater interest of the humanity. It widens the scope for self-discipline, which is the fundamental requirement of self-government or democracy. Here is the significance of human rights of each and every individual.

Human security in its broader perspective embraces healthcare services as its significant component. Like all human beings, physicians have rights as well as responsibilities and medical ethics has become increasingly important as physicians in many countries are experiencing great frustration, inconveniences, insecurity and harassment while practicing their profession. The reasons for these may be many, such as, limited resources, government interference, non-availability of work facilities and environment, heavy rush of patients, sensationalist media reports of medical errors and unethical physician conduct, or challenges to their authority and other healthcare providers. Similarly, patients' rights are also facing challenges like medical errors, negligence to duty, incompetence of service providers, corruption, unethical practices etc.

Further human values and accountability are the two basic tools of democracy. Man can create socio-political environment through adherence of human values in the society. These values may be transmitted to others through practice. Family, school, political party, NGO, intellectuals, social reformers etc. can play significant role in the process of transmitting these values to the young generations, which are reflected in their service life through practice.

In the book I underline the ethical or moral aspect of accountability. What is accountability? The accountability is an obligation of an individual or organization to account for its activities, to accept responsibility for them and to disclose the result in a transparent manner. Within an organization the principles and practices of ethical accountability aim to improve both the internal standard of individual and group conduct as well as external factors.

It is very clear that ethical failure begins soon after the service providers start hiding their acts of omission. This may also be called administrative or professional evils. This evil will certainly deprive the innocent people of their humanity—from small scale of assaults on a person's dignity to outright murder. Today's India is experiencing this kind of situation. And time has come to give a serious thought to it.

The moral foundation of any public service organization in a democracy requires that administrators and public officials to show a genuine care for their fellow citizens. Democratic values, such as equality, law, justice, right and freedom have moral connotations and demand an unwavering commitment from those who govern. Public servants are obliged to uphold these values. These values are enshrined in the Preamble to the Constitution of India itself. Democratic values warn us to view Governmental efforts as a moral endeavour.

The moral principles are derived from various religions and social cultures adopted by different nations. It is true with the progress of the society and modernization of way of life there emerges the ambiguity in the concept of morality. The co-existence of both tradition and modernity, abolition of the practice of modern, especially Western ways of living and at the same time valuing the age old tradition inwardly makes a man in modern India indecisive and creates confusing situation. One can feel the Gandhian flavour in the medical sciences which are rooted basically in Indian tradition and the major religions of the world. Therefore, I feel strongly that more we are inventing sophisticated technology in the field of medical care more is the need of adherence of ethical principles and human values to direct modern technology towards service to humanity and this is possible only when human power directs the application of modern technology for the service to humanity.

Basic Arguments: Today's India is heavily constrained by ethical vacuity causing emergence of all kinds of social ailments. Medical care and education are deeply rooted in the Indian culture and civilization which is based on humanity. Reference may be made to the university of Takshashila, the oldest university. Gandhi taught us truth and non-violence which are the basic tools of physician for effective functioning. But today we have submitted ourselves to the modern technology weakening our human power. We are failing to appreciate human values insisted upon in the traditional Indian society and trying to divorce ethical principles from religion.

The book is an attempt to establish that the expertness of the physician must be accompanied by adherence of ethical codes and honour to human values to be successful or to achieve the goals of medical care as desired by the World Health Organization and safeguard humanity in India. The application of sophisticated and modern technology cannot do away with the need of ethical and human values, rather their importance is increasing in the face of the progress of science and technology. The application of the modern techniques require control of manpower to achieve the goal of service to humanity. The Indian culture and tradition is flooded with these values.

Policies formulated by the Governments of a country must have human values orientation. Professor Bankowski, the Secretary General of the Council for International Organizations of Medical Sciences (C/O World Health Organization, 1211 Geneva 27, Switzerland) in his writing titled, *Ethics and Human Values in Health Policy*, published in World Health Forum, Volume 17, 1996) discussed about ethics and human values in health policies very effectively. To quote him, "Given the enormous power to medicine for both good and harm, the need for health policies is inescapable. The health policy of a nation or a community is its strategy for controlling and optimizing the social uses of its medical knowledge and resources. Human values are the guides and justifications that people use for choosing the goals, priorities and means that make-up that strategy. Ethics act as the bridge between policy and values. It examines the moral validity of the choices to be made, and seeks to resolve the conflicts between values which inevitably occur in the process. Ethics, therefore, orders human choices in accordance with normative principles.

A healthy policy thus reflects the fundamental beliefs and commitments of a nation or people. These commitments are its human values. Through their expression in health policies a community exerts its influence over the enormous momentum of technological advance. Ethics is itself grounded in socio-cultural, philosophical, or religious convictions. These convictions are a society's yardsticks for right and wrong, good and evil...."

Again Jean Martin, a Cantonal Physician for the Canton of Vaud referred in his writing titled, *Ethics and Health Services*: the debate continues published in above mentioned World Health Forum, about the guiding principles suggested by a Swedish Parliamentary Commission on which to base the decisions about priorities for the health policies as below:

- "*Human dignity*: all people are equal in this regard, whatever their characteristics or place in society;
- *Needs and solidarity*: resources should be allocated to the persons or services that need them most;
- *Cost-effectiveness*: there should be a reasonable relation between the cost of a measure and its effect, in terms of improvement of health or quality of life.

Interestingly questions which are very much related to the young generation of contemporary India was raised in the discussion, as mentioned by Martin are questions on the area of self-induced injuries, such as those caused by sport or reckless behaviour, or disorders resulting from consumption of alcohol, drugs or tobacco. The Commission decided that in principle lifestyle should not give rise to discrimination."

Two
Indian Culture
A Basis of Medical Sciences

India and '*Bharat*' denote the same country in our Constitution, but the two names do not evoke identical reactions in our minds, pointed out by S.R. Sharma, author of the book, titled, "*The Soul of Indian History*". India sounds Greek, foreign; but 'Bharat' is directly '*Vedic*': India from '*Indoi*' or inhabitants of the Indus region. It is also said that 'Indus' is from the "*Vedic Sindhu*".

Bharat is an abbreviation of '*Bharatvarsh*', the traditional Sanskrit name of India. By whatever name she is invoked, the image which ultimately emerges in the minds of Indians is that of 'Mother India'. Our national anthem, "*Vande Mataram* (Salutation to Thee, Mother) was sung generations before by Rabindra Nath Tagore gave us "*Bharata Bhagya Vidhata*" (Ordainer of Bharat's well-being). However, both evoke identical filial emotions:

> *Janani Janma-bhumischa Svargadapi gariyasi.*
> "Mother and Motherland are worthier of adoration than Heaven itself" is a very ancient sentiment of India. (Sharma: 1967)

The nature of Indian culture can be very precisely expressed by Radhakrishnan as below:

Humanism: India is well known for humaneness and calm nature of people without any harshness in their principles and ideals. Humanism may be defined as "any system of thought or action which is concerned with merely human interests." For humanism man is the highest type of individual in existence and the service of man is the highest religion. It believes that man is by nature good and evil rests in society, in the conditions which surround man, and if these are removed, man's goodness will emerge.

Tolerance: Gandhiji's principles of '*Satyagraha*' and '*Ahimsa*' are the basic tools of fighting freedom of India. Co-existence of different religions, languages and cultures in the country indicates it. (Radhakrishnan: 1961) As regards the values of tolerance, Prem Kirpal has pointed out several manifestations of tolerance. One of the forms of tolerance manifests curiosity and sympathetic awareness projecting a spirit of benevolence in cultural exchanges leading to fruitful contacts and active exchange for mutual understanding which demands the spirit of give and take. (Kirpal)

Unity: India is the home of men and women belonging to various castes and creed. It is a fusion of old traditional values and the modern principles. Throughout history religion has been a part of India's culture. Religious diversity and religious tolerance are both established in the country by the law and custom.

Secularism: India is a secular state as stated in the constitution. There is freedom of worship in the country without breaches or violations of any other's religious beliefs. The Hindus, the Muslims, the Christians, the Sikhs and the communities professing other religions share their thoughts and live together in spite of their religious differences.

Closely Knit Social System: The Indian society has a Closely Knit Social System based on Joint Family System, but for recently cropped nuclear families, in which grandparents, parents, sons and daughters share the same spirit, tradition and property. (Radhakrishnan: 1961)

What is Culture? The term 'culture' is generally used to refer sophisticated tastes in art, literature, or music. In various organizations, associations, institutions, especially in the educational institutions students are familiar with the usage of the phrases like, 'Cultural Function', or 'Cultural Show' and 'Cultural Procession, demonstrating folk dances, traditional dresses, social festivals etc. These reflect only a part of our culture. In other words, it is a narrow expression of culture.

The sociological use of the term is very comprehensive, for it includes the entire way of life of a society, and in this sense everyone participates in the culture of a society. To them culture consists of all the shared products of human society. These products are of two kinds—material and non-material. Material culture consists of all the art crafts or physical objects which human beings create—wheels, clothing, schools, factories, cities, books, spacecraft, and totem poles. Non-material culture consists of more abstract creations—languages, ideas, beliefs, rules, customs, myths, skills, family patterns, and political systems.

We create culture and culture in turn protects us. We are no longer the helpless victims of natural environment. We have explored and still exploring different ways to adjust in the changing situation. We make our own social environment inventing and sharing the rules and patterns of behaviour that shape our lives, and we use our acquired knowledge to change the natural environment as well. Our social life is based on the habit of sharing culture. The social audit, social monitoring and social control on the observance of social norms, behaviour pattern compel the members of the traditional society to be within the framework of the culture of the society.

We do not inherit our culture through the mechanism of birth. We acquire it from the social environment and through participation in different social activities. Obedience to elderly members of the family and family to the social leadership is another way to adopt social culture in the traditional society. It is an external force to regulate man's behaviour and social relationship. Robertson also stated that the contents of culture cannot be genetically transmitted. There is no gene that tells us to dance, to believe in a particular God, to build houses etc. Culture is thus a substitute for 'instinct' as a means of responding to the environment. Celebration of certain festivals, adherence of customs and traditions, maintenance of social relationship in a guided manner are the ideals or norms accepted by the society.

The codes are nothing, but norms to ensure that social life is peaceful and secured. For they give us guidelines within the framework of which individuals have to behave and these codes help establishment and promotion of mutual confidence in the social life. This social function of norms or ideals is so important that there is always strong social pressure on people to conform. However, one has to admit that all members of the society do not conform their behaviour and way of life to the social norms. It is also noticed that the same person changes his behaviour in different times and environments either to adjust himself with the new situation or to gain some personal benefits in the same social environment. Again it is found that all social norms are not rigid. Certain norms are changeable according to the changes in the environment. Society itself is not static, it is dynamic. Therefore, although the members of a society conform to the norms most of the time, it is difficult to deny the possibility of violations of these norms by some members while leading a social life. In the case of certain norms, the folkways, a fair amount of non-conformity may be tolerated, but in the case of certain other norms, the mores, very little scope for flexibility is noticed.

The norms of a society are ultimately an expression of its values—socially shared ideas about what is good, right, and desirable. The difference between values and norms is that values are abstract, whereas norms are behavioural rules or guidelines for people in particular kinds of situations. (Robertson: 1980)

Kirpal talks of three kinds of elements of culture—ideas, aesthetic forms and values. All these elements are to a great extent moulded by past tradition of a society and the aspirations for the future. Ideas shape or change habits and generate beliefs which are ultimately stabilized through institutionalization. The aesthetic forms reflect the artistic expression of a culture in its visual, arts, music and poetry. The values of a culture are formed by the interplay of both ideas and aesthetic forms and provide norms of conduct, standards of behaviours, and sources of faith and vision. (Kirpal)

The ancient Indian society dates back to the era of ancient Indian civilizations. The ancient India witnessed the evolution of different civilizations. Different communities had their distinctive cultures, religions, indigenous beliefs, customs and occupations. The remnants of the Indus Valley Civilization of Mahenjo-Daro and Harappa, dating back to the pre-Vedic period, are examples of one such civilization.

The evolution of the ancient Indian societies is well reflected in Sanskrit and Indo-Aryan Literatures. Besides, the Buddhist *Pali* works, particularly the *Jatakas,* and the *Jaina* works in *Prakrit* language and *Apabhramsha* that offer references of the ancient Indian societies. The *Rig Veda* is regarded as the earliest written record of Indo-Europeans. Ancient Indian societies also get reflected in other *Vedic Samhitas* are the *Yajur Veda, Sama Veda and Atharva Veda.*

While *Rig Veda* contains *Mantras* mainly about the various aspects of nature, conceived as deities and the *Yajur Veda* contains matters for ritual application of the ancient societies. *Atharva Veda* contains matters reflecting popular beliefs and practices that were prevented in the ancient societies. In it one can find the matters that were designed to prolong life, heal diseases, ward-off evils, counteract the venom of snakes etc. A considerable role is played by *Tantras* in the social life of India. They teach ways to liberation through enjoyment (*bhakti*).

Population pattern shows that the societies of ancient India comprised of people from different social groups. The main groups were Aryans or Indo-Aryans. There were also primitive tribes residing in hills and forests speaking different languages and dialects. (*http://www.indianetzone.com/49/ancient_indian socity.htm*)

Indian culture and civilization is as old as humanity. It is also deeply rooted in humanity. This was realized by Gandhi very well. Mahatma Gandhi, being the product of this culture, made life long sacrifice and efforts to humanize the Indian society. The long struggle to liberate India from British rule under the leadership of Gandhi tells us that the "service to humanity" is the only way to survive as human being and to create peace and tranquility in the world. It is a great social force for human progress along with the progress of science and technology and modernization of man's way of life.

India was the richest country on earth until the time of British in the early seventeenth century. The *Ayurveda* is the earliest school of medicine known to human. Charaka, the father of medicine, consolidated *Ayurveda* 2,500 years ago. To-day *Yoga* and *Ayurveda* are fast regaining their rightful places in our civilization. (Chowdhary: 2007)

More than 2700 years back a huge university known as Takshashila, existed in India where over 10,500 students from different parts of the world came for higher studies. This was the world's oldest university. This University was the IIT and MIT of the world. The students from all parts of the world used to come for attaining specialization in over 64 different fields of study: *Vedas*, Grammar, *Ayurveda*, Agriculture, Surgery, Politics, Archery, Warfare, Astronomy, Commerce, Futurology, Music, Dance etc. There were even curious subjects like the art of discovering hidden treasure etc.

The students were admitted in the University at the age of 16 after they had completed their basic education in the local institutions. Admission to this University was purely based on merit. The students had wide option to select subject of their choice for study and research.

Some of the prominent products of the University were Chanakya, Panini, Vishnu Sharma, Charaka and Jivak. Chanakya (was also called Kautilya). He authored the world's finest work till date on political duties, statecraft, economic policies, state intelligence systems, administrative skills and military strategy, called *Arthashastra* which consisted of 15 books. He was also serving the Great Mauryan Empire by guiding Chandragupta Maurya as a mentor.

It is said that Chanakya is known as the most famous management consultant in India after Krishna and Shakuni. Krishna occupies the top position for his successful advice to the *Pandavas* in *Mahabharata*. Shakuni is in the next position for successfully guiding the *Kauravas*.

Panini was another great product of this University. He was an expert in language and grammar and authored one of the greatest works of grammar ever written called *Ashtadhyayi*. Though it is very complicated one it is highly technical and specific in defining the rules of Sanskrit grammar.

Another great scholar from Takshashila was Vishnu Sharma, the author of the great book that teaches the art of political science in the form of simple beautiful stories called the *Panchatantra* (meaning with five techniques). It is said that Vishnu Sharma wrote these stories in order to convert three dumb princes of a King into able political administrators within a span of six months.

Charaka, the famous ancient Indian Ayurvedic physician was a product of Takshashila University. He originally authored the *Charaka Samhita* (simplifying an even older Ayurvedic work called the *Agnivesha Samhita),* which along with *Sushruta Samhita*, *Ashtanga Sangraha* and *Ashtanga Hridayam* forms the root of modern *Ayurveda*. Charaka said, "A physician who fails to enter the body of a patient with the lamp of knowledge and understanding can never treat diseases."

Another genius who came out of the Takshashila University was Jivak, a doctor and an expert in pulse reading. His areas of specialization were *Panchakarma*, *Marma* and Surgery. He was the personal physician of Buddha. He also invented a cure for Filariasis. There are over 15,000 handwritten manuscripts of Jivak's expertise passed on by generations to their children and are still preserved in India. (*http:/www.http.com/articles/history/takshashila-taxila-oldest-university; accessed on 7.6.2014*)

In ancient India, our systems of medicine and surgery were not deficient. Radhakrishnan mentioned in this context, "The ancient Indians were proficient in many surgical operations including what is now called *Rhinoplasty*." (Radhakrishanan: 1970)

India was known for the studies and contribution to the field of science, particularly through Takshashila University. But the Indians who had made significant contributions in the field of mathematics and natural sciences had been neglecting the sciences for several centuries, said Bipan Chandra. Their minds tied up with traditions. The minds of the common people were influenced by Superstitions to a large extent. Chandra was convinced that the struggle for power and wealth, economic decline, social backwardness, and cultural stagnation had a deep and harmful impact on the morals of a section of the Indian people. The nobles, in particular, degenerated in their private and public life. The virtues of loyalty, gratitude and faithfulness to their pledged word tended to disappear in the single minded pursuit of selfish aims. Many of the nobles were prey to degrading vices and excessive luxury. Most of them took bribes when in office. Significantly, the common people continued to exhibit a high degree of personal integrity and morality. Bipan Chandra quoted the comments of John Malcolm and another European Cranford as below:

John Malcolm said, "I do not know the example of any great population, in similar circumstances, preserving through such a period of changes and tyrannical rule, so much virtue and so many qualities as are to be found in a great proportion of the inhabitants of this country."

To Cranford "Their rules of morality are most benevolent, and hospitality and charity are not only strongly inculcated but I believe nowhere more universally practiced than amongst Hindus."

In the eighteenth century social life and culture was almost stagnated in nature and cultural diversity and existence of different ways of social life was noticed in the perspective of religion, geographical variation, language and caste.

Besides caste system two other major social ailments which existed in the eighteenth century India were the *Sati Pratha* and the status of widow amongst Hindus. Generally, the families of *rajas*, chiefs, *zamindars* and high caste people of Rajputana, Bengal and some parts of North India *Sati Pratha* prevailed under which a Hindu widow had to burn herself along with the body of her dead husband. Widows were not allowed to remarry. They had to observe various kinds of restrictions on dress code, diet, movement etc.

The relationship between Hindus and Muslims was cordial in the eighteenth century India. There existed religious tolerance. They used to cooperate with each other in the social and cultural affairs. There emerged composite culture in India. Hindu writers wrote in Persian while Muslim writers wrote Hindi, Bengali and vernaculars, often dealing with subjects of Hindu social life and religion, such as Radha and Krishna, Sita and Rama etc., the development of Urdu language and literature provided a new meeting ground of both the languages. (Chandra:1971)

The thirteenth century may be considered as a turning point in the history of north-east India. The Ahoms ruled Assam for about six hundred years. Their history also shed light on certain events in other parts of India besides throwing light on the socio-cultural aspect of the region. Sukapha, the chief of Ahom was the founder of Ahom Kingdom in Assam. The Ahoms restored the political unity of the Brahmaputra Valley which generated unity amongst different ethnic groups like Chutiyas, Kacharis, Morans, Barahis and Baro-Bhuyans.

The Ahom rulers were tolerant of all religions, Hinduism, Islam, Buddhism and tribal cults. They did not interfere with the freedom to enjoy by different communities of their own beliefs. Though their original forms of worship were of a primitive character based on the fertility cult, it was the policy of the rulers not to impose their own religious faith and practices on the non-Ahoms. Into their kingdom came Brahmin priests and poets from time to time from different parts of India beginning possibly in the early centuries of the Christian era. They also used to welcome '*pirs*' for the Muslims and granted for their maintenance lands called '*Pirpal*' grants. The extent of freedom, equality and justice which the ordinary citizens enjoyed, during Ahom period, fostered the growth of unity and integrity among different groups of people, irrespective of caste, creed and community.

In the annals of medieval Assam, inter-marriage occupied an important place as a means of achieving integration. In the social custom, there were instances of intermarriages, between the Ahoms and the non-Ahoms and non-Ahom tribes and race. Sukapha, the founder of Ahom kingdom in Assam, married Borahi and Moran princes, Siva Singha, son of Rudra Singha, married a non-Ahom girl, named Phuleswari, belonging to a '*nat*' family. Rajeswar Singha married Manipuri Princess Kuranganyayani. A large number of Manipuri people accompanied the bride in the marriage ceremony and settled down near old Ahom capital Garhgaon, in the district of Sibsagar.

Muslim settlement in Assam can be traced from twelfth century. The number of Muslims increased with even successive attacks on Assam during the reign of Mughals. In 1198 A.D. Md. Bin Bakhtiyar Kheljee entered Kamrup, on his way to attack China. Mirjumla invaded Assam in 1662 A.D. The Muslim historian Shihabuddin Talish, accompanied Mir Jumla in his invasion of Assam. He made mention about amity and solidarity between the indigenous Muslim and the Assamese Hindus. Many of the soldiers, later on, settled at Maligaon and Jalukbari areas. They accepted Assamese culture and language, took part in its promotion.

For the first time, during the period 1254-56 A.D. Muslim Saint Gyasuddin Aulia visited Assam to preach the message of the prophet of Islam. He established a prominent Muslim Shrine, known as *Poamecca* at Hajo, in the district of Kamrup.

During 1635-42 A.D. another Muslim Saint Syed Shah Milan Ajmiri Bagdadi, known as Azan Fakir composed some devotional songs known as 'Zikirs' in Assamese language and sung in the tune of Hindu religious Hymns, with similar expression, verse and tune of 'Bargeet' composed by Sri Sankardeva and Madhabdeva. He occupied a significant position in the Assamese society by composing and popularizing Assamese Zikirs in such a way which was hardly attempted by any other Muslim Saint. The lofty ideals of Zikir, not only be remembered as a treasure of Assamese literature, but will also be regarded as unifying force in the Assamese society. Ahom King, Pratap Singh provided him several facilities. The great Vaishnavite Saint Sankardeva had one Muslim disciple Chand Khan by name who took lively interest in the religious discussions also. (Dutta: 1990)

The great epic, *Mahabharata* and sacred text *Bhagavad Gita* teach us that survival must be on the basis of quality of life. These provide a framework of human values. Here let me pick up one or two examples in support of it. (Sharma: 1967)

Values or Virtues in *Mahabharata* are mentioned by as, Chapter VI –fearlessness, control of senses, truthfulness, absence of anger, kindness, peace, sacrifice, valour, absence of malice; chapter VII—control of mind, dutifulness, lordliness, service, contentment; Chapter XII—compassion, equanimity, purity, self-control, devotion; chapter XIII—non-violence, freedom from hypocrisy, forgiveness, straightforwardness and non-attachment. (Gupta: 1995)

The 'Unity in Peace' is the cry heard in the cultural history of India. Even Duryodhana ostensibly seeks the same. There is no parallel to the noblest among the epic heroes—Yudhishthira, also called *Dharma raja*—whose character mirrod in action, not mere slogans. The war they were about to engage in was *dharma yuddha* (righteous struggle); the combatants were first-cousins; among the commanders were teachers like Drona and Grandsires like Bhisma. These relations baffled Arjuna and provoked Sri Krishna to preach *Gita*. To a great surprise Yudhishthira sought benediction from his elders—Bhisma and Drona—who were pledged to destroy the Pandavas (the enemy). He said, "Grandsires, we dare to oppose you, but we seek your blessings for our victory." Bhisma, in a very dignified way responded "Child", "born of the race of Bharata you have acted worthily and in consonance with our code of conduct. It gladdens my heart, indeed, to see you respecting our noble traditions. Fight and you will win. I am not a free man, and am obliged to serve my king; but you will not be defeated. Drona, Kripa and Salya, too, repeated the benedictions of Bhisma. This is the uniqueness of the culture of India.

Krishna simply argued Arjuna into sense and action. That it meant war, involving killing of kinsmen, was due only to the accidental context.

"Self-reliance and fulfillment *Svadharma,* surrendering all consequences to God was the core of teachings." (Sharma: 1967)

N.L. Gupta in his book, *Education and Values in the Mahabharata* while explaining the system of values stated that *Mahabharata* propounds "primarily spiritualistic and yet realistic, humanistic and individualistic and yet socialistic and universalistic, ancient and yet dynamic and progressive" system of values. No society whatever modern it is can ignore these values for its very survival. He quoted what Dr. A. Sengupta said, "the social outlook in *Mahabharata* is essentially humanitarian as the social ideal is to awaken in man all human excellences which he will make him fit for the realization of his own infinity and bliss." It is only when a man attains moral qualities that his mind is elevated to a higher level, and of an embodied soul." *Mahabharata* is a treatise on philosophy, religion, ethics, politics, morality etc. (Gupta: 1995)

Yoga, the *Gita* declares, "is skill in action". But it is not merely the physical adroitness of the acrobat. It is rooted in the tranquillized and harmonized mind. The *Gita* gives very detailed instructions for the attainment of this mental poise.

Yoga is equipoise: "Not attainable by him who eats too much, nor one who starves himself: not by him who sleeps too little, nor by one who sleeps too long."

Here reference may also be made of King Asoka, who held that the greatest conquest is not of lands by arms, but of men's hearts by love. Hence, he has been hailed as the greatest monarch known to history, especially because of his attitude towards war. Professor H.C. Rawlinson remarked, "Two hundred and fifty years before Christ, Asoka had the courage to express his horror and remorse at the results of a successful campaign and deliberately renounce war as a means of policy, in spite of the fact that his dominions included the unsubdued tribes of the north-west frontier; and was able, in practice, to put an end to cruelty to man and beast, and establish complete religious toleration throughout India. Asoka fulfilled Plato's ideal of the state in which "Kings are Philosophers and Philosophers are Kings".

The empire over which Asoka ruled (270–236 B.C.) extended from Kabul to Kamrupa (Assam) and from Kashmir to Kurnool. The thirty seven years of Asoka's reign constitute a lustrous epoch in Indian annals because of the emperor's earnest efforts to govern his vast dominions on the noble principles of Buddha. He had extraordinary courage to launch his idealistic experiment on a plane hardly attempted by any ruler before and since. After more than twenty five centuries of all sided development, we are still dreaming of a peaceful co-existence without trust in the efficacy of *Ahimsa* as advocated by Buddha, Asoka and Mahatma Gandhi. Both Buddha and Asoka averred that "the chief conquest is the conquest of Right not of Might". They also held with *Mahabharata* that "a King should first subdue himself and then seek to subdue his foe. How should a King who has not been able to conquer his own self be able to conquer his foes?"

Asoka started his reform with himself. His war with Kalinga, which involved great slaughter, brought about a change of heart in him. He, thereupon, avoided violence as far as possible in his public as well as private life. To him there is no higher duty than the welfare of the whole world.

Asoka undertook pious pilgrimages to holy places like Kapilavastu, Gaya, and Sarnath, instead of hunting-excursions involving cruelty to animals. He gradually reduced the slaughter of birds and animals for food, in his own household as well as by the public. "All men are like my children", declared Asoka, "and just I desire that they may obtain every kind of welfare and happiness both in this and the next world, so do I desire for all men." The extension of his humanity towards all living creatures was demonstrated by the establishment of hospitals for them all over his dominions. Wells, tanks, *serais* and avenues were maintained for the convenience of travellers. Quinquennial surveys were undertaken to ascertain the condition of the empire, and to check-up the regular reports of the official informers. Finally, people were encouraged to make personal representations to the emperor himself: "At all hours and in all places,—whether I am eating or in the parlour....... on horseback or in the orchard, the reporters may report people's business to me."

His educational policy is reflected in his inculcation that children should obey and respect their parents, teachers and elders in general. Thus, Asoka's ideas are flooded with moral principles needed for the development of a human society. Asoka emphasized the essential truths underlying on all faiths and discouraged the many trivial and worthless ceremonies. He urged that, most self-exertion behooved all men, small or great, and that self-examination of one's deeds—Good or bad, and reflection thereon were helpful to moral life. The mastery of the senses, purity of thought, steadfast devotion, *satya, daya* etc. are also inculcated. (Sharma: 1967)

It is noticed that the Vedic literature, the foundation of Indian culture and civilization advocates unity and solidarity of our universe, of which doors are open to noble principles from all directions. The spiritual broad base of this philosophy helped India to unite all sections of people together. This culture of unity in diversity believes in the basic human values. The philosophy of *Vedas* remind us that Truth is one, but it is called by different names. Indian thought, philosophy and culture have been promoting the feeling of universal brotherhood for centuries.

Our *Rishis*, Saints and Sufis dedicated themselves to the above philosophy in spite of great upheavals faced by our society. They inspired us to develop a feeling of oneness across the world. This philosophy has been flourished in our country through the practice of tolerance, compassion and dignity of human life without discrimination of big or small.

The *Bhagavad Gita,* a famous religious book lays emphasis on ethical and moral principles in life, "You shall not do to others what you do not want to be done to yourself. It enjoins all to do actions to meet the obligations and duties of life in the perspective of the larger interest of humanity."

In recent times Gautama Buddha, Bhagwan Mahavira, Guru Nanak Dev, Saint Kabir, Swami Dayananda Saraswati, Aurobindo, Ramkrishna Paramahamsa, Swami Vivekananda, Mahatma Gandhi contributed remarkably for promotion of dignity of life, universal brotherhood, harmony and unity amongst religions.

The ethics and morals of all religions are an integral part of Indian culture. The study of major religious scriptures helps us to identify several common areas which bring humanity closer to each other. These are: belief in God and love of God for mankind, compassion, tolerance and universal brotherhood. Indian literature, music, architecture and arts are symbols of our common heritage and culture.

Akbar, the great Mughal Emperor (1555-1605 A.D.), consolidated his empire in India by tolerance and compassion. His courtiers included Muslims and Hindus who were treated with equality in the royal court. The debates were free and frank without prejudice of religion. Epics of all major religions were translated for royal library, which were read to the emperor when in conference with his advisers.

Sufism became an accepted religious order to both Muslims and Hindus. Hazrat Khwaja Gharib Nawaz won the hearts of people through his love and message of God that we should help each other. His message of unity, fraternity and equality made him the leader of spiritual leaders. Hazarat Nizamuddin Aulia and his follower Amir Khusro gave birth to new culture around Delhi by which Hindus and Muslims worked to carry out his message to all sections of the society. Urdu, which is now a part of our culture and heritage, took birth here. Indian culture attracted European scholars who were Christians. Father Hanleden lived in Malabar from 1699 to 1732 and compiled the first Sanskrit-English grammar. Coeourdoux was a famous scholar of philosophy who could see the linkage between Sanskrit and European languages. Sir William Jones, a civil servant during Warren Hastings time (1783-94) and later a judge of Supreme Court at Fort William, Calcutta worked for Indology and Asiatic Society and he became a scholar of Sanskrit Persian, Hebrew, Turkish and Chinese.

Wilkins translated the *Bhagavad Gita* in 1784, the *Hitopadesha* and *Gita Govinda* in 1789 and 1792 respectively. His book, *Institutes of Hindu Law* was published posthumously in 1794. Sir William Jones and Wilkins worked tirelessly to discover India and established the Asiatic Society of Calcutta. Many other Europeans, like Henry Colebrook (1765-1837) and Horace Hayman Wilson (1789-1860) and the French scholar Anqutil Duperro, were devoted to the cause of Indology and worked as a link between the two cultures.

The philosophy of *Upanishads* attracted several European philosophers to the study of Sanskrit. The French Government founded the Ecole des Languages Orientals Vivantes in France. In 1814, the Government offered first Sanskrit Chair at the College de France. Friedrich Schlegel introduced the study of Sanskrit in Germany. The East India Company started Sanskrit teaching at Hartford in 1805. The Universities of Cambridge and Edinborough also established Sanskrit Chairs. French Societe Asiatique was founded in 1821 followed by Royal Asiatic Society in London in the same year.

At a time when Greek and Roman classics were dominating Europe, German scholars put forth Indian cultural literature before the West. This literature, mainly based on the philosophy of the *Upanishads*, dealt with self-realization and identification of *Atma* with *Brahma*. Friedrich Schlegel's "Essay on the Languages and Wisdom of India" stated that Sanskrit represents the beauty and soul of Languages of the world. He indicated that the ancient Indian people lived in close communion with nature and social harmony.

Thus, India has a rich and diverse philosophical tradition dating back mainly to the composition of the *Upanishads* in the later Vedic period.

The modern Indian philosophy was developed during the period from 1750 to 1947. Let me refer to Swami Vivekananda (1863-1902) and a few others who have made significant contributions to Indian philosophy. To Swami Vivekananda, man is a part of the *Paramaatma* or universal soul. From this he drew certain conclusions, such as, first, man is not inherently bad. He is essentially pure and divine. It is wrong to think that man is weak, evil and sinful; second, the association of man with *Paramaatma* leads to the concept of equality of man and unity of mankind. *Vedanta* preaches the message of universal love and service. As love and service demand the spirit of sacrifice and renunciation, the message of *Vedanta* also insists on it. As a strong believer of *Vedanta,* Vivekananda found real essence of India's religion and spirituality in the observance of love, service, sacrifice and renunciation. No nation can be strong by making material progress and enacting good laws. It is the strength of the character of her people, which makes her great and strong. Vivekananda was realistic enough to realize that the truths of *Vedanta* would have little appeal for a hungry man.

Vivekananda placed before the mankind some significant features of religion; first, origin of religion is rooted in the innate struggle of human mind to transcend the limitations of human senses, and not the nature worship or ancestor worship; religion is neither word nor doctrine: it is realization. It is not hearing or accepting. It is being and becoming.

Vivekananda considered freedom not only for maintaining religious harmony among various religious faiths and for realizing the spiritual life by individual, but he also thought that the individual freedom was equally indispensable for the realization of his personality in the social and economic spheres. He, therefore, wanted to make freedom as the natural possession of all individuals. He inspired that every individual must cultivate a free body, mind and spirit. He defined his concept of freedom as, "Liberty does not certainly mean the absence of obstacles in the path of misappropriation of wealth etc. by you and me, but it is our natural right to be allowed to use our own body, intelligence or wealth according to our will, without doing harm to others...."

Swami Vivekananda, speaking to the historic Parliament of World Religions in Chicago, said,

> "To the Hindu, then, the whole world of religion is only a travelling, a coming up, of different men and women, through various conditions and circumstances to the same goal. Every religion is only evolving a God out of the material man, and the same God is the inspirer of all of them. Why are there as many contradictions? They are only apparent, says the Hindu. The contradictions come from the same truth adapting itself to the varying circumstances of different natures. It is the same light

> coming through the glasses of different colours. And these little variations are necessary for purposes of adaptations, but in heart of everything the same truth reigns.... holiness, purity and charity are not exclusive possession of any church in the world, and that every system has produced men and women of the most exalted character. In the face of this evidence, if anybody dreams of the exclusive survival of his own religion and destruction of others, I pity him from the bottom of the heart, and point out to him that upon the banner of every religion will soon be written in spite of resistance: "Help not Fight". The help of a physician with devotion and wholeheartedness is required for the quick recovery of any patient suffering from disease. Similar is the case with regard to a teacher who comes forward to build up the character of the students and to help them to develop their thinking capacity and widen their horizon of reasoning power. In both the cases mishandling, lack of dedication, devotion to the profession and lack of accountability to one's own reason will cause unrepairable damage to the country and the world humanity. They must be well equipped with comprehensive knowledge of their tasks entrusted to them as well as human qualities. These are the two services on which dependence of the human society for its survival is found. Each and every religion is reminding us since its beginning through the ethical principles incorporated in them with clear concept of the serious consequences of the failure to adhere it. The Ancient Indian tradition instructed us in very terms about it through the concept of *Dharma.* (Bharadwaj: 2007)

Besides *Vedanta*, Vivekananda's faith in international unity and brotherhood was also strengthened by his understanding of the role of science. He said, "if modern science is proving anything again and again it is this that we are one—mentally, spiritually and physically." Science is bringing the world together and accelerating universal unity. He pointed out that "The old lines of demarcation and differentiation are vanishing rapidly. Electricity and steam power are placing different parts of the world in inter-communication with each other..." He firmly believed that neither the *Vedanta* nor science negates the existence of different nations. He affirmed international unity and brotherhood through national diversities and religious and cultural varieties.

Bal Gangadhar Tilak is another thinker who contributes significantly to the cultural life of India. Referring to the changes in the society he was convinced that it was inevitable, but to direct the changes or to remake India in the right way there is the need of philosophy. He wrote, "It is difficult to see the way in darkness without light or in thick jungle without a guide." He was of the opinion that mere common sense without faith in religion is of no avail in searching for the truth. In the era of religious and philosophical renaissance of the *Bharat-dharma,* Tilak sought out the guidance of India's own philosophy.

In his private life itself Tilak attempted to rediscover the Indian philosophy. He picked up religion and custom to search for values that had built the Indian civilization. He realized that Hindu religion was not fragile as the custom. Otherwise it would have been leveled to the ground long back. It has lasted because it is based on everlasting truth. He also regarded spiritual truth as the basis of social good. He wrote, "The structure of faith collapses with the collapse of faith in the existence of the soul. The doctrine of soullessness removed the need of faith. When the faith thus ceased to be an organic force binding society together, the society was bound to be disrupted and the individuals living in a community were sure to find their own different paths to happiness. The ties which bind society in one harmonious organization would be snapped, and no other binding principle would take place. Moral ties would loosen and people would fall from good moral standards."

To Tilak reform must begin from within the individual and it must be based on the value system of the people. He believed in popular education which must be initiated with an understanding of classical values and must proceed to recreate the vitality of those values in the form of social order. His belief on the inner strength of man for reform led him to undertake the task of reawakening India to her past to base her future on her past glories. He also realized that real progress could be made through self-governance only, just as moral progress is possible only by decision based on morality. Thus, Tilak's ideas are based on solid moral values.

He taught *dharma* of action which he drew from *Gita*. He reminded the people that India had not become a great nation through negativism and indolence, but through a dynamic willingness to meet the problems of the day and to solve them morally. This was the need of the day. He also reminds us that no one can expect the providence to protect one who sits with folded arms and throws his burden on others.

Along with the *dharma* of action, Tilak taught the *Dharma* of unity to the people. The unity of India, the unity of the Indian civilization, is the *Bharat-Dharma,* spiritually-based and spiritually dedicated way of life. The spirit of orthodoxy was a serious hindrance to the way of life. It had divided the people and inimical to the feeling of common heritage and common cause. The true spirit of *Varnashrama-dharma* was harmony and cooperation and unity. (Gupta: 1963)

Dr. Bhim Rao Ambedkar's concept of democracy provides first priority to social democracy to political democracy or self-rule. He did not contribute to the view that to reform the society one requires political power. Ambedkar in his book titled, '*Ranade, Gandhi and Jinnah*' that it would be a serious mistake to believe that social democracy would follow political democracy and asserted that rights must exist first before power is set-up. What Ambedkar believed cannot be rejected when one looks into the existing state of political and administrative worlds of India. The contemporary trend of social changes and the values asserted by the individuals as members of the society have contributed to a great extent the existing deteriorating political and administrative situation in the country. Effective and healthy political democracy can flourish only in a society which is governed by democratic and ethical principles. (Doctor: 1997) In ancient India people practiced democracy in spirit instead of dissecting its implications. The village affairs were conducted by the principle, "what concerns all must be discussed by all".

The word *Dharma* comes from the Sanskrit root *dhri,* meaning to 'uphold' or to 'sustain'. From this perspective, the best way to think of *dharma* is to say, "that which upholds or sustains the positive order of things: the nation, the community, the family and ultimately even the universe." At the social level, every individual has a particular *dharma* according to his or her position in life. Children have a *dharma,* parents have a *dharma,* teachers have a *dharma,* the police have a *dharma* and even the head of the nation has a *dharma.* One of the *dharmas* of a child is to obey parents and to study, parents have a *dharma* to protect and look after children, to make sure that they are educated, fed, housed and trained. A head of a state has a *dharma* to protect the country and provide secure environment to the citizens. If everyone performs his or her *dharma:* children obey parents, parents look after children, citizens uphold the laws of the land, the police enforce law, the head of state protects the nation, then the family, the community and the nation are "upheld" and there can be prosperity. This is *dharma,* and it all follows from the idea of *dhri,* to uphold.

The opposite of *dharma* is *a-dharma.* If children fail to obey parents, if parents fail to protect, if the head of state fails to act in the interest of the nation, then *a-dharma* exists, and when there is too much *a-dharma,* there will be break down of the family, society and the nation. The nation, the community, the family and even individuals cannot prosper when too much *a-dharma* reigns. There is a saying, "protect *dharma* and *dharma* will protect you."

The ancient Hindu social system was called *Varnashrama Dharma* and the great epics of India, the *Ramayana* and *Mahabharata* are built on this system. In the *Ramayana,* Rama exhibits the ideal of execution of *dharma* as son and King, Sita, his wife, illustrates the *dharma* of the ideal woman and wife. Hanuman, the divine monkey, exhibits the *dharma* of a devoted servant in the way he serves Rama. The evil Ravana, the villain, is the very personification of *a-dharma* as he kidnaps Sita and tries to usurp Rama's Kingdom. In the end *a-dharma* destroys Ravana. In the *Mahabharata*, a great war takes place as *dharma* and *a-dharma* collide in a cosmic struggle over good and evil. In the end good triumphs over evil. *Dharma* always rules over *a-dharma.* This is the way of the universe. (*www.sanskrit.org/www/Premier/dharma.html*)

Dharma is a path of righteousness and living one's life according to the conduct as described by the Hindu scriptures. Hinduism describes *dharma* as the natural universal laws whose observance enables humans to be contended and happy, and to save himself from degradation and suffering. *Dharma* is the moral law combined with spiritual discipline that guides one's life. Hindus consider *dharma* as the very foundation of life. *Dharma* is the 'law of being'. (*Hinduism.about.com/od/basics/a/dharma.htm*)

The word *dharma* is also used in different ways within Hindu philosophy that can also be understood from the root *dhri.* Every constituent of matter: liquid, metals, gases, fire and so on have different *dharmas.* For example, the *dharma* of water is liquidity and wetness, The *dharma* of ice is solidarity and coldness. The *dharma* of fire is heat and light. (*www.sanskrit.org/www/Premier/d arma.html*)

Here mention may be made of *Vaishnavism*, both *tantric* and *puranic,* which was known to and practiced by a section of Hindu population. Mass people could not involve themselves directly in any of the major three religious faiths—*Saktism*, *Saivism* and *Vaishnavism* without the intermediary service of Brahmin priests or religious *gurus*. As a result, common masses could not derive the pleasure of the sense of participation in religious observances. Direct participation in worshipping and religious festivities, was facilitated by Sankaradeva through his new creed of *neo-Vaishnavism*, which he introduced in early decades of the sixteenth century.

It is said that a great man's appearance on the stage of history is hardly an accident and an isolated event. The *Bhagavad Gita* has rightly propounded the theory that whenever there is a decay of spiritualism on the face of the earth leading to the growth of sin and evil God reveals himself through an incarnation to protect the righteous and to re-establish the Law of Piety. Batadrava (Bardowa) in Assam hailed the advent of Sri Sankardeva, the great exponent of the *'Dasya'* school of *Bhakti*, who ushered a new epoch of lasting importance in the history and culture of eastern India. Mahendra Mohan Choudhury, who was a Chief Minister of Assam during 1971-72, wrote, in his foreword in the booklet, titled, 'Culture and Civilization of Assam', "It is indeed difficult to think of Assam and her cultural life without remembering the *Vaisnavite.* Revival of the sixteenth century brought about by Sri Sankardeva and the band of scholars and devotees that flocked round him carried out his mission. Besides spreading the "*Dasya*" school of *Bhakti* amongst large section of the people inhabiting the vast region from Sadiya to Cooch Behar in eastern India, he was also inspirer of a rich literature in Assamese which formed the foundation of modern Assamese literature. The movement he began, gave a strong impetus to the growth of the arts of music, painting, dance and drama that contributed to the all-round cultural development of the people. In other words, Sankardeva was a reformer, spiritualist poet, dramatist, stage actor and playwright all in one. He as all this and much more for he set the pattern of the cultural life of the people as a whole and also established institutions like *Sattra* and *Namghar* to give it a permanent footing.

Assam has suffered in the estimation of people outside due to insularity of her position in the easternmost corner of India. Not much is known of her history, culture and civilization in other parts of India.

Here mention may be made of one or two instances of Sankardeva's miracles and magnanimity. As an extraordinary physical power possessor, Sankardeva at his young age could cross and re-cross mighty Brahmaputra river by swimming. On another occasion Sankardeva, while passing through a jungle he saw a bird enmeshed in a hunter's net struggling to be free. In a boundless compassion of his heart, he immediately set the poor creature free, but simultaneously, he felt that he was depriving the hunter, who was not on the spot, of the means of his livelihood, and he left in the place of the bird in the net a coin tied to a piece of cloth. The King Nara Narayana of Cooch Behar desired to test the genius of Sankardeva and asked him to reduce the *Bhagavata* to a concise form within one night. The sage achieved a sort of miracle by producing next morning the *Guna-*

Mala containing the essence of *Bhagavata*, encased in small casket. The miracle was found when the King wanted to initiate into *Nama-Dharma.* Sankardeva declined to do that on the ground that it would not suit the grandeur of royalty. But the King insisted and one day the Saint asked the King to remain prepared for the next day. And on that particular day news was brought to the King to his deep distress and sorrow that the Saint had passed into a *Samadhi* when his soul parted from his body.

The time of Sankardeva's arrival on the scene of fifteenth and sixteenth century Assam was facing chaotic condition. In the later part of fifteenth century, the ancient kingdom of Kamrupa was facing disintegration both politically and religiously. This ancient kingdom, out of which later emerged the state of Assam, was being ruled from Kamatapur near Cooch Behar by a succession of rulers who could not preserve the boundaries of old kingdom intact. In the east the Ahoms, Mongoloid people expanded control over many tribal and feudal principalities. The situation was full of vague possibilities and permeated by underlying currents of hatred and strife.

As in the sixteenth century Europe, spiritual poverty and moral degeneration set the stage in Assam, as in any other parts of medieval India, for a movement for reform—a movement for recovery of lost ideals in their pristine purity. Sri Sankardeva (1449-1568 A.D.) emerged as patron saint in Assam. He directed the religious emotion towards one Supreme God, Sri Krishna also known as Vishnu. However, it is stated that the cult of Vishnu or Vaisnavism was not a new faith enunciated by Sankardeva and his contemporaries. It had already formed an essential component of Hindu religious philosophy. Sankardeva and others like Chaitanya and Ramananda only re-stated the principles and revived the tenets of this noble faith for the welfare of the society. The movement was not guided by priestly class, but by non-Brahmins. The religious and cultural history of India has many instances of non-Brahmins assuming spiritual leadership with great success. The neo-Vaisnavite movement that Sankardeva ushered in Assam could reduce the evils of ceremonialism and blind formalism and exposed the barrenness of soulless rituals.

Sankardeva gave first priority to the field of religion as it needed very badly new light or reform. He enunciated the doctrine of "*Ekasarana Dharma*" or the religion of single minded devotion to the One Supreme God based on '*Dasya*' relationship of man to God. The '*Dasya*' conception implied complete surrender of man to the Will of God like that of a servant to his master. The teachings of Sankardeva reflected his great erudition in the ancient scriptures and wide experience gained by northern India and contact with holy men associated with the Vaisnavite revival. The essence of his teachings comprising the philosophy of his cult was derived from *Bhagavad Gita* and *Upanishads*. Sankardeva is undoubtedly one of the foremost religious leaders of India and the system he expounded, though rooted in the sacred lore of the Hindus, has traits and characteristics of deserving to be compared with other systems, not only in respect of its abiding effects as a sectarian creed within the fold of Hinduism, but also in respect of the organizational and institutional set-up through which it has worked for centuries retaining all its freshness and vigour.

The *neo-Vaisnavite* Bhakti movement initiated by Sankaradeva marked the advent of a new age, an age of Renaissance, in the history of north-eastern part of India. The success of a movement depends mainly on the genuineness of the cause and the character and tenacity of the leaders. The cause of Sankaradeva was true religion and purity of conduct on the part of God's devotees. Naturally, he could mobilize a group of followers with religious emotion, who by their devout zeal and instinctive understanding of the popular mind, could swept the clouds of superstition and corruption from the social life. They possessed, just as Sankardeva did, a background of Sanskrit learning for their devotional outpourings, and had command of thought and language and technique of poetry and music for making an emotional approach to the people. The soil was thus fertilized for a luxuriant vegetation of literary and cultural exuberance and moral and ethical perfection.

The first fruit of the movement was the growth amongst the people of a consciousness of spiritual equality above all social distinctions as enforced by the caste system and other usages and institutions. The creed formulated by Sankardeva had a universal appeal. It declared in emphatic terms the universal brotherhood of man and oneness of God, and recognized the spiritual equality of all men irrespective of caste and social status. The problem of untouchability which assumed hideous aspects in the parts of India in modern times receded to the background in this part of India more than five hundred years ago. Even Muslim and tribals were accepted by Sankaradeva as his disciples. The teachings of Sankaradeva were simple. For example the conception of spiritual equality or equality of all men before the eye of God, like the conception of the equality of all citizens before the eye of law, had the effect of liberalizing the conception of caste privileges. The dignity of the human soul was recognized above earthly limitations of man in the society.

The growth of the vernacular Assamese literature was a direct outcome of the *neo-Vaisnavite Bhakti* movement that swept Assam. The literature was mostly in verse and comprised works of translation or adaptation from the ancient scriptures, mainly the *Bhagavata*, the *Gita* and the *Upanishads*. The ancient stories which the people loved were made the instruments of a great religious revival. The old ballads found in the Epics and *Puranas* were rewritten, supplemented and so overlaid with didactic matter that works like the *Kirtan-Ghosa* and the *Dasama* of Sankardeva became the *Vedas* of the masses. The *Nam-Ghosa* of Madhabdeva which acquired the same status is essentially a poem of a thousand verses in recitation of Holy Name. It also contains masterly exposition of the philosophy of the *Upanishads* in terms of *Bhakti.*

Sankardeva himself was a prolific writer. He composed more than thirty treatises on religious themes, the most important of which was the *Kirtan-Ghosa* containing gleanings from different scriptures. His compositions, though translations and adaptations in the main from scriptural texts, bear a stamp of originality in them. The *Bargeets* and the One-Act-Plays are significant contributions of Sankardeva and Madhabdeva to the Assamese literature. The *Bargeets* are divine songs which, when sung to tune set by the Masters, are capable of giving ecstatic pleasure to the hearers. The One-Act-Plays are a unique feature of the sixteenth century Assamese literature. Sankardeva also evolved the popular stage where the '*Bhaowna*' or dramatic presentation of divine themes was made to attract the people and evoke their religious sentiments. Sankardeva himself painted the screens with heavenly scenes and took part in the dramatic show as an actor.

Another very interesting part of his writings was their multiplication as there was no printing or Xerox machine during his time. Writings were done on the leaves of *Sanchi* tree or barks of *Sanchi* trees. The barks were cut to size and smoothed out by a special process. All copies had to be made by the scribe. Though the work was laborious thousands of such manuscripts were found their ways to the homes of devotees.

Two institutions created by Sankardeva—*Sattra* and *Namghar* contributed a lot for the maintenance of disciplined social and moral life amongst the people in general and *Vaisnavas* in particular. The term *Sattra* is derived from Sanskrit root '*troi*', means to protect with prefix *'Sat'*, meaning good. Here Guru and *Bhaktas* reside together devoting themselves to religious practices, study and discussion of sacred literature. The campus of the *Sattra* is held sacrosanct and within it are to be found a *Namghar* or prayer house with annexures, and residential cottages for the Guru and the *Bhakta*. Even today *Namghar* is working as an institution to provide social and religious guidance to the people (Dutt: 1956).

Ramanuja launched the *Bhakti* movement in the southern part of the sub-continent, in the eleventh century A.D. in order to fight the perversions and debaucheries in the name of religion, which were eating into vitals of the society. He emphasized on monotheism and *Bhakti* or devotion as the real way to worship God. One of his disciples, Ramananda, who established a sect at Varanasi, brought the message of *Bhakti* to northern India. Gradually, through the pioneering works of Kabir, Nanak, Mirabai and other Saints, the doctrine of *Bhakti* permeated the Indian society.

In the similar way, Sankardeva introduced a creed, adhering to the main principles of *Bhakti,* preaching a doctrine of 'Universal social brotherhood,' which revolutionized the entire face of the life of the people and lead to the formation of a broader society. It had united the diverse tribal communities of the region and gave a culture, to be identified later as Assamese culture. Even Islam was not looked upon as an alien element. Mir Jumla's chronicler was surprised with the assimilation of the Muslim with the indigenous people. Hindus pays homage to the Muslim Peers and the Muslims participated in *'Nam-Kirtanas'*.

Sankaradeva taught qualified monotheism of absolute surrender to one God and advocated the *Dasya* attitude of *Bhakti,* in which the votary is to consider himself as the servant of God. The religion that Sankardeva propounded is based on four principles. These are:

The comprehension of *Parama Brahma* (the all pervasive Supreme Being) in the form of Vishnu as extolled in the *Vedas*. *Ek Sarana* (absolute and undivided devotion to the Supreme Being) in the form of Krishna as extolled in the *Gita*; *Sat-Sanga* (the company of pious divine) as enjoined in the *Bhagavata Purana* and *Nam-Kirtana* (divine services in the form of prayer). These four principles in the condensed form are *Guru, Deva, Bhakta* and *Nama.* Since his teachings were mainly based on the *Bhagavad Gita* and the *Bhagavata Purana*, his creed was called *Bhagavata Dharma* or *Ek Sarana Naam Dharma,* as Sankardeva was recognized as *'Maha-purusa'* or 'God-incarnate'. Sankardeva taught equality of all human beings and accepted disciples from amongst the tribesmen and the Muslims, whom he placed on equal footing.

Sankardeva introduced the system of distributing *'prasad'* after '*Naam-Kirtan'* ceremony is over at the places of religious congregation, composed of pulses like gram, and *mung* or green gram, available seasonal fruits, ginger, betel leaves and areca nut, coconut, sugarcane etc. Since each family had homestead land, where these crops were grown, the *Mahapurusa* took this advantage for social good and his followers put in extra efforts for increasing the production of these items. (Rajkhowa:)

While talking about *Dharma* let me explain it with the help of Hinduism as a way of life. Four goals of life are enjoined by Hinduism to be observed within the span of our life from birth to death. The *Karma,* i.e. work is human life, not merely life. It is more true to the profession of teaching and medicine. However, this does not mean that the other professions are not enjoined with *Dharma.* To me these two professions are occupying top priority in the list of services to humanity, for the simple reason that if these services are entrusted to inhuman, inefficient persons, human society will certainly face the threat of survival. The only difference between the two services is that in the case of medicine the result is immediate and even an uneducated person can feel the negative result without delay. On the other hand in the case of education the negative result on the humanity is not felt immediately. Interestingly large section of the society is failing to realize it and some are insensitive to it.

What are the four goals of life as advocated by Hinduism to be pursued? These are *dharma* (fulfillment of all obligations), *artha* (wealth), *Kama* (fulfillment of desires), and *moksha* (realization of the Divine). The last of these goals is with the domain of religion and spirituality mainly, while the other three are essentially individual with social responsibility. Hinduism is not against acquisition of wealth or pursuit of passion and desire. But such activities must be governed by *dharma,* according to Hinduism. To be governed by *dharma* one needs the power of self-restraint. It is on this ground the Hinduism is giving importance on the cultivation of certain personal qualities which again are required to be an efficient physician in the world of medicine.

The rules for the observance of *dharma* as incorporated in the *Manusmriti* (chapter VI, verse 92) are cited by Dr. B.K. Modi as below:

- *Dhriti* (Endurance, fortitude, steadfastness): A commitment to doing one's duties in every situation is the basis of *dharma.* One should not be cowed down by obstacles or temporary setbacks but move resolutely towards one's destination. One must have patience.
- *Kshama* (Forgiveness): The capacity to accommodate another's fault or mistake or different point of view… an unforgiveness person defiles himself with enormous complexities. On the other hand forgiveness frees a person from the need to get even, or harbour thoughts of revenge. Forgiveness is choice, not an emotion.
- *Dama:* (Self-restraint, self-control): A mature and well-integrated personality having developed the capacity to have control over

the faculties of mind does not disintegrate or dissipate his energy and channelize all potentialities for chosen higher goals. Such a wise person who has gradually and quietly freed himself from the inner conflicts shines in his purity, tranquility and completeness.

- *Asteyam* (Non-convetousnesness, non-stealing): Desire for acquisition of material goods, particularly of money, is very compelling. Money is seen as a source of power, security, happiness, which can give social status. It is a resource that helps overcome calamities. However, when man's pursuits become targeted towards fulfilling his endless desires, unmindful about his *dharmic* obligations, one naturally remains acquiring wealth and his needs become greed. One should earn money through righteous means and after meeting own requirements, share the surplus back with the society wherefrom he has got it and focus on supporting those in need. This also results in social responsibility.
- *Shaucham* (Purity, cleanliness): This is both external and internal. A clean body, cloths, dwelling place and environment is a daily focus. Inner cleanliness calls for dealing with undesirable feelings or impurities of mind, like *kama* (lust, endless desires), *krodha* (anger), *lobha* (greed), *moha* (attachment), *ahankara* (false ego, pride), and *vishaya* (jealousy). The fire of wisdom and balanced intellect is expected to burn these impurities.
- *Indriya Nigraha:* (Control over the senses): Sense organs are like horses and man's mind is the charioteer, who will not allow them to be rebellious but give them direction.
- *Dhi* (Wisdom, discrimination, inborn instinctive intellect): A wise person sees himself as a part of a wide scheme of creation.
- *Vidya* (Self-knowledge, learning): Knowledge by itself does not produce possessions or pleasures. Actions are required for the same. Knowledge shapes that effort for making it as a valid, effective and appropriate action.
- *Satyam* (Truthfulness): Truthfulness starts with the understanding of things as they are, without imagining or colouring and then speaking and actions based on that understanding.
- *Akrodh* (Absence of anger): A wish unfulfilled, an expectation not satisfied, undue interference in one's affairs, humiliation, ingratitude etc. provoke one's anger. To control the same, one must understand that one's anger is a reaction and not a deliberate

action. One also needs to understand that things do not necessarily go the way one wants. One who gains mastery over anger, where mind is tranquil and free from agitation, stands tall in the society like a mountain.

- *Maitri* (Friendship): A true friend is consistent, honest and willing to share his thoughts and feelings without being subject to conditions of pride, jealousy or rivalry. The openness and reciprocity in friendship allows one to have a mature relationship (Veeranghavan: 2007).

Manu further writes, "Non-violence, truth, non-coveting, purity of body and mind, control of senses are the essence of *dharma.*" Therefore, *dharmic* laws govern not only individuals, but all in the society.

*(Hinduism.about.com/od/basics/a/*dharma.*htm)*

Karuna (Compassion): Trying to avoid hurting others by means of speech, thought or action is a great value. A sensitive or alert person goes beyond non-injury and sees the entire world as an expression of the Divine. (Veeranghavan: 2007)

Dharma refers to the religious ethics as propounded by Hindu *Gurus* in ancient Indian scriptures. Tulsidas, author of *Ramcharitmanas*, has defined the root of *dharma* as compassion. This principle was taken up by Lord Buddha in his immortal book of great wisdom, *Dhammapada.*

(*Hinduism.about.com/od/basics/a/dharma.htm*)

Dharma is a concept of central importance in Indian philosophy and religion. It is difficult to provide simple and concise definition for *dharma,* as the word has a long and varied history and straddles a complex set of meanings and interpretations.

Referring to Law in the universal and abstract sense, *dharma* designates those behaviours considered necessary for the maintenance of natural order, and that justice, social harmony and happiness require that people discern and live in a manner appropriate to the requiring that order.

The idea *dharma* as duty is found in India's ancient legal and religious texts. The guidelines and rules regarding this accumulated in a body of literature called *Dharmashastra.*

(en.wikipedia.org/wilki/Dharma #Definition_and meaning)

Radhakrishnan, the great philosopher, statesman and former President of India has described what *dharma* is as: *Dharma* is that which binds society together. That which divides society, breaks it up into parts and makes people fight one another is *Adharma* (non-religion). *Dharma* is nothing more than the realization of the Supreme and acting in every small act of our life with that Supreme is in our mind. If we are able to do so we are performing *dharma.* The real believer in God has his heart always lifted to *Dharma.*

The words religion and *dharma* are synonymous and interchangeable. Religion literally means that which leads one to God. *Dharma* is derived from the Sanskrit word "*dhri*" which means "to hold together". It has a wider meaning than the word "religion".

(Hinduism.about.com/cs/basics/a/aa0630303.htm)

Gradually in India many of these values are adhered only by poorer and uneducated classes. Many among the educated in the modern form or style have given up these values at least partially. (Veeranghavan: 2007)

What is Karma? The Concise Oxford Dictionary defines it as the "sum of person's actions in one of his successive states of existence, viewed as deciding his fate for the next." In Sanskrit *Karma* means "volitional action that is undertaken deliberately or knowingly." It also provides self-determination and strong will power to abstain from inactivity. *Karma* is the differentia that characterizes him from other creatures of the world. The law of cause and effect forms an integral part of Hindu philosophy. This law is termed as *Karma*, which means to act.

The theory of *Karma* harps on the Newtonian principles that every action produces an equal and opposite reaction. Every time we think or do something, we create, which in time will bear its corresponding effects. This cyclical cause and effect generates the concepts of *samsara* (the world). It is the personality of a human being—with its positive and negative actions that causes *Karma.*

Karma could be both the activities of the body and mind, irrespective of the consideration whether the performance brings fruition immediately or at a later stage. However, the involuntary or the reflex actions of the body cannot be called *Karma.*

According to the ways of life chosen by a person, his *Karma* can be classified into three classes. The *Sattvika Karma,* which is without attachment, selfless and for the benefit of others; the *Rajasika Karma,* which is selfish and where the focus is on gains for oneself; and the *Tamasika Karma*, which is undertaken without heed to consequences, and supremely selfish and savage.

(Hinduism.about.com/od/basics/a/karma,htm)

Coming to Indian Philosophy it is noticed that India has a rich and diverse philosophical tradition dating back to the composition of the *Upanishads* in the later Vedic period. According to Radhakrishnan, the oldest of these constitute the earliest philosophical compositions of the world.

The Indian thinkers of antiquity viewed philosophy as a practical necessity that needed to be cultivated in order to understand how life can best led. It became a custom for the Indian writers to explain at the beginning of philosophical works how it serves human ends. Recent scholarship, as shown that there was a great deal of intercourse between Greek and Indian philosophy during the era of Hellenistic expansion.

Indian philosophy is distinctive in its application of analytical rigour to metaphysical problems and goes into very precise detail about the nature of reality, the structure and function of the human psyche and how the relationship between the two have important implications for the human salvation.

Jain *Tirthankars* find exclusive mention in the *Vedas* and the Hindu epics. During the Vedic age, India had two broad philosophical streams of thought: The *Shramanas* philosophical schools, represented by Buddhism, Jainism, and the long defunct and Ajivika on the one hand and the *Brahmana/Vedantic/Puranic* schools represented by *Vedanta, Vaishnava* and other movements on the other. Both streams are known to have mutually influenced by each other.

Bal Gangadhar Tilak has described Jainism as the originator of *Ahimsa* and wrote in a letter printed in *Bombay Samachar*, Mumbai on 10th December, 1904, "In ancient times, innumerable animals were butchered in sacrifices. Evidence in support of this is found in various poetic compositions such as the *Meghaduta*. But the credit for disappearance of this terrible massacre from the Brahminical religion goes to Jainism." Swami Vivekananda also credited Jainism as one of the influencing forces behind the Indian culture. Jainism is a religious tradition in which all life is considered to be worthy of respect and Jain teaching emphasizes this equality of all life advocating the non-harming of even the smallest creatures. Non-violence is the basis of right View, the condition of right Knowledge and the kernel of right Conduct in Jainism.

Buddhism shares many philosophical views with other Indian systems, such as belief in *Karma*, a cause and effect relationship between all that has been done and all that will be done. Events that occur are held to be the direct result of previous events.

Modern Indian philosophy was developed during British occupation (1750-1947). The philosophers in this era gave contemporary meaning to traditional philosophy. Some of them were Bal Gangadhar Tilak, Bankim Chandra Chattopadhyaya, Raja Ram Mohun Roy, Sri Aurobindo,

Mahapandit Rahul Sankrityayana, Debiprasad Chattopadhyaya, M.N. Roy, Indra Sen, Haridas Chaudhuri, Swami Sahajanand Saraswati, Ananda Coomaraswamy, Ramana Maharshi and Sarvapalli Radhakrishnan.

The political philosophy most closely associated with India is the one of *Ahimsa* (Non-violence) and *Satyagraha*, popularized by Mahatma Gandhi during the Indian struggle for independence. It was influenced by the Indian Dharmic philosophy, particularly the *Bhagavad Gita*, as well as secular writings of authors like Leo Tolstoy, Henry David Thoreau and John Ruskin. In turn it influenced the later movements for independence and civil rights, especially those led by Martin Luthar King Jr. and to lesser extent Nelson Mandela.

(en.wikipedia.org/wiki/Indian philosophy)

India gained independence on 15th August, 1947 from colonial rule after a long struggle under the leadership of Mahatma Gandhi, whose ideals of non-violence is well respected throughout the world even now. The process of the struggle for independence of India may be traced with the efforts of Mahatma Gandhi to fight for human rights in South Africa. Throughout the long struggle he devoted to the cause of the human rights of the Indians through *Satyagraha* and Non-violence. He could mobilize even the Indian women to come out of the four walls of their habitation to participate in the movement. The non-cooperation movement which was a major component of the freedom struggle could embrace even the young students of the country.

The old values which were adhered by the Indians during ancient, medieval and initial stage of independent India continued to play a significant role in the socio-political life of the country. However, with the spread of education, development of communication facilities, recently with the development of information technology, emergence of globalization cause change of values in our society. More weightage is attached on enhancement of material possession and money power. While enriching money power man does not care to set aside the standing values like doing no harm to others, showing due respect to human dignity, to avoid unethical activities etc. The main reasons for this state of affair in the country may be—power of money in occupying respectable position in the society, to secure employment, to get admission in the professional institutions for study people do not hesitate to adopt all kinds of unethical devices and to distort old Indian values required for the establishment of peace and harmony in the society and to make progress of the nation. The concept of *Dharma* as enshrined in the *Manusmriti* and other ethical values constituting the core area of each religion of the world has been dethroned from the world of religion. The superfluous rituals in the religious occasions have become very strong commanding force to attract the people of all ages in the country.

The leaders of freedom struggle like Dadabhai Naoroji, Gopal Krishna Gokhale, Lokamanya Bal Gangadhar Tilak, Lala Lajpat Rai, Bipin Chandra Pal, Surenda Nath Banerjee, Pandit Madan Mohan Malaviya, Motilal Nehru, Sardar Vallabhbhai Patel, Maulana Abul Kalam Azad, Dr. Rajendra Prasad, Jawaharlal Nehru etc. were men of eminence and strong personality. In the beginning of the twentieth century, the great "freedom fighter" Balgangadhar Tilak gave voice, "Swaraj is my birthright and I shall have it". Ultimately, the British went away and we gained independence on 15th August, 1947.

The British left India leaving severe negative impact on the country. However, they also left scope to pick up some positive impact on us. Here mention may be made of Lord William Bentinck (1828-35) for his humane prohibition of *Sati* (self-immolation of widows on the dead husband's pyre) in which he was heartily assisted by Raja Ram Mohun Roy—the Morning Star of modern India. He also took very bold step to reverse the anti-native policy of Cornwallis in respect of Government employment in responsible offices. Among the pioneers of this liberal policy were also British civilians like Sir Thomas Munro, Sir Charles Metcalfe and Sir John Malcolm. Lord Dalhousie (1848-56), the last great Governor General of India under the Company's regime had as great a flair for administrative advancement as he had for territorial annexations. There is not a sphere of activity, in which he did not leave the impress of his personality. Another person to be remembered is Lord Ripon, an Irish and Catholic, the only non-English- or-non-Protestant, to rule India (1880-84). Ripon's constructive measures for extension of local self-government. "What I want to secure by extension of local self-government", Ripon explained, "is....gradual training of the best, most intelligent, and most influential men in the community to take an interest and an active part in the management of their local affairs.... What I am trying to do is not to impose an English system on India, but to revive and extend the indigenous system of the country. That indigenous system we have done a great deal to destroy, but the remnants of it exist to a greater or lesser extent in most parts of the country, and it is upon those remnants that I hope to build up the edifice of local self-government".

Mahatma Gandhi, leader of the movement stated clearly that *Swaraj* is to be gained by educating the masses to a sense of their capacity to regulate and control authority.

Jawaharlal Nehru also gave tremendous value to individual freedom. The purpose of a democratic society was essentially to provide necessary conditions of creative development. Explaining the reasons for accepting the democratic process in India, Nehru observed: "It is not enough for us merely to produce the material goods of the world. We do want high standard of living, but not at the cost of man's creative spirit, his creative energy, his spirit of adventure, not at the cost of all fine things of life which have ennobled man throughout the ages. Democracy is not merely a question of elections."

Nehru also insisted that a scientific approach be accepted as the guiding principle of life and as a process of thinking regarding our problems. Nehru seems to have a profound sense of history and deep respect for India's heritage. He wanted the Indian people to be free from the shackles of the past. At the same time he urged them to recondition their mind equipping themselves with the problems of the present and perspective on the future. This is possible through humanism and scientific spirit. Despite an apparent conflict between the two, there was a growing synthesis between humanism and scientific spirit, resulting in a kind of scientific humanism. Nehru expressed his mind very clearly in the last chapter of *The Discovery of India* as, "The modern mind, that is to say, the better type of the modern mind, is practical and pragmatic, ethical and social, altruistic and humanitarian....It has discarded to a large extent the philosophic approach of the ancients, their search for ultimate reality, as well as the devotionalism and mysticism of the medieval period. Humanity is its god and social service, its religion."

In the language of Radhakrishnan gaining independence has been a simpler task compared with the one of administering the country in a clean, decent way. This seems to be more formidable task. For it we require selfless leadership, an honest and competent civil service. We require a disciplined military and police force. We require expert industrial managers and skilled workers and good agricultural peasants. Our ordinary citizens should have civic sense and national feeling.

All these things cannot be achieved in a day. What we are attempting to do to our best of our power is to take some steps towards developing a sound administration, a stable Government and a healthy nation. We cannot say that we are satisfied with what we have done. There are things happening in different parts of the country which make us feel sad, depressed and ashamed of ourselves. What is necessary is the strong sense of patriotism. It is true that we developed a negative kind of patriotism when we struggled to rid of the country of foreign rule. (What we do not want: Foreign rule) But a positive patriotism, a dynamic fellow-feeling, a sense of belonging to this country, of being proud to belong to it, these things yet to come. We have to build these in the minds and hearts of men. (Radhakrishnan: 1992)

We fought for independence with a desire to develop a democratic set in the society. Democracy has three basic dimensions—political, economic and social. Political and economic democracy are rooted in social democracy. Social democracy has been said by Mahatma Gandhi as a way of life. It is not merely a way of life, but an ethical way of life. Nobody could deny it and recently the Indian scholars have started discussing about good governance in the country. The government did not make any explicit pronouncement of it nor the course of actions of the government reflects it till recently. Only the government led by Narenda Modi as Prime Minister made explicit pronouncement of it when it said, "Minimum Government and maximum governance". Here lies the need of ethical way of life. As Radhakrishnan said, Democracy is a faith. It is a faith on human power as well as intellectual power. The concept of maximum governance also demands freedom which means restraints. Once a man restraints himself from encroaching upon other's freedom there emerges humility of man which is the core element of good governance. Good governance is nothing but democratic or self-governance.

Those who won freedom for India and created its constitutional systems were, like the founding fathers of the United States Constitution, men of rare talent and dedication. One point of similarity, and perhaps the greatest, between the constitutions of the world's two largest democracies is their high moral tone. Acharya J.B. Kripalani spoke eloquently in the Constituent Assembly on 17th October, 1949, "I want this House to remember that what we have enunciated are not merely legal, constitutional and formal principles, but moral principles; and moral principles have to be lived, whether it is in private life, or it is public life, whether it is in commercial life, political life or the life of an administrator. They have to be lived throughout." (Palkhivala: 1997)

The Constitution of India reflects the Indian culture very well. It was formulated at the instance of galaxy of eminent Indians under the chairmanship of Dr. Rajendra Prasad. Dr. B.R. Ambedkar was the Chairman of the Drafting Committee. Under their leadership other eminent Indians participated in the task of preparation of the Constitution. The Preamble to the Constitution focuses on moral and human values and inclusiveness of all in governance of the country through the phrase, "We, the People of India." The Preamble may be read as,

> "WE, THE PEOPLE OF INDIA, having solemnly, resolved to constitute India into a SOVEREIGN SOCIALIST SECULAR DEMOCRATIC REPUBLIC and to secure all its citizens:
> JUSTICE, social, economic and political;
> LIBERTY of thought, expression, belief, faith and worship;
> EQUALITY of status and opportunity;
> And promote among them all
> FRATERNITY assuring the dignity of the individual (unity and integrity of the nation)
> IN OUR CONSTITUENT ASSEMBLY this twenty-sixth day of November, 1949, do
> HEREBY ADOPT, ENACT AND GIVE TO OURSELVES THIS CONSTITUTION. (Bakshi: 2004)

Thus, the Preamble to the Constitution of India lays emphasis upon the maintenance of the dignity of the individual for establishment of fraternity or brotherhood. Towards this end fundamental rights of the citizens have been provided so that each individual can get an opportunity to be developed as human person. The violation of fundamental rights invites a serious threat to human dignity. It is also noticed that the framers of the constitution realized that it is not enough to make the fundamental rights justiciable unless he is free from economic wants and misery. Dr. Radhakrishnan in his speech at a seminar on Parliamentary Democracy on 25th February, 1956 said, "Poor people who wander about, find no work, no wages and starve, whose lives are continual round of sore affliction and pinching poverty, cannot be proud of the constitution and its law." As a result of it the Directive Principles of State Policy have been incorporated in the Part IV of the Constitution of India, exhorting the State to shape its social and economic policies in such a manner that all citizens, men and women equally, have the right to an adequate means of livelihood, just and humane conditions of work and a decent standard of life and full enjoyment of leisure and social and cultural opportunities. (Agarwal : 1986)

Unfortunately, in India the divisive forces on the basis of caste, community are assuming alarming nature. The social, political, administrative institutions which have to take the leading role in establishing mutual faith in establishing harmony amongst social groups professing different religious faiths, practicing different social cultures, speaking different languages, are almost collapsing and not in a position to command the confidence of the citizens of independent India and the question of taking the leading role in establishing peace, harmony, mutual faith in the society does not arise. In other words, India's glorious past with rich culture and civilization is in threat of disappearing.

Here mention may also be made of what Guy B. Adams and Danny L. Balfour talked about ethical failure in their article, titled, "Ethical Failings, Incompetence, and Administrative Evil". Incompetence and greed are the two major sources of ethical failure in public administration. Both of them made an attempt to bring out a relationship between incompetence and ethical failure by saying that both combining together may lead to serious wrong things (Adams and Balfour: 1984).

Gandhi's principles provided the scope for acquiring moral strength of the people during struggle for freedom of the country. His style of living and social relationship and committed service to the freedom of the individuals as well as the nation remind us every moment that mere material progress cannot bring human progress. Human progress must be grounded on human values. Gandhi realized it and accordingly he made human approach for bringing social change.

Here mention may be made of what Herbert Spencer thought of social change. To him social progress is divergent, moving in different directions touching different areas of man's life. In this process each element of change gives birth to new elements inviting new approach or modification of existing approach. Naturally, there arises multiplicity of changing elements making social life complex day-by-day. The process of social reform must address all the elements. Because each element is active in its own way in the society and different persons may give different weightage to these elements according to their personal or individual interest overlooking the social interest. To Professor Ellwood the material as well as moral development emerges only from this process. But the problem of modifying the social life is essentially a problem of modifying habits in the masses of individuals and therefore, our efforts have to be made in the direction of combined growth of individuals as well as the masses. Gandhi also realized that to uproot exploitation from the society the exploiter must change his heart. He preferred social service as an instrument for establishment of an exploitation free society and if it fails then one should take the help of *Satyagraha* (Bharatiya: 1987). Religion is an inalienable of part of social culture and therefore let us have a look to the major religions in India as below:

Hinduism: Like all other religions Hinduism provides enough space for ethical principles. Selfless actions for the good of others is the way to liberation according to Hinduism. Hinduism recognizes three paths as below:

1. Path of Knowledge (*Jnana Marga*)
2. Path of Action (*Karma Marga*)
3. Path of Devotion (*Bhakti Marga*)

All the three paths are interdependent. *Bhagavad Gita* envisages that either by following the path of knowledge or by following the path of selfless actions or again following the path of devotion to the Lord, one can attain liberation.

The path of knowledge helps identification of one's own inner self with that of others; the path of action invites performance of selfless service to others and the path of devotion requires sincerity in action self-confidence. For being successful in all these three paths *Yoga* and *Sadhana* are the two strong devices.

Hindu morality has its roots in *Vedas* and *Upanishads* themselves, although *Vedas* are generally regarded as a treatise of rituals and *Upanishads* as treatise of *Jnana*. The central concept of morality comes from *Rig Veda* itself. Further, the virtues like truth, charity, liberty etc. are much emphasized in the *Vedas* themselves. In the *Upanishads,* the lesson of *Jnana* to the pupils instructs them to practice virtue, to speak truth, to cultivate modesty, humility etc. which are needed for liberation. The Hindu society has been divided into four broad classes—*Brahmana, Kshatriya*, *Vaishya* and *Sudra*. Duties of each class is well defined and every member of each class is expected to perform his own duties. Such duties of the individual are known as *Varna Dharma.* The *Bhagavad Gita* enumerates the following duties to each class as below:

1. *Brahmana*: Self-control, austerity, purity, forbearance, uprightness, wisdom, knowledge and faith in religion.
2. *Kshatriya*: Heroism, Vigour, steadiness, resourcefulness, not fleeing from the battlefield, generosity and leadership.
3. *Vaishya*: Agriculture, tending cattle and trade.
4. *Sudra*: Service to all the above classes.

The general duties to be performed by everyone irrespective of his *Varna* are differently conceived by different thinkers. According to Manu they are the following:

1. Steadfastness
2. Forgiveness
3. Application
4. Non-stealing
5. Cleanliness
6. Restraint
7. Wisdom
8. Learning
9. Truth
10. Freedom from anger

The duties and virtues were abridged into the following five only by Manu himself:

1. Non-Violence
2. Truth
3. Non-stealing
4. Cleanliness
5. Restraint of Senses

The '*Panchamahavrata*' of Jainism and '*Panchasila*' of Buddhism are the symbols of these virtues.

Non-Violence or *Ahimsa* negatively refers to abstention from injury or harm to any living being in any form, but positively, it refers to the virtues of love, kindness and compassion towards all beings.

Truth refers to abstention from telling lie or speaking harsh and unpalatable language.

Non-stealing implies abstention from taking away anybody's property without his consent. Taking undue profit in business, restraining someone from earning the gains of his legitimate rights etc. all come under stealing and these must be avoided. *Brahmacharya* refers to a life of purity, celibacy, non-adultery etc. *Aparigraha* is a general attitude of non-attachment towards worldly objects. We have seen that attachment towards worldly objects is at the root of all vices according to Hinduism and therefore, it must be avoided. Thus, Hinduism, in general, emphasizes the virtues of love, kindness, compassion, truth, purity, celibacy, self-restraint, non-attachment etc. as virtues to be inculcated and cultivated.

Prashatapada provides a more comprehensive list of virtues and duties as below:

1. Moral earnestness or regards for *Dharma*
2. Non-Violence
3. Seeking good of all creatures
4. Veracity
5. Non-stealing
6. Celibacy
7. Purity of Motive
8. Restraint of Anger
9. Personal Cleanliness
10. Non-eating of impure food
11. Devotion to the recognized deity
12. Fasting

Buddhism: The sixth century B.C. constitutes an important epoch in the history of ancient India. The period was the "light of Asia, that perfect embodiment of knowledge, courage, love and sacrifice." The religion which Buddha founded covered the whole of India. It even crossed the boundaries of India to Ceylon, Burma, Siam, Malaya, Java, Sumatra and then again to Nepal, Tibet, Mangolia, Korea, China and Japan. It continues to be a living force. It is again the religion of the Buddha which laid the foundation of Asian unity.

Buddhism, in its original form, is a practical religion of pure ethical discipline. It is basically a man-centred religion, totally humanistic in its outlook, approach and aim. In its essence, Buddhism gives us a way of life with universal character or applicable to all human beings. It advocates eightfold path to get relief from all kinds of suffering. Every man is a saviour of himself. The present miserable condition of human life can be transcended by the sincere efforts of himself. Man is not to seek the grace of any power superior to him. He is himself sufficient for improving his condition and that is by the adoption of the eightfold path:

1. *Right View or Right Understanding*: This primarily refers to a clear understanding of the four noble truths as propounded by Buddha—(a) Concerning the nature of suffering, (b) concerning the origin of suffering, (c) concerning the removal of suffering and (d) concerning the state of *Nirvana*.
2. *Right Thought*: The Right Thought requires that our mind should be pure, free from lust, ill will etc. Further, we must avoid anything that impedes our onward march.
3. *Right Speech*: This consists of refraining from telling a lie, back

biting, harsh talks and idle gossip. Moreover, our speech should be free from ill will, selfish interest, dogmatic assertion etc.

4. *Right Action*: This generally consists of observing the five precepts (*Panchashila*) in both their negative and positive aspects–
   (a) Not to kill but to practice harmless and compassion to all.
   (b) Not to take that which is not given, but to practice charity and generosity.
   (c) Not to commit sexual misconduct, but to practice chastity and self-control.
   (d) Not to indulge in false speech, but to practice sincerity and honesty.
   (e) Not to practice intoxicating drinks or drugs, but to practice restraint and mindfulness.
5. *Right Livelihood*: This advises for a just, honest earning. One must avoid adopting any means of livelihood which deprives others from their just rights. This includes counsel for abstaining from inclinations towards undue hoarding, unjust money making etc. The traditional trades from which people are asked to abstain are—(a) dealing in arms; (b) dealing in living beings; (c) dealing in flesh; (d) dealing in intoxicating drinks; and (e) dealing in poison.
6. *Right Effort*: The right effort is nothing, but sincere effort to avoid evil habits and cultivate good habits. It therefore, comprises of the following four constant efforts:
   (a) The effort to prevent the arising of evil which has not yet arisen;
   (b) The effort to eradicate that evil which has already accumulated;
   (c) The effort to induce good which has not yet arisen; and
   (d) The effort to cultivate that good which is already present.

   By sincerely practicing these, one is expected in Buddhism to cultivate the following higher ethical virtues such as—generosity, morality, renunciation, wisdom, energy, patience, truthfulness, determination, loving kindness and equanimity.
7. *Vigil*: This consists in one's having a constant vigil over the body, the feelings, the mind and the ideas to prevent them going astray.
8. *Right Concentration*: The right concentration provides perfect rapture.

Of the eightfold path mentioned above, the first two constitute what is called *Prajna* in Buddhism, the next three constitute what is called *Shila* and the last *Samadhi.* So, in one way of taking things, *Prajna*, *Shila* and *Samadhi* are three broad ways through which one can achieve final salvation. Sometimes order changes and the three are put as *Shila*, *Samadhi* and *Prajna,* which implies that after practicing morality, mindfulness and concentration, a right understanding about the nature of things arises. All are interrelated.

Sikhism: Man occupies a very high position in Sikhism. He is rather the highest being in the creation. "Man is blessed with the light of reason and discrimination."

But man in his present state is in a degenerated condition. He is constrained by various kinds of evils which are indicated in "*Haumai*" in Sikhism as—lust, anger, covetousness, attachment to the worldly objects and pride. Due to these evils man has become degenerated and lost his true nature.

The principal vice according to Sikhism is self-centredness or egoism and this consists in being attached to the five evil passions. Hence, Sikhism is way of cleansing the mind to be free from above five evils. For this Nanak has propounded a path of *Sadhana.* Through *Sadhana* one can realize that God is present in all creation, particularly in human *atma* and he is the only reality to be adored. When one fully recognizes this fact and becomes fully conscious of its truth, then he is to proceed towards meditation, which will cleanse his mind.

Islam: Islam as a religion is unique in its rigorous discipline of daily life that it prescribes for its followers. The religion takes God as the supreme Lord and man's duty towards Him is an unconditional and absolute submission. Consequently, much of Islamic discipline consists of teaching its people definite ways of sincere devotion and prayer to God. However, it also consists within itself elements of self-purification and liberality. Islamic discipline may be taken both as a religious and ethical discipline simultaneously. It consists of the following five duties known as the "Five Pillars" prescribes of Islam.

1. *Repletion of Faith in the absolute oneness of Allah*: As a strict monotheistic religion, Islam prescribes it to be the basic duty of every Muslim that before every prayer he should repeat the following words—"*La ilaha illa Uahu, Muhammad resulu uah*" (There is no God, but Allah and Muhammad is his prophet).
2. *Daily Prayer*: The observance of set of prayers five times a day—

at day break, at noon, at mid afternoon, at sun set and at early night is another important pillar of Islam. Every Muslim is expected to take as his basic duty of praying to God unfailing five times a day at the appointed hours. These prayers follow a set of formula of devotional postures. According to A.C. Bonquet, the innate psychological skill with which these devotional prayers postures are planned is remarkable and the nearest parallel is to be found in the system of *'yoga'* postures in India.

3. *Alms giving*: Giving alms to the poor and the needy is another essential duty of all the Muslims. It was recommended by Muhammad from the very beginning as a mark of piety and liberality towards the poor, but later on it took the form of, a regular religious tax, called *Zakat* for the support of the poor and other state purposes. Various formulas for the giving of gifts have been worked out in Islam. Sometimes, 1/10th and sometimes 1/20th of one's land income is required to be gifted. Additional gifts by the able are regarded as signs of greater religious merit. As regards the merit of the gifts, it has been related in the *Quran*, that a man served God for seventy years and then committed a sin which cancelled the merit of his entire service. Afterwards he gave a loaf of bread to a poor man and God pardoned his sin and gave him back the merit of his entire service.
4. *Fasting:* Another important religious rite to be observed by a Muslim is fasting during the whole month of *Ramajan*, i.e. the ninth month every lunar year. This consists in refraining from any kind of food or drink between sunrise and sunset. Eating is allowed at night. But taking wine and practicing such other impurities are forbidden for all times during the month. This fast of *Ramajan* is strictly to be observed by every Muslim. However, children, the sick and the travellers are made exceptions. It is believed that this fasting remits all kinds of sin committed during the whole year.
5. *Pilgrimage*: For every able bodied Muslim who can take journey pilgrimage to Mecca at least once during life time is regarded as an essential religious duty. No religious rite does more to unite the Muslims than this pilgrimage, which is taken by thousands from all corners of the sacred month of *Dhul-Hijja*. Although the observance of the above essential duties in utmost sincerity

seems to be sufficient guarantee in Islam for the attainment of heaven, it does not nevertheless vacuum in ethical virtues and duties of every Muslim in his dealings with others. Muslim ethics is, therefore, social. Hospitality is one of the greatest virtues that Islam teaches. It also preaches the ethics of brotherhood and service to humanity. Furthermore, virtues like obedience to parents, avoidance to adultery, cheating and lying, refraining from stealing, murder etc. are also emphasized. Islam forbids fighting except for the cause of religion or self-defense. It also teaches certain virtues for individual guidance. Use of powerful oil and various sorts of intoxicating drinks are forbidden in it. The virtues of renunciation and non-attachment towards worldly objects are taught to be cultivated by the individual.

Judaism: The basic principle of conduct in Judaism is the imitation of God. It means imbibing in oneself the attributes of God. Judaic God is imbued with essentially such ethical qualities as justice, mercy, righteousness and holiness. The basic ethical virtue therefore, consists in the cultivation of these qualities. To be more specific, Judaism counsels its followers to do such acts as clothing the naked, visiting the sick, comforting mourners, burying the dead and so on. In essence, it teaches acts of love and kindness. The *Torah* begins with an act of love and kindness and ends with an act of love and kindness. Besides, the qualities of modesty, humility etc. are also much emphasized, "Let all your words be gentle and let your head be bowed, let your eyes be directed to the ground and your heart on high...." It asks men to avoid the following because God hates them—pride and arrogance, lying, shedding innocent blood, devising wicked plots, creating mischief, presenting false witness and sowing the seed of misunderstanding amongst brethrens. As is well said in the proverb, there are six things which Lord hates:

- "Haughty eyes, a lying tongue,
- Hands that shed innocent blood,
- A heart that devises wicked plots,
- Feet that are swift to run to mischief,
- A false witness that utters lies; and
- And one that sows discord among brethren."

Similarly, Judaism disapproves three things: Speaking one thing from the mouth and entertaining something else from the heart; Knowing of evidence in favour of someone, but keeping silent over it and testifying alone against someone for disgraceful thing in him. According to the Judaic thinking, a minimum of two witnesses are required to prove someone guilty; only one witness merely gives the defendant a bad reputation. Judaism is very much against charging interest for money from someone.

A clear-cut mandate has been given for the Jewish way of life in the form of the ten moral precepts, known as the Ten Commandants. These are:

1. Thou shalt have no other God before me;
2. Thou shalt not make any graven image;
3. Thou shalt not take the name of the Lord thy God in vain;
4. Remember the Sabbath day (i.e. Saturday on which all Jews are required to refrain from all kinds of work and join the Divine worship)
5. Honour thy father and mother;
6. Thou shalt not kill;
7. Thou shalt not commit adultery;
8. Thou shalt not steal;
9. Thou shalt not bear false witness against thy neighbour; and
10. Thou shalt not covet thy neighbour's wife, man servant, maid servant, ox, ass etc.

Jaina Discipline: Basically, Jainaism teaches a threefold discipline, called the discipline of here jewels, following which one can get rid of bondage and attain liberation. This threefold discipline consists of:

1. Right Faith
2. Right Knowledge
3. Right Conduct

Moksha is a function neither only of faith, nor only of knowledge, nor again of morality alone. It is a joint product of all the three. Again, three are interconnected. Right knowledge is not possible without right faith and right conduct is not possible without right knowledge.

Right Faith: There seems to be controversy regarding the exact connotation of right faith. Some define it as faith in the *dharma* devoid of violence and in the way of life prescribed by *Jins* and *Kevils* etc. Umaswami defines right faith as faith in the greatness and efficacy of knowledge. However, in general it seems to mean having a pro-attitude, a sense of respect and regard towards Jaina principles. In following a disciplined path towards *Moksha,* the Jainas believe that the first requisite is to have a faith in the spiritual principles taught by the *Jins* and other *Siddhas.* If one is skeptical about all these, no effort on his part can be successful. So before attaining right knowledge, or having allegiance to right knowledge or having allegiance to right conduct, some faith in spiritual truths and principles necessary. Of course, in the context of Jainism, this faith means faith in the spiritual truths as taught by the *Jaina Tirthankaras* and Jaina Scriptures. But in no case by teaching right faith, Jainism wants to teach blind faith in authority. It leaves for personal thinking and realization. Right knowledge means personal realization and right faith and right knowledge go hand in hand.

Following eight essentials are given in Jainism for right faith:

1. Absence of doubt about the scriptures.
2. Absence of desire for worldly pleasure.
3. Absence of doubt about the attainment of spiritual path.
4. A clear and unconfusing vision about the ideal.
5. Augmentation of spiritual qualities.
6. Re-establishing deviations from truth.
7. Sense of affection towards followers of right knowledge.
8. Preaching the importance of truth.

Right Knowledge: Right knowledge is very essential for *Moksha* according to Jainism. To it ignorance is the root cause of our problems. It is *Karma* done with passion which bind and such *Karma* is the result of ignorance. By knowledge, Jainism does not mean mere intellectual and scriptural knowledge. Knowledge means here inner realization. A man having the inner knowledge sees things for himself and is therefore, never in the danger of being attached again. Right knowledge is that which helps in controlling the mind and purifying the self and this is possible only by the knowledge which is self-realized, which is attained in one's inner intuition or vision.

Right Conduct: Mere right faith or right knowledge is not sufficient for liberation. Right conduct is also necessary. Jainism mentions five vows which constitute the necessary ingredients of the behaviour of everyone whether he be a householder or a monk. These are known as "*Panchamahavrata*". These are:

1. *Non-Violence*: It is the greatest rule of conduct in Jainism, Violence in any form is strictly prohibited. The *Vedas* and *Upanishads* of Hinduism also recognized it as a great moral virtue. But the *Vedas* did not forbid *himsa* in the context of sacred rituals. It is the uniqueness of Jainism that it strictly forbids *himsa*. To cultivate this virtue in its strict sense and spirit, Jainism sometimes go to the extreme of non-burning light or cooking meal after sunset and Jaina monks walk by brushing the path with a smooth brush in their hand so that not a single worm should come under their feet. *Ahimsa* is understood and practiced in Jainism in a very wide connotation. Violence or injury or harm caused to any living being in any form is *himsa*. So *ahimsa* is to be practiced not only in deed, but also in thought and words. Keeping ill will against someone in thought or speaking harsh words to anyone is an example of *himsa* as inflicting any bodily injury to any.
2. *Truthfulness:* Generally speaking, this rule of conduct enjoins abstinence from giving false statements or telling a lie. But mere statement of fact is not truth. Truth, if it is harmful to others, should be avoided. It must be spoken with a beneficent intentions. Exaggeration of fact, finding fault with others, using indecent speech etc. are all examples of untruth according to Jainism and therefore must be avoided. Speaking in a noble, beneficent and balanced manner and with a peaceful mind upholds truth and hence it must be practiced. According to Amritachandra, the following are the examples of falsehood and they must be avoided–
   (a) Denial of existence of thing.
   (b) Asserting the existence of a non-existent thing.
   (c) Representing a thing as something else.
   (d) Reprehensible Speech.
   (e) Sinful Speech.
   (f) Unpalatable Speech.
3. *Non-Stealing*: Generally speaking this means abstention from taking a thing from someone else which is not given. But as a Jaina rule of conduct, it is much more comprehensive and includes within it the avoidance of all sorts of dishonesty and conceit. Buying a valuable article at low price, appropriating something that has been forgotten by someone's possession whose ownership is doubtful etc.

4. *Brahmacharya:* This vow has been much emphasized in Hinduism and Buddhism in general, *Brahmacharya* also means abstinence from excessive desire for any sort of sense enjoyment.
5. Avoidance of desire for such possession.

Every religion consists of certain beliefs and practices. In many respects it is found that different religions contain certain similar types of beliefs, though in many others they differ too. Generally, in respect of the practices, the differences seem to be more glaring than similarities. The ways of prayer, the observance of various rituals and ceremonies and such other religious practices sometimes sharply differ from one religion to another. However, there is an underlying similarity in spirit and that is that all these practices in their own distinctive ways are directed towards God or Gods to secure their grace, so that, man may find himself out of suffering he faces in the world and may strive for a better destiny. Differences in the actual nature of these practices are bound to be there, because men coming from different geographical and cultural traditions cannot all be expected to observe exactly the same set of practices. What is to be wondered at is not that there are differences, but that there are a few striking similarities. For example, fasting is taken as a very important religious practice in all such religions as Hinduism, Buddhism, Jainism and Islam. Similarly, very secret fire-worship is regarded as very sacred in both Hinduism and Zoroastrianism, pilgrimage is given a great religious value in both Hinduism and Islam. There are striking similarities between Islam and Judiaism on the one hand and Judiaism and Christianity on the other in respect of many other religious practices. Again, reciting of religious texts is regarded as a very important religious duty in almost all the religions. Similarly, every religion gives credence to the erection of religious temples and shrines where people go either individually or in groups to pay their respect and devotion to God. Even religions like Buddhism and Jainism which originally did not believe in any God have found place such temples. Thus, even if there are not exact similarities in the various details of the various practices of different religions, there are definitely similarities of a general nature in different religions.

There is, however, a very clear and definite similarity in the nature of the ethical practices that the different religions prescribe. There is no such religion which teaches enmity with others, teaches excessive attachment to worldly objects as desirable. On the other hand, every religion without exception teaches the observance of such ethical virtues as liberty, humility, chastity, purity, love, kindness, truth etc. to be the sacred duty of every religious man. All religions without exception teach universal brotherhood. Similarly, all of them teach abstention from cruelty to creatures. There may be the difference of emphasis, but that does not affect the inner similarity of conviction. Sometimes, the similarity is very direct and obvious. The three religions tradition—Hinduism, Buddhism and Jainism—assert with equal emphasis on the desirability of the observance of five ethical virtues—non-violence, truth, celibacy, non-stealing and non-attachment. An obvious similarity may be marked between the religious of Indian tradition on the one hand and Zoroastrianism on the other in as much as all of these equally emphasize the need for observing rightness of thought, speech and action all together. (Tiwari)

The study of the religions shows that almost all the religions spell out ethical principles in very clear terms. These principles are necessary for the physical and mental health of the individuals as well as the society. These are very strong threads to tie up different communities together and to move towards the same direction with different modes of movement. These ethical principles are the devices used by different religions to assert human values in a society and these may also be considered as motivating factors to render service to humanity. Humanism is the supreme religion—religion of all the religions. It is also a significant part of Indian culture. The religions are the torch bearers to direct activities and thought of a man towards service to humanity. The welfare of mankind requires guidance or control of human power over the application of modern sophisticated technology. Survival of mankind depends only on the authority of human power over the application of technology for the progress of human society. The unique position of medical services cannot be denied in this respect.

However, the humanism may be distinguished from religion. Though man is a religious animal, both religion and humanism view man's life from different angles. Humanism is defined in the *Oxford Dictionary* as "any system of thought or action which is concerned with merely human interests or with those of the human race in general. For humanism service to man is the highest religion as man is supreme in existence in the world. It believes in the good life, in moderation, harmony, balance. Humanism believes that man is by nature good and that evil rests in society, in the conditions which surround man, if these are removed, man's goodness will emerge and progress will be achieved. Religion on the other hand, believes in the radical insufficiency of human nature.

Humanist revivals occur when religions disintegrate and fail to attract men's attention. It was also in ancient Greece, Protagoras' work on *Truth* has a striking saying, which finds an echo today: "Concerning the Gods, I have not been able to ascertain whether they exist or not; the obscurity of the subject and the brevity of human life have hindered me from finding it out".

The leaders of the eighteenth century enlightenment had an optimistic attitude to life. They insisted on ethics of enthusiastic devotion to human welfare. Humanism became the secular religion and its practical results were seen in the Declaration of the Rights of Man and the French Revolution.

Professor G.E. Moore in his book, *Principa Ethica* published in 1903 insisted on the intrinsic value of human relations and exhorted his disciples to multiply instances of his two most valuable things, friendship and beauty, and not the pursuit of personal power and success.

Humanism is a legitimate protest against those forms of religion which separate the secular and sacred, divide time and eternity and break-up the unity of soul and flesh. Every religion should have sufficient respect for the dignity of man and the rights of human personality. (Radhakrishnan: 1961)

One of the classic expressions of humanism is to be found in the ethics of Aristotle (384-322 B.C.) Son of the physician to the Macedonian King, Aristotle acquired the empirical interest of the medical profession; he regarded ethics as an art, like medicine, although the former was concerned with the health of the soul rather than a body. He was greatly influenced in his ethical concepts by Plato, whose student and assistant he was for twenty years. Like his master, he believed that the good is the harmonious development of human capacities, above all the capacity to reason. After the death of Plato, Aristotle spent four years on the coast of Asia Minor, engaged in biological research; then for several years he acted as tutor to prince Alexander of Macedon. In 335 B.C., he returned to Athens, where he spent twelve very productive years as head of a school of his own founding, the Lyceum. Finally, he was accused of impiety, and fled to the island of Euboea, where he died after a year later.

His conception of ethics was essentially humanistic. The knowledge of man, he believed, is the basis of establishing norms and values. Ethics is based upon psychology and not upon theology or transcendental metaphysics. It is a branch of practical science and apart of politics. The business of the ethical philosopher is to determine the qualities in human life that the educator and the statesman should cultivate in the people. Its principal object is to find out what is man's highest good.

In the opening paragraph of "*The Nicomachean Ethics*," Aristotle pointed out that the various practical arts are to be distinguished by the ends they serve. Health is the aim of medicine, vessels of shipbuilding, victory of military strategy, and wealth of economics. The ends and corresponding arts form a hierarchy, some being subordinate to others. (Rader: 1964)

Man is a social animal. It is known to all of us. But he is also a religious animal as stated by C. Joseph Barnabas in his article, *Religious Freedom and Human Rights.* It is generally conceded that only humans are religious. In providing satisfaction of biological drives, animals appear to have good life, but for humans biological needs are not everything. It is said by J.A. Hutchison, "A conscious relation to the wider human world, including the world of ideal possibilities, becomes a fundamental need for man." This is precisely the function of the ultimate values of religious experience. Through religious tradition, humankind in the past experienced and communicated humanism to the younger generation. He cited an example—among the Anglo-Saxons, certain religious traditions were followed in order to give weightage to human life and human values. If a family lost an adult because of murder, the man who killed was to pay the dead man's price to the bereaved family: a nobleman's price was fixed at 1,200 shillings, a lesser nobleman at 600 shillings, and a peasant at 200 shillings. The 200 shillings of the late seventh century works out to an average value of Rs. 1 lakh today. For that amount, one could buy one hundred sheeps and sixteen bulls. It is in these aspects that the idea of protection of human rights and freedom as a whole developed and over time was identified as religious freedom based on texts. From religious freedom gradually evolved ideas of personal, political and social freedom. Freedom has meant not only 'freedom from', but also 'freedom to' and 'freedom for'. (Barnabas: 1999)

The tradition of Indian society is flooded with many such instances through which people are sensitized to humanism—Guest to the family is honoured like God or Goddess, service to old and disabled is considered as service to God, not to deprive any beggar who comes to our house, not to ill-treat parents under any circumstances etc.

Referring to religion and social relations Radhakrishnan said that religion is confused with the mechanical participation in the rites or passive acquiescence in the dogmas. Many of those who observe the forms of religion, the gestures of faith, the conventions of piety do not model their lives on the precepts they profess. To-day it is found that many people visit temples, celebrate religious festivals, offer prayer to Gods and Goddesses of their faith, but their behaviour in daily life or in social relationship the spirit of religion is not reflected. The modern Indians in most cases are moving towards rituals instead of going to the depth or the core meaning of the religion they profess. This is very common among the youths.

Religions, at their best, insist on behaviour more than on belief. Orthodoxy is not confined to the defining of faith. It includes the living of it. Definition is the means and not the end. A vehicle is not more important than the goal to which it is to take us. We must live religion in truth and deed and not merely profess it in words. There is a difference today between our belief and behaviour. Once we develop faith in any principle we must take care to see that it is reflected in our day to day lives. Otherwise it will remain in lips only without having any impact on our lives. This kind of situation cannot help the society to be transformed towards humanism.

St. Paul has rightly pointed out: "Do not be conformed to this world, but be transformed by the renewal of your mind, that you may prove what is the will of God, what is good and acceptable and perfect." If religion is not dynamic and pervasive, if it does not penetrate every form of human life and influence every type of human activity, it is only a veneer not reality.

Today man lacks patience as well as time to observe norms or principles necessitated by traditional society in observing both social and religious festivals. Science has induced us to simplify the ways of getting things done in the modern society. One gets information about the happenings in the world in a moment within the four walls of his habitation. Most social activities can be performed without having face to face relationship. Even in the administration the e-governance and IT system have made the modern life comfortable and speedy.

To Radhakrishnan social organization rests on a series of decisions taken by human beings as to the manner in which they and their followers shall live. These decisions are matters of spiritual discernment while actions to implement them require technical knowledge and social sense.

While realizing the significance of what Radhakrishnan's statement on social relationship what one is experiencing today is just opposite. Today's Indian society is constrained by several serious ailments—hypocrisy among political and administrative leaders and social and religious reformers, emotional blackmailing of unemployed youths and their parents and poor people's aspiration for financial security, involvement of greedy persons in establishing fake financial and academic institutions, various corruption cases, emotional exploitation of voters at the time of election, inhuman treatment etc. It appears that in most cases the decisions taken by the decision makers of today's India are deviated from the interest of humanism.

It is true that religion is not a social reform movement. But a man's life can be viewed only in the face of social life only. Even in modern life people do not or cannot give up the human tradition of judging good or bad or determining norms of human society. A civilized life is a democratic life grounded in the stable social order. Religion is a social cement, a way in which men express their inspirations and find solace for their frustration.

We cannot build a society of nations by fostering economic and political ties alone. We have to give to the society a psychological unity, a spiritual coherence. To sustain a world community we need unity.

All religions insist on compassion to the suffering. Christianity, for example, asks us to do good to them that hate us and despitefully use us. There is nothing special in loving those who love us or who are themselves lovable. Jesus asks us to love our enemies in the hope of reawakening their humaneness, their potential capacity for love. We are called upon to remove from the enemy's heart the fear of our own hateful intentions. (*en.wikipedia.org/wiki/Indian philosophy*)

Experience in contemporary India shows that a person who is incompetent for a particular position, but is aware of the facilities, power and prestige attached to it tries desperately to reach that position by all possible means. Similarly, a greedy person irrespective of his position desperately attempts to exploit every situation for his own benefit. In both the cases aspirants do not care to throw out all the laws and ethical values to the dustbin. In most cases they take the help of 'middlemen' or 'linkmen" to hide their intention and effort in order to safeguard their image before the public. This act of hiding their evil activities and intention gives birth to ethical failure and ethical failure brings evils in the service to humanity.

What is Evil? Oxford English Dictionary defines evil as antithesis of good. Elias Staub, while analyzing the roots of evil defined evil in a comprehensive way as—"Evil is not a scientific concept with an agreed meaning, but the idea of evil is a part of a broadly shared human cultural heritage. The essence of evil is the destruction of human beings...." Fred Katz provides a behavioural definition of evil as, "behaviour that deprives innocent people of their humanity, from small scale assaults on a person's dignity to outright murder..." This evil behaviour of man is harmful to others.

In Independent India, the strength of vulnerable population is increasing instead of decreasing in spite of spread of education through various formal and non-formal devices. A vulnerable man is one who is unable take care of himself or protect himself from harm or from being exploited. Generally people become vulnerable due to various reasons, such as having mental health problems, physical disability, age or illness, poverty etc. In other words, vulnerability refers to those individuals or groups who due to age, ill-health, infirmity, minority status or otherwise are in the disadvantageous position.

There are also examples of even the youths with university degrees are being exploited by fake financial and educational institutions, fake employment agencies. Besides, trafficking of women and children has become regular news. In addition, large numbers of youths are the victims of drug addiction and alcoholism causing serious mental tension and financial problems to the families.

What is an abuse? It is an act or word of one or more people which makes a person feel upset or frightened. It may also be mistreatment by one or more people that violates a person's human and civil rights. There are also a large number of cases of it. (Staub: 1992)

Many of the existing problems in Indian society—corruption, breakdown of law and order, abuse of power by institution, growing inequalities in wealth and income, extreme poverty, large scale unemployment, inability to provide education in the true sense, hypocrisy amongst educated, social and political leaders, emotional exploitation of ignorant people by the power hungry leaders in each community rooted mainly in the deterioration of Indian cultural values and negligence of ethical dimension of religions.

The Indian society is also constrained by the emergence of globalization and privatization in the process of development of the country. It is true that development of a country is not possible in isolation. At the same time one cannot afford to ignore ethical principles and human values while climbing up in the escalation of development. In contemporary India, it is noticed that in most cases possession of wealth and fulfillment of personal desire are occupying a dominating place in the value system adhered by an individual. Under this situation, there is the possibility of change of the status of man, from "man of need" to that of "man of greed", provided ethical principles are ignored or human values are not honoured while planning for development strategies. Because under such situation the strength of the human power may be neutralized to the zero level and he may be the victims of irrational elements, like, *Lobha, Moha, Kama,* and *Krodha* etc. The position of such a person is no better than that of an elephant whose all the four legs are tied up by iron thread.

However, religion like Hinduism is not against the goal of a man as consumer. The man as consumer provides space for development of employment market. But one has to be careful to see that the consumerist goal of a man does not do any harm to others. In the contemporary Indian society media focuses very frequently the problems faced by the families due to the consumption of drugs and alcohol by their young members. Laws are being formulated to get rid of it, police and military forces are strengthened and trained with new techniques for regulating crimes and to maintain law and order in the country. But experience shows that criminalization of politics and administration is increasing day by day. Corruption has its easy way even to public health and education sectors of administrators. It is not only illegitimate, it is also unethical and anti-religious.

In such a situation, a reformer should not confine his eye only to the nature of the problem that comes to the surface and the problem creators. One must look beyond it. Family atmosphere, the trend of social change, education system, impact of science and technology etc. Above all, the state of power of *Dharma* in the society is also an important factor to be studied. The decline of the power of *Dharma* means rise of evil elements of the inner person of an individual like anger, greed, ego etc. The attitude and mental status of such kind of individuals are described in a very precise form in the *Bhagavad Gita* 3000 years ago. Let me quote it as stated by Veeranghavan in the following words:

1. There are two creations of beings in this world: the divine and the demonical.
2. The creations under demonical group do not know when to act and when to desist from action. They have no truthfulness, nor purity nor right conduct.
3. They assert that the universe is Godless, without truths and without moral foundation.
4. Holding fast to this view, these lost souls of feeble wit and of fierce deeds, come forth to destroy the world as its enemies.
5. Resorting to insatiable passion, full of hypocrisy, pride and arrogance, they act with impure vows through delusion.

6. Beset with countless worries that last until death, they become immersed in gratification of desires, convinced that, that is all.
7. Bound by hundred ties of hope, given wholly to passion and anger, they seek, for sensual gratification, to amass wealth by unlawful means.
8. "This I have earned to-day, this desire I shall gain (next): this is already mine, more riches will come in future."
9. "That enemy has been slain by me; and I shall kill others too. I am the master, I am the employer, I am successful, powerful and happy."
10. "I am rich and noble birth, who else is there equal to me? I shall sacrifice, give alms and rejoice"—so they think deluded by ignorance.
11. Bewildered by many such thoughts, caught in the web of delusion, and addicted to sensual enjoyments, they fall into foul hell.
12. Self-glorifying and stubborn, drunk with wealth and pride, they offer sacrifices in name only, with orientation, not conforming to scriptural injunctions.

Following are the Divine values to imbibe in man:

1. Fearlessness, purity of mind, steadiness in Yoga and Knowledge, charity, self-restraint, sacrifice, Vedic study, austerity, uprightness.
2. Non-injury, truthfulness, absence of wrath, relinquishment, tranquility, non-calumny, compassion for creatures, lack of greed, gentleness, humility, absence of fickleness.
3. Vigour, forgiveness, fortitude, cleanliness, absence of envy and pride. (Veeranghavan: 2007)

S.R. Mohnot in his article, "Relevance of Hindu Philosophy to Understand India" stated that at the base of all the maladies is the pollution of mind—extravagance, unlimited lure for money and consumerism, rivalries, insatiable hunger for wealth, position and fame.

To reduce all pervasive criminalization in all forms ethical aspect of all religions must be brought to light and the children must be made aware of it through theory and practice of education process of the country. The moral code should be emphasized in all institutions to make them effective in rendering service to humanity. Since in the ultimate analysis of institutions there remains the human beings and morality is the human related problem. The ethical principles and human values contribute significantly to make a nation strong (Mohnot: 2007).

Realizing the gravity of this kind of trend in change which is dangerous to the global humanity United Nations of Organization initiated instructing the nation states to safeguard human rights of the people through establishment of Commissions and provision for human rights education to the children. India is also responding positively to the instruction of the United Nations.

The 2nd October in each year is observed as Non-violence Day. It is being the human power, can work as a noble and strong force to achieve global unity, irrespective of geographical, cultural, lingual and religious diversity amongst the nations of the world.

K.R. Narayanan, warned the Indians on the eve of assuming the office of the President of India as:

> "Indian civilization has had the unique honour of demonstrating to the world that man does not live by bread alone. Cultural, moral and spiritual values have always formed the fundamental underpinning of our society. Today there are signs of the weakening of the moral and spiritual fiber in our public life with evils of communalism, casteism, violence and corruption bedeviling our society."

Indian culture taught us to respect the views of others and to be the listener of it with patience. The Indian society was not touched by the diversity of religion and culture. Any enlightened man can realize that *Vedas* and *Quran* are the two different ways towards one Almighty, who govern the universe. Christianity infused on us the spirit of service to humanity and love of God in our culture. The Buddha built his *Sangha* on the same principle. Mahavira gave the eternal message of non-violence to our society.

The possession of noble principles of the *Vedas* and *Vedanta*, Islam, Christianity, Buddhism, Jainism, Sikhism, Zoroastrianism, Sufism and other faiths help establishing unity in diversity.

If we repent for our sins and change our behaviour, God takes note of it and assists us in our endeavour to improve. To Radhakrishnan heaven and hell are not physical areas. A soul tormented with remorse for its deeds is hell, a soul with the satisfaction of a life well lived is in heaven.

We have to keep up our struggle against the inertia and evil in us. All our enemies are within us. The impulses which seduce, the flames which burn, spring from the inner region of ignorance and error in which we live. Man's glory is not in never falling but in rising every time he falls. Professor A.N. Whitehead says, "religion is a force of belief cleansing the inward parts. For this reason, the primary religious virtue is sincerity, a penetrating sincerity. Religion is art and theory of the internal life of man. The way from passion to peace is by self-conquest. There is a nobler life than that of sinning and suffering. The measure of a man's saintliness is judged by the degree to which he has been able to overcome the frailties of his nature. Religion is not a way out of life, but a way unto life. The general assumption that Hinduism negates social values and sacrifices material and cultural needs to a world—negating spiritual quest is not correct. It is true that when we have the vision of reality, we feel that we are strangers in the outer, visible, alien world of appearance. We do not feel at home.

In a new society we need a new universal reliance of religion. By it we mean not a uniform religion but a religion of awareness and love, of wisdom and compassion, of truth and love. Religions must be cured of their provincialism and made to reveal their universality. This does not mean spiritual vagueness or ambiguity.

Tolerance implies an elementary right belonging to the dignity of every man. The right to believe like the right to live a free, unfettered life, is fundamental to the concept of brotherly love. We have had in our country peaceful co-existence of different religions. It is not mere passive co-existence but an active fellowship, a close inter-relation of the best of different religions. We have not adhered steadfastly to these ideals and have suffered often. Yet the ideal has been kept in view and supported by great leaders like Ram Mohun Roy, Ramakrishna, Tagore and Gandhiji.

Each religion is unique so far as its form is concerned. We can hold that our particular formulation is valid formulation of truth without denying the validity of other forms. We must develop those loyalties to the free mind and spirit which transcend the narrower loyalties to the caste or class, race or nation. Whatever progress we make at the cost of these values is morally wrong.

True religion is not the religion of routine which we adopt as a matter of habit. It is the aspiration of every human soul, that which unfolds within oneself, that which is built by one's life blood. It is the fulfillment of our nature in which overflows into the world's service. (Radhakrishnan: 1970)

The Constitution of India stands for a secular state. The state has no official religion. Secularism pervades its provisions which give full opportunity to all persons to profess, practice and propagate religion of their choice. The constitutions not only guarantees a person's freedom of religion and conscience, but also ensures freedom for one who has no religion, and it scrupulously restraints the state from making any discrimination on grounds of religion. A single citizenship is assured to all persons irrespective of their religion.

Dr. Radhakrishnan, has explained secularism in his book, titled, "*Recovery of Faith*" as,

> "When India is said to a Secular State, it does not mean that we reject the reality of an unseen spirit or the relevance of religion to life or that we exalt irreligion. It does not mean that secularism itself becomes a positive religion or that the State assumes divine prerogatives.... We hold that not one religion should be given preferential status......... This view of religious impartiality, or comprehension and forbearance, has a prophetic role to play within the National and International life."

The significant components of secularism are:

(i) *Samanta* (equality) is incorporated in article 14;
(ii) Prohibition against discrimination on the ground of religion, caste, etc. is incorporated in articles 15 and 16;
(iii) Freedom of speech and expression and all other important freedoms of all citizens are conferred under articles 19 and 20;
(iv) Right to practice religion is conferred under articles 25 to 28;
(v) Fundamental duty of the State to enact uniform civil laws treating all citizens as equal is imposed by article 44;
(vi) Sentiment of majority of the people towards the cow and against its slaughter was incorporated in article 48.

India is a secular state. However, religion plays a very significant role in the day to-day life of an Indian. The development of science and technology and modernization of way of life are not hindrances to it. I have found that the visit of religious temples even by the educated youths in large number on religious occasions is a common sight even today. For example, the political leaders from President down to the Chief Ministers of different states of the country use to visit religious temples, especially the world famous Kamakhya temple situated in Assam for the blessings of the Goddess and this is found in other places of the country also. What I want to bring to light is that religion is still a force to play a significant role in the life of a man in India. Every child character is equipped with the faith in God or Goddess at the family itself basically from the parents. Gradually, it becomes a part of their habit which is reflected in his behaviour while rendering service to the people in any capacity. The physicians are not an exception to it. The ethical dimension of religions cannot be considered as a digression in any profession or organization of man. Melanie Phillips and John Dawson, in their book, "Doctors' Dilemmas" stated that an attempt to reassert the importance of religious ethics in the modern way of life does not denigrate a modern man. For many people in our society, moral codes of Roman Catholicism, Protestant Churches, Judaism or Islam will provide moral guidance in the field of medicine just as they do in other aspect of social life. (Phillips and Dawson: 1985)

It may also be said that religion, as it is understood, is opposed to the spirit of science. The method of science is empirical while that of religion is dogmatic. Science does not rely on authority, but appeals to communicable evidence that any trained mind can evaluate. Science does not admit any barriers to freedom of thought and inquiry. It welcomes new knowledge and experience. A true scientist does not take refuge in dogmatism. His outlook is marked by modesty, self-criticism and readiness to learn from others. It is incompatible with authoritarianism, which is the dominant feature of religion.

Besides, there is an element of universality about scientific views, which is not to be found in religious doctrines. Scientists recognize no national or geographical boundaries. They exchange information with fellow workers in other lands. Secrecy is repugnant to the spirit of science.

However, it is difficult to deny that in a technological civilization, in a mass society, the individual becomes a depersonalized unit. Things control life. Statistical averages replace qualitative human beings. Therefore, it is essential to realize that to be human is to be trusting, to be kind, to be cooperative, to be sympathetic and responsive. It is to be democratic and not be afraid to exchange opinions even with those who differ from us. It is to trust our neighbours and magnanimous to our enemies. If we recover our humanity, we will refuse to submit to arbitrary authority and help nations to recover from the state from the collective paranoia into which some of them have fallen. But the technological organization of modern society in which individual counts less and less fosters a fundamental skepticism and negation of the spirit of man.

All religions insist on compassion to the suffering. Christianity, for example, asks us to do good to them that hate us and despitefully use us. There is nothing special in loving those who love us or who are themselves lovable. Jesus asks us to love our enemies in the hope of reawakening their humanness, their potential capacity for love. We are called upon to remove from the enemy's heart fear of our own hateful intentions.

Religion requires us to appeal to the higher instincts of man, reason, cooperation, love, and not fear, greed and hatred. Religion assumes that human nature, however depraved, will always respond to the power of goodness.

There are two sides to scientific activity, the discovery of facts and the construction of an intellectual pattern which will explain it, taking into account other known facts. While facts are established, interpretations are provisional. Again, facts are not judgements of value. When we interpret facts as a whole and pronounce judgements of their meaning and value, we get beyond science.

A physician, as a scientist, to be a good one must have knowledge in his field. Simultaneously, to serve the humanity with commitment one must have clear understanding of human dignity and human nature. His position is that of a teacher in the educational institutions. To be a successful teacher he/she must understand the subject to be taught, at the same time he/she must also understand the students because lack of understanding of the students may cause failure to the teacher. What is needed here is the urge to know about the students at least about their strengths and weaknesses for adjusting the ways of explaining lessons and maintaining healthy teacher-student relationship. Similarly, a physician must have command over the subject as well as knowledge of the condition of the patient. The knowledge about patients and students can only be sought if a physician/teacher has certain qualities, such as absolute sincerity, singleness of purpose and honest humility, that is always ready to acknowledge mistakes. Here exists the need of ethics. The values acquired by an individual at home during childhood and in the educational institutions in student life are reflected in his or her service life.

Experience shows that the student-culture is changing very fast in India with the improvement of information technology, increase of unemployed educated youths, distortion of traditional family pattern, development of communication facilities etc. These require constant and sincere efforts of the teacher to adjust with the changing situation through innovative strategies to help the students to learn lessons and to guide them to acquire human qualities. It is the teacher who can create human culture in the school just as the parents at home and leading personalities in the society, civil servants in the administration, the political leaders in politics and religious leaders in temples. Involvement of teacher in unethical activities will bring gap between teacher-student relationship and similar is the case in other fields also. Here begins constraints in their relations which are unwelcome in the process of socialization of the students in the greater interest of building a human society or service to humanity. Human culture was created in ancient India by the *Guru* when the disciples stayed in his house for learning lessons. However, due to various factors, such as, increase of student-population and progress of science and technology, change of social values and culture old traditional ways of maintaining *Guru*-disciple relationship cannot or need not be maintained. But this does not mean that the human relationship and human values have lost its significance in the days of science. In the ancient times scriptures were written with hand, later manual typewriter came followed by electronic typewriter and computer. Teachers, students and other writers accordingly adjusted to the changes. However, in the case of the process of socialization of the children drastic changes have been noticed in the major agencies, especially in the family. In the traditional Indian society there existed joint family system and in the process of transformation of the agricultural society to the modern society there appears nuclear family system. The act of socialization in the joint family system addressed a very wide area of child's life and it helped the child to learn human behaviour, adoption of certain standards of social relations with family members of different age groups, obedience to family authority, responsibility to the members, accountability, sharing of essential things for example food, shelter, household facilities in the day to day life, the family environment generated scope for mutual help and respect to each other, entertainment of guest etc. This informal learning process begins at home and went on spreading over the social life, especially in helping the neighbours or villagers at the time of distress and observing social, religious and family festivals. The elderly members took utmost care to see that their children develop good habits and never pick-up bad habits of the elders in the family. In social life or in the professional life the children exhibit these habits. The peer groups could not do harm to each other as there was face to face contact not only with the friends, but also with the parents of their friends as the personal visit was the only way to meet each other. Gradually, the social values, moral or ethical principles, family structure and functions and responsibilities of the parents have been affected by several external factors from outside the family. The modern information technology, media and also international and national laws are gradually influencing heavily the process of socialization of children in India. What is found today is the annihilation of the authority of the teachers and even of the parents over the children. Human environment is disappearing from family as well as from the school. Educational institutions have become almost training institutions to train the children to acquire technique of appearing in the competitive examinations with goal of getting job. While appreciating the efforts of the schools or educational institutions to produce employable candidates through appropriate syllabi, it must be admitted that human aspect of human being has been neglected totally on the ground that moral/ethical principles have no value in modern India. Money power has been valued most. Of course there are reasons to believe this because in competitive examinations for job money is valued more than performance in the examination, money and material possession can give social status, public opinion at the time of election can be manufactured by money, money has become the moving wheels of files in the administration, criminals have been empowered to represent people, fake educational and financial institutions have been established very comfortably to award higher degrees and fixed deposit financial certificates to the customers. Gradually, most people are realizing with heavy heart the worst consequences of all these. People have started raising voice against dysfunctions of the government mechanisms.

There is no denying the fact that the people in India also value health by giving top priority in their needs. They have become conscious of their health rights. Medical professionals in recent years are facing conflicting situation very frequently. The patients' trust in them has lost its ascriptive character. The ethical vacuity in the services may be one of the major reasons for it (Rao: 1980).

Philips and Dawson have rightly indicated that every service has inalienable ethical implication. Though the nature of the service demands different kinds of ethical principles there are also several meeting points. The ultimate goal of all services is one, i.e. service to humanity. The nature and requirement of each service differs depending upon the immediate goal of each service. For example, the immediate goal of the medical service is to take care of patient, that of education service to impart education to the students and of police personnel to maintain law and order etc. The situation and the nature of beneficiaries demand different kinds of behaviour or attitudes of the service providers. But the ultimate goal of all services is to serve the humanity. (Phillips and John Dawson: 1985)

Every man has the capacity to develop human qualities like love, affection, fellow feeling, tolerance etc. At the same time he has vulnerability to be exploited by anger, emotion, greediness, aggressiveness, selfishness etc. Thomas Hobbes in his book *'Leviathan'* showed the dark side of man's nature while narrating the state of nature. To him man has restless desire for power. Every individual strives for the gratification of his appetites. He considers man as essentially selfish, stupid and egoistic. He possesses the faculty of reasoning and at the same time absurdity. Man is moved to action not by his intellect or by reason, but by his appetites, desires and passions. What Hobbes thought about human nature cannot be summarily throw into the dustbin. To control the negative aspect of man's nature one has to do certain things and be refrain from doing some other things. (Rao: 1980)

Another issue is the concept of privatization which is emerging in the domain of public service in India, especially the privatization in the fields of medical sciences and education is drawing more attention of the public in the country. In these two sectors private institutions are providing more than 30 per cent of the services to the public. In the field of higher education most colleges were established in India at the initiative of the public. For example, in the state of Assam Henry Cotton established the Cotton College in 1909 itself and it was followed by two more Colleges in the Hill districts of North Cachar Hills and Karbi Anglong District of Assam. All other colleges were established at the initiative of the people of the state. Today the Government schools are gradually closed down due to non-availability of students, as the parents prefer private schools for the education of their children. This preference is due to efficiency and discipline maintained in the private school and for solution of the problem of language in the perspective of job market at the national as well as international level. On the other hand, a large number of private hospitals are coming up in the later part of twentieth century in the country. Unlike the education sector, the people prefer to go to Government hospitals due to its service efficiency and monetary benefit. But they go to private hospitals due procedural delay and redtapism in the Government hospitals and overcrowd of patient population in the Government hospitals.

The normative theories justifying privatization as a direction for public policy draw their inspiration from several different visions of a good society. By far the most influential is the vision grounded in *lasses-faire* individualism and free market economics that promises greater efficiency, a smaller Government, and more individual choice if only we expand the domain of property rights and market forces. The second vision, rooted in a more socially minded conservative tradition, promises return of power to the communities, through a greater reliance in social provision on families, churches and other largely non-profit institutions. Privation in this way means a devolution of power from state to ostensibly non-political and non-commercial forms of human organizations. Third perspective sees privatization as a political strategy for diverting demands away from the state and thereby reducing Government 'overload'. (*www.princeton.edu/~starr/meaning.html*)

Privatization has a close relation to the theory of New Public Management, as it encourages movement of managerial responsibility from the public to private bodies. It reduces the scope of Government bureaucracy. The process of privatization provides freedom and flexibility which are generally absent in the Government control such as, Ministerial obligations, restrictions on the rights and code of conduct etc. It is expected that this freedom will enable the service providers in the private sector to maintain efficiency and flexibility in the administrative process. Due to these reasons in 1970s, privatization of public services was welcomed by many European countries, Australia, New Zealand and even developing countries. India welcomes private institutions in large number in different sectors. In this regard health and education occupy a prominent position. The private healthcare services constitute not less 40 per cent of the total service in this sector.

Once responsibility of the state is shifted to the private organizations with the assumption that people's power is being returned for effective administration, in practice it does not happen in India. These services are beyond the people's control, the Government do not have effective mechanism to ensure accountability of the private service providers, in ultimate analysis most of these organizations are guided only by profit making motive or selfish interest. In India whole problem is arising due to devaluation of human values.

References

Adams, Guy. B. and Danny, L. Balfour: Ethical Failings, Incompetence and Administrative Evil (Lessons from Kartina and Iraq) *Ethics and Integrity in Public Administration: Concepts and Cases*; edited by Raymond W. Cox III, M.E. Sharpe, New York, 1984.

Agarwal, R.C. *Constitutional Development of India and National Movement*, S. Chand & Company, Delhi, 1986.

Bakshi, P.M.: *The Constitution of India*, Universal Law Publishing Company, Delhi, Fifth edition, 2004.

Barnabas, C. Joseph: Religious Freedom and Human Rights, *Human Rights in India*: ed. by Chiranjivi J. Nirmal; Oxford University Press.

Barnett, John H. 1985: Action and symbolic Viewing (An investigation of the *Gita* and Executive Ethics: published in the *Journal of Gandhian Studies*, Institute of Gandhian Thought and Peace Studies; Gandhi Bhawan, University of Allahabad, Volume 12, No. 46, January 1985.

Bharadwaj, H.R.: *Heritage of Unity, Harmony and Peace: Understanding India*, ed. by Subhash Chandra Kashyap and Abhaya Kashyap, Vitasta Publishing Ltd., New Delhi, 2007.

Bharatiya, L.K.: *Prospect of Change on Gandhian Lines*; *Journal of Gandhian Studies* in 1987 by Institute of Gandhian Thought and Peace Studies, Gandhi Bhawan, University of Allahabad, Allahabad.

Chandra, Bipan: *Modern India*, National Council of Educational Research and Training, 1971, New Delhi.

Chowdhary, T.H., *Relevnce of Hinduism,* National Council of Educational Research and Training, New Delhi.

Doctor, Adi H.: *Political Thinkers of Modern India*; Mittal Publications, New Delhi, 1997.

Dutta, Sashi Dhar, Chairman, *National Integration Committee*, National Integration, 1990.

Dutta, Keshab Narayan: *Culture and Civilization of Assam*, Mahendra Kumar Barua, Shrimanta Sankar Krishi Bikash Samiti; 1st edition, 1956.

Frankiln, D. "Relevance of Gandhi for our Time" Souvenir, Gandhi Centenary Celebration Committee for Assam.

Gupta, R.C.: *Great Political Thinkers: East and West*, Lakshmi Narain Agarwal, Agra, 1963.

Gupta, N.L.: *Education and Values in Mahabharata*: Concept Publishing Company, 1995.

Kerridge Ian, Michael Lowe and Camerun Stewart: *Ethics and Laws for the Health Professionals*, Federation Press; Australia, 2009.

Kirpal, Prem, *Culture and Development,* Har-Anand Publications, 364-A, Chirag Delhi, Delhi-110017.

Khatami, Seyyed Md.: President of the Islamic Republic of Iran: Chapter 2: *Deepening Democracy by Tackling Democratic Deficits: Human Development Report*: 2002; UNDP.

Monhot, S.R.: "Relevance of Hindu Philosophy to Understand India", *Understanding India*, ed. by Subhash Chandra Kashyap and Abhaya Kashyap, Vitasta Publishing Ltd., New Delhi, 2007.

Philips, Melanie and John Dawson: *Doctor's Dilemmas: Medical Ethics and Contemporary Science*; Harvest Press, 1985.

Rader Melvin 1964: "*Ethics and Human Community*" Hott Rinehart and Winston, 1964, USA.

Rajkhowa, J.P.: *Sankardeva: His Life Preachings and Practices*, Rupsmita Rajkhowa, Guwahati, Assam.

Rao, V. Venkata: *A History of Political Theories*: S. Chand & Company, New Delhi, 1980.

Radhakrishnan, S., 1961: *Recovery of Faith*; George Allen & Unwin Ltd.

Radhakrishnan, S., *The Present Crisis of Faith,* Orient Paperbacks: A Division of Vision Books Pvt. Ltd., New Delhi, 1970.

Robert Ian: *Sociology*; Worth Publishers.Inc. 7th edition, 1980.

Staub, E., *Roots of Evil: The Origin of Genocide and Other Group Violence*, New York, Cambridge University Press, Katz F., 1993.

Tiwari, Kedarnath, *Comparative Religion*; Motilal Banarasi Dass, Delhi.

Treadwell, Donald and Jill B. Treadwell: 2005, Public Relations Writing; Second edition; Response Books; A Division of Sage Publications, New Delhi, pp. 57-59.

Veeranghavan, J., "*Dharma:* The Values that Sustain", *Understanding India*, ed. by Subhash Chandra Kashyap and Abhaya Kashyap, Vitasta Publishing Ltd., New Delhi, 2007.

THREE
Gandhian Flavour in Medical Sciences

Gandhi's ideas, many may consider as outdated in the face of modern India which is developing fast in almost every walk of life since the country attained Independence on 15th August, 1947. One cannot deny the progress of science and technology, education, standard of living and several reforms in the socio-economic and political life of the Indians. In almost every front of public services noticeable changes have taken place. Simultaneously, however, corruption, violation of human rights, hypocrisy, unethical activities, severe frailness of human power to control violent activism of money and muscle power, lack of serious thought to the consequences of the politicization of public services, buying and selling of job, massive growth of fake financial and educational institutions exploiting the poor and innocent Indians' hard earned money and helpless unemployed youths by all possible means may be considered as a serious threat to the nation. Under this situation Gandhi's ideas, I feel, will certainly help to a great extent to relieve the nation from various kinds of ailments. In the words of Mahatma Gandhi himself let me forward an argument in favour of my feeling as below:

> Gandhi said, "......it is not my purpose to attempt a real autobiography. I simply want to tell the story of my numerous experiments with truth, and as my life consists of nothing, but those experiments, it is true that the story will take the shape of an autobiography. But I shall not mind, if every page of it speaks only of my experiments. I believe, or at any rate flatter myself with the belief, that a connected account of all these experiments will not be without benefit to the reader. My experiments in the

> political field are now known, not only to India, but to a certain extent to the 'civilized' world. For me they have not much value; and the title 'Mahatma' that they have won for me has, therefore, even less. Often the title has deeply pained me. But I should certainly narrate my experiments in the spiritual field which are known only to myself and from which I have derived such power as I possess for working in the political field. If experiments are really spiritual, then there can be no room for self-praise. They can only add to my humility. The more I reflect and look back on the past, the more vividly do I feel my limitations."

Now, the question arise, are we failing to adhere or acquire knowledge from the well established or ancient human culture of India while delivering or receiving service in modern Indian state? Is it true to say that there is nothing to learn by a modern Indian from the past history?

While discussing the relevance of his ideas on medicine or health it is found that Gandhi had strong faith in nature cure and diet for good health, though he depended upon medicine in Durban during his illness. He said, "with the growing simplicity to my life, my dislike for medicines steadily increased." But he admitted, while practicing in Durban, he suffered from debility and rheumatic inflammation. Dr. P.J. Mehta, who had come to see him, gave him medicine, and he got well. At the same time he used to be troubled with constipation and frequent headache. While at Johannesburg he kept himself fit with occasional laxatives and well regulated diet. He was not healthy and tried to get rid of laxative medicine. Then he started regulating diet. He said, "...I read of the formation of a 'No Breakfast Association' in Manchester. The argument of the promoters was that Englishmen often ate too much, that their doctors' bills were heavy because they ate until midnight, and that they should at least give up breakfast, if they wanted to improve this state of affairs. Though these things could not be said for me, I felt that the argument did apply in my case. I used to have three square meals daily in addition to afternoon tea. I was never spare eater and enjoyed as many delicacies as could be with vegetarian and spice less diet.... I, therefore argued if I also dropped the morning breakfast, I might become free from headaches. So, I tried the experiment. For a few days it was rather hard, but the headache entirely disappeared. This led me to conclude that I was eating more than I needed.... Though I have had two serious illnesses in my life, I believe that man has little need to drug himself. Nine hundred and ninety nine cases out of a thousand can be brought round by means of well regulated diet, water and earth treatment and similar household medicines. He who runs to the doctor, Vaidya or Hakim for every little ailment, and swallows all kinds of vegetable and mineral drugs, not only curtails his life, but by becoming the slave of his body instead of remaining its master, loses his self-control and ceases to be a man" (M.K. Gandhi: 1989).

Today, however, the expert advice is, "eat breakfast like king, lunch like prince and dinner like pauper". Considering the difference of weightage on breakfast, lunch and dinner, one can come to the conclusion that heavy eating throughout the day is not desirable and one can take care of food considering time and workload to maintain good health. This is true to each one of us. The saying of Joan Robinson, "The problem of survival is not only to eat, but also to avoid being eaten away" may be referred in support of the above. Further very rightly he pointed out that our feelings are as rooted in a biologically determined apparatus require a certain degree of detachment. For example hunger. We think that we desire to eat because food is necessary to life, but it is by no means so simple. We desire to eat because we have endowed with an apparatus that makes us feel hungry, and we are endowed with that apparatus because a species that lacked it would not have survived. In some illness the patient suffers a total absence of appetite; then to push external substance inside oneself seems not merely boring but actually abhorrent. An intellectual perception that food is necessary for life is not enough to get it down (Robinson: 1970).

Gandhi in his book, '*Key to Health*' wrote about health as, "He is a healthy man whose body is free from all disease; he carries on his normal activities without fatigue. Such a man should be able with ease to walk ten to twelve miles a day, and perform ordinary physical labour without getting tired. He can digest ordinary simple food. His mind and senses are in a state of harmony and poise. A man with extraordinary physical strength is not necessarily healthy. He has merely developed his musculate, possibly at the expense of something". A happy working of the human machine depends upon the harmonious activity of the various components of the body (Gandhi: 1948).

History of every civilized nation is full of experiments from which each can be empowered to give effective steps in the escalation of the nation's progress. Today human security is the significant factor in the paradoxical global situation. It is more true in a developing country like India with the increase in ailing population. The health security is the primary component of human security. The rapid development of medical sciences in various dimensions provides enough scope to think of relevance of ethical values to the medical services embracing ailing population of the country in the face of turbulence of commercialization and globalization of public services. Food security is, again a main component of health security. Here let me refer to an article, titled, *Prevention of Malnutrition*, published in *The Assam Tribune*, a daily newspaper, written by Dr. Nalini Kanta Dutta. The Food Security as defined by the World Food and Agricultural Organization (FAO) means access of all people at all times to sufficient, safe and nutritious food to meet their dietary needs and food preferences for an active and healthy life.

Nutrients in food are the contributors for body growth, development and maintenance. Nutrients constitute proteins, vitamins, minerals and amino acids. Prevalence of healthy lives through consumption of nutritious foods can abolish nutrition deficiency diseases such as protein energy malnutrition, endemic goiter, nutritional anemia, nutritional blindness, and diarrhea diseases. Nutritional science has also detected the links of nutrition with infection, immunity, fertility, maternal and child health, family health and community health. The nutritious food includes cereals and millets, pulses, vegetables, animal food, nuts and oil seeds, fruits, fats and oils, sugar and juggery, condiments and spices and miscellaneous foods. With a view to mitigate the nutritional deficiency, a balanced diet is preferred. A balanced diet is one which contains a variety of food in such quantities and proportions that the need for energy, amino acids, vitamin, minerals and fats, carbohydrates and other nutrients are adequately met for the maintaining health, vitality and general well-being with extra nutrients. There are many nutritional problems which affect a vast section of Indian population. The major ones are low birth weight, protein energy malnutrition, dry eye (exophthalmia), nutritional anemia, iodine deficiency disorders, endemic fluorosis and lathyrism. Diet also in many situations can help curing the heart diseases, specially coronary heart disease, diabetes, obesity etc. Most of the problems of food security can be solved with cheap and easy ways through diet based on naturally available and cultivated vegetables, fruits and several foodgrains easily accessible to the most people. However, purchasing power of the people has to be enhanced. Mahatma Gandhi was also aware of food security and his ideas on health related diet cannot be rejected even to-day.

We are neglecting his ideas while moving towards modernization and industrialization of our lives. However, even the British who had to leave India due to pressure by the Indians under Gandhi's string leadership, honoured his ideas. For example, let me mention the Gandhi centenary celebration in London in 1969 (*The Assam Tribune*, 29th April, 2013).

The British, against whom Gandhi led the freedom struggle, remembered him with honour for his principles which he practiced in the life. Here mention may be made of the Gandhi Centenary Celebrations in London in 1969. The Gandhi Centenary tribute was arranged in the Royal Albert Hall under the auspices of the United Kingdom Gandhi Centenary Committee presided over by Lord Mount Batten. The British Prime Minister, Harold Wilson in his address stated that because of the very genuine respect and admiration of the British people for the principles of Gandhi both enunciated and practiced His Royal Highness, the Prince of Wales was present on the occasion. The Indian Education Minister Dr. V.K.V. Rao also attended the celebration.

Harold Wilson said, "Mahatma Gandhi's connections with this country extend back into the nineteenth century. It was 81 years, in 1888, when Mr. M.K. Gandhi first visited Britain. He came here as young student of 19 on his first journey outside his native land to study and to qualify in law. Three years later, in 1891, he left this country not only as a qualified Barrister but also, through his experiences here in these formative years of his life, strengthened and reassured in his moral principles and with a friendship and understanding of the British people—an abiding friendship and understanding which was to endure throughout all the long and difficult days which were to come in his relations with successive British Governments and the Government of India.

For during these three years in London he not only learned to study by himself and to make up his own mind on many problems of ethics and religion, he also learned a great deal about the ordinary people of this country—how they lived their daily lives, their prejudices and the working of their minds and what really interested them. In the years which were to come this enabled him to look behind and through the official façade to the Britain and the ordinary British people whom he had come to know so well in his years as a student.

On his first visit to this country, Gandhi was introduced by his British friends to new concepts of his philosophy and religion. It was, while he was in London and in the company of English friends that he first read in full, in Sanskrit, the Hindu scriptures, the *Bhagavad Gita*, which was to become the foundation of his philosophy of non-violence which he later developed and practiced. He also became familiar with Christianity, and although he always remained firmly Hindu, Christianity had a profound influence on him and later in his life he acknowledged how much his philosophy owed to Sermon on the Mount.

Even at this early stage of his life it is possible to trace the beginnings of his iron self-discipline which he imposed on himself through the rest of his life. There was his unshakable resolve to remain a strict vegetarian and never to touch meat, the frugal life he led in London, walking long distances through our streets and cooking his own meals—and his refusal to drink alcohol on any occasion" (Harold Wilson: 1969).

While in London Gandhi read Henry Salt's book, "*Plea for Vegetarianism*". Till then he had been vegetarian by custom and tradition but from the moment he read Salt's book he became a vegetarian by choice. The reason was the growing sense that flesh eating is a cruel, disgusting, unwholesome and wasteful practice (Guha: 2013).

H.R.H., the Prince of Wales while speaking on the occasion said,

> "Many of you may think it strange that I should be standing here in order to speak about a man who died almost a year before I was born, in a distant country, who was one of the chief architects of Britain leaving India, who took tea with my great-grandfather wearing just a loin cloth and sandals, and who succeeded where no one else had in helping to replace my grandfather's title of Emperor of India with that of Head of Commonwealth. And yet, just before the transfer of power, when the engagement of my parents was announced in 1947, one of the first messages the Viceroy received was from Mahatma Gandhi. It asked for his best wishes to be conveyed to them. Later he regretted he could send no wedding present because he had no personal possessions beyond his sandals and *dhoti* and a cheap watch on a piece of string. However, Lord Mountbatten suggested, he might make something and he duly set to work on his spinning wheel to produce a small tablecloth. This was sent together with a magnificent diamond necklace from the Nizam of Hyderabad to Buckingham Palace. Recently, the British Museum asked to include the cloth in their Gandhi exhibition, but it could be found nowhere until the Queen produced it from a place where some of her most treasured belongings are kept.
>
> It does seem strange, to me, and yet if Mahatma Gandhi had lived, I doubt it would have seemed strange to him. But having heard so much from the last Viceroy about Gandhi's life and being fascinated by India herself, I am honoured to speak in the

> memory of a man who achieved such astonishing things for India without bitterness or hostility and who by his own magnetic personality, prevented the terror of bloodshed in Bengal. How fortunate was India to have a man like that at one of his most critical periods in her history, when the situation was so tense that civil war throughout the whole sub-continent could so easily have flared up" (HRH, the Prince of Wales: 1969).

Gandhi may be considered as the incarnation of truth and non-violence in modern India. The physicians are also the true agents of truth and non-violence. Both are the seekers of truth. Both adopt non-violent means to achieve the goal of human security. A surgeon uses sharp knife on the human body with the noble mission of giving relief to the sufferer. His act of using knife is an act of non-violence. On the other hand, a dacoit also uses sharp knife on human body, but his act is an act of violence. It is not the weapon which makes the difference between the two, but it is the inner motive which makes a difference between them. A dacoit's act is guided by animal power whereas that of a surgeon is guided by the human power. A dacoit is a threat to man's life, but a physician is a saviour of man's life and a creator of peace and happiness in the life of a man. A physician deals with physically ailing population of the society while Gandhi's ideas address the mentally ailing population of the society.

Till recently physicians could claim unquestionable faith of the people. They did not face any violent and suspicious attitude of the patients. However, today the earlier trust on physicians has become shaky. Various factors are responsible for this state of affairs. Besides external factors, there are internal factors such as, corruption, weak social relationship, administrative challenges, medical errors, commercialization of services etc. within the domain of medical services which are also responsible to a great extent for it.

In India social values are changing very fast. The old traditional values are considered by the modern Indians as outdated and they feel these should be discarded. They find them hindrances in the modern way of life and start giving interpretation or arguments in favour of their statement according to their convenience or advantage. Various reasons may be assumed for this—impact of science and technology, commercialization of social relationship, various developmental programmes undertaken by the Government etc. The negative impact of the replacement of Joint family by nuclear family system may also be considered as a factor for erosion of social control over individual and frangibility of social relationship. Love, affection, sympathy, fellow feeling, sense of belongingness etc. are measured in terms of financial benefits or by selfish interest. The elderly members of the family who cannot earn and need financial, physical and healthcare are considered as burden by the members of the modern nuclear families in most cases.

Interestingly, a modern man neglects the elderly and old people on the plea that there is always shortage of time in very busy life. Further, corruption and crimes have become omnipresent. Mutual distrust, hatred towards each other, violation of human rights, exploitation through fake financial and educational institutions, hypocrisy, etc. as mentioned above have become common problems in modern India. The cities or urban areas are full of exploiters, dacoits, violators of laws in the country causing deterioration of the law and order situation to a large extent. Threat is occurring to the survival of human society as well as the animal world. In every field of life (whether public or private) corruption is rampant. Media focuses almost every day involvement of high officials and top political leaders in huge financial corruption cases. The cases of domestic violence against women, youth unrest caused by alcoholism, drugs addiction, heavy television viewing are increasing in the society very rapidly. Parents, very frequently confess their inability to have effective control over their children. It is difficult to deny the contribution of ethical vacuum to this kind of social situation in modern India in addition to other factors. The Gandhian way of life may be a way of solution to most of our problems in the contemporary society. Because it is Gandhi who cares for human conscience and creativity and gives impetus to non-violent resistance to evils.

Gandhi believed that relation of individual with individual must be based on truth, benevolence, cooperative spirit and amity. Truth embraces each and every domain of man's life. One must lead a self-disciplined life. But average modern Indians move other way round. The multiplication of wants, unnecessary craze for material and physical comforts, useless consumption expansion, accumulation of huge property etc. are the major impediments on the path of justice, morality, ethical principles etc. Because desire multiplication is an unending process leading to end of life itself.

Nobody can deny that no social group based on violence, exploitation, corrupt practices, aggressive behaviour can be truly dignified or is honoured in a human society (Gopalakrishnan: 1985).

Since every service provider reaches to that status after passing through the stages of the process from being to becoming. During childhood and youthhood he/she learns many things through socializing process in which family and educational institutions play a significant role as primary agents. What he or she learnt from these social institutions, mainly from the parents and family community environment and social values are reflected in his or her attitude and behaviour as service provider to the society. The attitude and behaviour of the service providers are very deeply rooted in the social and family culture. Significantly, they are also influenced by the changing social values and culture. The appearance of corruption, unethical activities, inhuman treatment etc. in the services are found mainly due to several sociological factors like these, besides other factors. Failure of the socializing agencies in achieving their goals brings failure of human power to control other external powers and an individual in this situation may become the slave of any destructive power or activities. They start losing the reasoning power. Here begins the self-abasement as human being. From whichever direction wind comes they will be blown easily because they cannot be firm on their feet as they have lost the human power. They forget their identity as human being and allow animal power to function.

Another aspect of Gandhi's social philosophy is his concept of truth. The pursuit of truth does not admit of violence being inflicted on one's own opponent, "for what appears to be truth to the one may appear to be error to the other. The adversary is opponent, not enemy, and he is to be won by patience and sympathy." And patience means self-suffering which comes to mean "vindication of truth not by infliction of suffering on the opponent, but on one's self". Gandhi understood suffering to be neither negative nor a necessary evil. Rather he understood it to be a positive force in its own right, and even more powerful instrument than violence. "Real suffering bravely borne melts even a heart of stone. Such is the potency of suffering and *tapas*. And there lies key to *Satyagraha*. As against it, violence is intended to achieve an end through the exploitation of fear. It strengthens the elements of passion and compulsion. But suffering appeals to a man's moral nature. It brings out the elements of love and compassion. It was Gandhi's firm conviction that "human nature in its essence is one and therefore unfailingly responds to the advances of love. And success is the certain result of suffering of the extremist character, voluntarily undergone" (Grover: 1977).

Gandhism, as it is said by many, is not a set of doctrine nor a set of rules or regulations, but a way of life led by Gandhi himself. His way of life is a mirror where the ancient Indian tradition and philosophy are reflected. The Indian tradition, philosophy and religion provide a strong foundation for flourishing the culture of peace. In Indian tradition, a person's spiritual enlightenment is measured in terms of his capacity to lead a life of calmness, desireless, non-attachment and self-control. All these are qualities of a *Karma Yogi*. The culture of peace is the highest spiritual and ethical value in India. It is a practical ethics. It can be the basis of co-existence of the diverse points of view, attitude of understanding and tolerance in one concerning the other's ideology and value and unconditional rejection of force in all interpersonal and international dealings and brotherhood among all without any injury to the dignity of each (Sinari: 1978). It may be said that a man's way of life is partially a product of social culture and it is not imposed on him but internalized through socialization. Gandhi's way of life itself is an example for it.

Gandhi's actions sprung from the inner recesses of his soul. Human life was his laboratory, love his instrument, and appeal of the human heart his language. In the words of Erikson, Gandhi had achieved "an identity of two identities—personal identity and the identity located in the core of his communal culture." His social philosophy is based on the spirit of identification with humanity as a whole, on the basis of love, dignity, personal responsibility and solidarity.

Gandhiji bridged the gap between individual and social ethics and regarded social reality as a counterpart of man's inner reality. To him individual freedom had a value, but one must not, he said, "forget that man is essentially a social being. He has risen to present status by learning to adjust his individualism to the requirements of social progress" (Tripathi: 1980).

It made a heart felt appeal not only to the enlightened people of the country, but also illiterate and innocent people of all parts of the country during freedom movement. To Gandhi there must be non-violence in the private life itself. He lived in an atmosphere of non-violence from the Jainist traditions of non-violence, his saintly mother, disciplined father and tolerant wife. It is that helps one to develop the inner strength, the soul force necessary for the *Satyagrahi*. A *Satyagrahi* is a man of peace. Positively, a *Satyagrahi* will always try to overcome evil by good, anger by love, untruth by truth, *himsa* by *ahimsa*.

It is also a way of group life. *Satyagraha* fights violence among groups. Because of this it has its techniques of organization, leadership, discipline, training and strategy. Gandhi points out that "anything that millions can do together becomes charged with a unique power." A

Satyagraha needs a leader, he is the very soul of mass *Satyagraha*. The leader should have sterling qualities. The most important of these are:

(a) Sincerity and all-embracing love,
(b) Culture and dignified bearing,
(c) Self-control,
(d) Selflessness,
(e) Pursuit of non-possession,
(f) Rooted in the soil of and having the spirit of *Swadeshi;* and
(g) Faith in God which is synonymous with truth should be unshakable (Quartey).

To be a true servant of the human being he must be the possessor of above qualities. Because these qualities make a man human. Human society can be served effectively only by a human being not by a half-human being or by an animal, just as only the democrats can make democratic way of life successful (Verma: 1978).

To-day's socio-political situation in India induces a researcher or a social scientist to think that the way of life of an Indian has to be grounded in the Indian tradition and philosophy to make the country strong and suitable for living with human dignity. While adjusting with the changes in the modern world he must be well acquainted with the Indian tradition and philosophy to serve the country successfully. Mere expertness or knowledge on a particular issue or modern equipment are not enough unless the user of these is selfless, moral and sympathetic to the people The author makes an attempt to bring to light the relevance of Gandhian way of life to the medical services. The medical services constitute a very significant component of public services in any country. It has its uniqueness in dealing with the ailing people who are vulnerable and surrender themselves to the physicians the right to life, the primary human right of a person.

It may be noted that at a time when many people in Ghana and Africa had a doubt about the need of study of the philosophy of Non-violence as advocated by Gandhi Francis Ofosu Quartey, Secretary of Gandhi Brotherhood League, Ghana expressed his personal feeling that it was necessary for the following reasons:

1. "It is the most original contribution of India to political thought and practice;
2. *Satyagraha* was the life long study and practice of Gandhi. To know Gandhi one must know what *Satyagraha* is; and

3. *Satyagraha* formed the philosophical background of the struggle of India for independence. To understand the meaning of the struggle and present institutions of India one must know the meaning and the body of ideas which constitute *Satyagraha.*"

The evolution of *Satyagraha* by Mahatma Gandhi has made him the most significant figure in the world. Non-violence in social life is not peculiar to Indian people. History is replete with leaders who have advocated non-violence. However, India is unique in having a tradition of non-violence and it is India's greatest contribution to world thought. There is in India the belief that "all life is one". Gandhi lived in an environment in which non-violence was the norm. Let us examine some of the influences that might have swayed him to the ideas of non-violence.

In the *Bhagavad Gita* we find a commendation of non-violence as:

> "When the body is obedient, when the senses are mastered, when man knows his *atman* is the *atman* of all creatures, then let him act untainted by action."

In Jainism, a religion of India, we have a negative side of non-violence in which no life is to be destroyed.

In Buddhism, the Buddha taught non-violence. In a famous admonishment to his followers he pointed out—

> "if a man by causing pain to others, wishes to obtain pleasure for himself, he, entangled in the bonds of selfishness, will never be free from hatred. Let a man overcome anger by love, let him overcome evil by good; let him overcome greed by liberality, the liar by truth. For hatred does not cease by hatred at any time; hatred ceases by non-hatred, this is an old rule. Speak the truth, do not yield to anger, give, if thou are asked; by these steps thou will become divine. Lead others, not by violence, but righteous and equity."

Gandhi was the product of the thoughts of China and Japan. In China, there is a long tradition of non-violence as embodied or found in Confucianism, Taoism and Buddhism. Thus, Confucius advocated that men should not do to others as they do not want done to themselves.

We find the influence of John Ruskin on the thinking of Gandhi, Ruskin's work *Unto His Last* influenced Gandhi greatly. Gandhi liked

Ruskin's idea of the importance of manual labour, that the good of the individual rests on the good of all, that the engineer's work has the same value as that of the labourer as all have the same right of earning their livelihood from their work.

Tolstoy, an advocate of non-violence also influenced Gandhi. Gandhi, himself pointed out "Next to the late Rajachandra, Tolstoy is one the three moderns who have exerted the greatest spiritual influence on my life, the third is Ruskin."

The aim of Gandhi was to seek truth. In seeking truth he wanted to see how he could be of the greatest use to humanity. He pointed out several times that the "greatest good of all" and not the "good of the majority" is to be sought. To Gandhi means and ends must be pure. The reason is that end grows out means. That which is achieved by chicanery, bribery, deceit, is transitory. Good means, alone, it was believed by Gandhi, can achieve lasting peace and progress. But a question that arises is how can this be achieved. Gandhi said:

"1. Self-realization in which the individual examines himself,
2. Self-purification, and
3. Ethical discipline in which the individual follows certain laid out principles. He points out, "he who is not prepared to order his life in unquestionable obedience to the laws of morality cannot be said to be a man in the full sense of the word." Therefore, he advocated certain moral vows. (Quartey)

Gandhi's ideas or his way of life influenced the India's freedom movement as well as the framers of the constitution and the rulers of the country in the beginning of the administration of India. The culture of the Indian society has also governed the policies of the Government of India both within and without the country. For example, *Panchshila* (five Principles) formed by Pandit Jawaharlal Nehru and Chaou-en-lai at the conclusion of latter's three day visit to India on 26th June, 1954 may be cited here as below:

1. Mutual respect for each other's independence,
2. Mutual non-aggression,
3. Mutual non-interference in each other's affairs,
4. Equality and mutual benefit, and
5. Peaceful co-existence.

As regards domestic policies one may put his or her finger on the Preamble to the Constitution of India which is a standing reminder to all the Indians for leading a peaceful human life and progress of human society. The very structure of the Indian society is unique in the sense it has diversity of culture, diversity of language and diversity of religion which nobody can do away with or deny it as the reality of Indians' life (Verma: 1978).

Truth and Non-violence are the key elements of Gandhi's way of life, just as 'power' is the key element of politician's way of life and addition, subtraction, multiplication and division are the elements to mathematicians' way of functioning. Truth was the fundamental vow adopted by Gandhiji and he instructed others to know truth, to speak truth and to work according to truth (Ghosh: 1985).

Both Gandhi and a physician may be called as the seekers of truth. Similarly, truth and non-violence are the basic elements of a physician's way of service life. He is, like Gandhi is the seeker of truth. Both Gandhi and a physician are analysts of man—Gandhi analyzes the inner person while a physician analyzes the animal body of a man. But both of them meet at the area of interdependence of body and mind. Truth precedes non-violence and peace. A physician tries to make correct diagnosis of the disease of a patient with the aim of curing the patient by administering right medicine so that he/she can regain healthy body and secure peace of mind. To do so the doctor must have peace of mind and free from all kinds of tension.

Truth and non-violence form the bedrock of goodness in human being. Peace at personal level is an undisturbed state of mind, a state of serenity and tranquility with a love for fellow human and sub-human species. It is non-violence and reverence for all life and nature. Gandhi envisioned a dynamic form of peace to be embedded in the heart of every human being. Gandhi said, "I believe in peace. But I do not want peace that you find in stone; I do not want peace that you find in grave; But I do want peace which you find embedded in the human breadth, which is exposed to the arrows of a whole world, which is protected from all kinds of harm. To Gandhi one should be peaceful in thought and intent, while maintaining peace with hand one must also keep the tongue clean. It is not possible to maintain peace without avoiding anger from one's mind" (Government of India: 1966).

Non-violence is the greatest force at the disposal of mankind. Violence is the mightiest weapon of destruction of mankind. Destruction is not the law of humans (Prabhu and Rao: 1945).

Thus, truth and non-violence are the foundation of peace. Truth indicates existence and it signifies peace. Gandhi's concept of non-violence has wider perspective embracing love, self-discipline and positive attitude towards peace. The negative connotation of it implies non-war, non-exploitation and non-violent action against social injustice. Non-violence is an effective weapon to be used against diverse forms of violence. It demands necessary training for self-discipline.

In social relationship peace is a state of freedom from direct and structural forms of violence between human beings. It confines not only to a small group, but may be extended to national and international levels.

Self-suffering and non-violent activities are the two important components of *Satyagraha* and these may be considered as substitute to violence. These two components liberate both the oppressor and the oppressed from violence. To make *Satyagraha* effective the non-violent actor must have courage (Government of India: 1966).

The term '*satya*' comes from the word '*sat*' which means 'to exist'. What exists in this world is truth or *satya*. It is praiseworthy for a man who shows his respect to an entity that exists. Therefore, Gandhi advises mankind to show respect to truth and to be true in their thinking, speech and action. If someone, after hiding his own true nature talks or works with others for having some benefits from them, he will be treated as a man of complex nature. He may be called a hypocrite.

Naya, to Gandhi, meant both "truth and justice". It is the function of *Naya* to reveal the object as it is, i.e., true nature of the object. To find out truth through reasoning is called *Naya*. Where there is *Naya* there is truth.

The Law and the law giver are one for Gandhi, since the law giver is none other than truth itself. This has been interpreted by Dr. Raghunath Ghosh in the light of *Advaita Vedanta*. Laws are truth because all pervading truth remains in it. Where there is no truth there is no law. The maker of the law may also be called law giver. So, the term "truth" may be used both as law and law-giver just as the term "justice" is used both in the sense of law and the person dealing with law (Ghosh: 1985).

Dr. R. Gopalakrishnan, while referring to Gandhi's concept of truth, said that truth may be of two kinds—absolute truth and relative truth. Absolute truth has absolute value and it is always preferable. One cannot go beyond the absolute truth. Another classification of truth is—1. Objective truth and 2. Subjective truth. Exhaustive knowledge of anything and everything embodies the objective truth which is constant. It is the real nature of anything. Subjective truth is the best knowledge of anything possessed by anybody. It is the *ad hoc* standard of truth we use in measuring the truth of relevant truth. Another classification of truth is—1. Truth as it is, and 2. Truth as achieved so far. The fourth classification of truth is—1. Empirical truth, 2. Moral truth, and 3. Metaphysical truth. Empirical truth is reflected in natural and physical sciences. Moral aspect of truth is reflected in our thoughts, words and deeds. Metaphysical aspect of truth is the highest reality. *Upanishad* propounds as the highest reality. *Upanisadic* sages exposed 'To be true is to become divine' Buddha says, "truth is the image of the eternal". *Mahabharata* declares that there is no religion higher than truth. Vinobaji gives Vedantic interpretation of it as, "Truth brings knowledge and bliss." Truth begets truth. Life is meant for truth. So, the whole of mankind and its allied pursuits are in search of truth.

According to Gandhiji lying does not justify the noble cause. It is a complex phenomenon in two ways—1. every lie is intentional by nature. Since, it is intentional by nature, every lie becomes complex; 2. every lie gives a distorted report about a particular fact.

No special effort is needed to speak the truth, but special effort is needed to tell lie. There is no scope for contradiction in the statement of truth. But there is a lot of possibilities for contradiction in the statement of untruth. A lawyer fighting for the victory of truth is a good sign of moral progress. A lawyer fighting for the victory of untruth is nothing but a moral degradation.

Agustine and Immanual Kant were not in favour of telling lie under any circumstances. They sincerely believe that a lie may not be told even for an urgent purpose. In Gandhiji's opinion also lying is an evil. It should not be encouraged, in any circumstances. If we have to save humanity from destruction and promote morality on earth, lying should not be treated to justify a noble cause. (Gopalakrishnan: 1985) As regards the medical sciences it is found that there is a little bit deviation from this view of Gandhi. In certain cases, the doctors may not tell the truth to the patient so that no harm takes place through truth telling to him and sometimes they conveyed the sad message indirectly to the attendants. The indirect message carries the hints that the patient will not be cured.

The essence of entire content of Gandhian philosophy may be conveyed in a single word: *Satyagraha*. It is also the word that has the entire Gandhian technique of action as its core. *Satyagraha* is essentially the art of confronting the opponent with a moral challenge and socio-psychological situation. It is logically impossible to deny Gandhi's contention that *Satyagraha* is the only means which can preserve and promote the values of liberty, equality and fraternity. A *Satyagrahi* is constantly training himself for assuming profound moral responsibility of changing social relationship and institutions; and in doing so he is not only refusing to violate the liberty of his adversary, but subjecting himself alone to all the suffering involved in the act of *Satyagraha*. He is thus acting as a free agent with individual moral responsibility as well as allowing his adversary to act in a similar manner. Secondly, since the whole basis of *Satyagraha* is the recognition of the relativity of values and the essential equality of all human beings, it preserves and promotes equality in a very real sense. The *Satyagrahi* confronts his adversary fearlessly, to the extent of sacrificing his life in the confrontation, and looks him in the eye as equal, not as inferior or superior. Finally, fraternity and wider love is the very essence of *Satyagraha*. *Satyagrahi* covers neither power nor dominance either for himself or for his party or class, but is interested solely in securing justice, and is constantly training himself not to bear ill will for the adversary, he is an embodiment of fraternity although he is determined to extinguish the system for which his opponent is responsible. Indeed fraternity is the first principle of *Satyagraha* and all other considerations are secondary.

Erikson said, "In a period when arrogant statesmen could speak of a "war to end war"; when the super policeman of Versailles could bathe in the glory of a peace that would make "the world safe for democracy"; when the revolutionaries in Russia could entertain the belief that terror could initiate an eventual "withering away of the state"—during the same period, one man in India confronted the world with the strong suggestion that a new socio-political instrument, endowed with a new kind of religious fervour, may yet provide man with a choice" (Tripathi: 1980).

Like Gandhi a Physician is also a seeker of truth. He must understand the true nature of the diseases as well as the patient to prescribe right medicine for curing the diseases. He cannot but know the truth even for his survival in the professional. It is a professional demand. To know it without distortion or exactly today several modern equipment have been invented. However, to have the knowledge of the sources of the suffering or the environmental factors the physician has to depend on the conversation with the patient. Here, however, absolute truth may not emanate from the conversation as all the patients may not be in a position to communicate effectively to him about the background of his suffering. While communicating the nature of treatment to be administered or other related matters he has to communicate to the patient only to the extent which helps the patient understand it. It is not speaking the untruth, but speaking the truth with some restrictions or setting aside technical issues from the process to make the patient understand the situation. In no other profession pursuit of truth in such detail as is the case in the medical sciences is found or needed (Gopalakrishnan: 1985).

Just a physician tries to cure a patient and save his life, Gandhi also tried to inculcate strength to a man who is ailed by his animal power. Gandhi never believed that a man can be wholly wicked and ignoble. His concept of human nature is the basis of his entire socio-economic and political thought. The individual is the main consideration. If man is regarded as essentially evil, it is not only an insult to the whole human race, it is also a counsel of despair. To Gandhiji the only difference between the good man and the wicked man is that in the case of latter the good is dormant. He wrote, "There is an innate nobility even in an apparently ignoble man." To him man's heart is good at the core. It may get rusted on the surface due to various factors, but its goodness remains always the same whatever its outward appearance. To Gandhiji traits of character may be acquired by means of teaching, practicing, habit and proper education. So, he believed that man can be changed. Man has in him the capacity of responding to noble impulses. So, to change the society he wanted to change the individual through Ashram Vows.

The impact of Gandhiji's Ashram Vows on us is invisible. But this invisible impact does wonders whenever there is demand for it. To gain this impact six weaknesses of human mind are to be eradicated. According to Indian Ethics the six weaknesses are—1. Passion, 2. Anger, 3. Greed, 4. Infatuation, 5. Pride, and 6. Jealousy. Gandhiji called these six weaknesses as deadly enemies. These may also be called as deadly diseases of mind. Similarly, there are certain deadly diseases of human body for prevention or cure of these diseases the physician take extra care (Gopalakrishnan: 1985).

Truth rules out prejudice, evasion, secrecy and deception as well as exaggeration, suppression or modification of reality. Another principle advocated by Gandhiji was to speak the truth, but it should not be bitter. Because bitterness offends against the principle of fundamental unity; truth without non-violence is not truth, but untruth. The non-violent truth does not mean hypocrisy; even the most harsh truth can be uttered courteously and gently. Essential components of *Satyagraha* as described by Gandhiji are—a view of reality, belief in the ethical principles, right action, keeping the purity of means, strict and austere discipline and constructive programme (Dogra: 1978).

Surendra Verma in his article, '*Modern Search for Peace: Gandhian Way*' discussed the concept of peace at different levels—such as Environmental, Personal, Interpersonal, Group and Social levels. At environmental level peace means silence or quiet and is free from noise.

Peace at personal level is an undisturbed state of mind. It is a state of serenity, or tranquility. Search for such a peace was the main concern of the ancient *rishis* of India. They developed many techniques to find such an undisturbed state of mind. *Yoga* was one of them. Gandhi who followed the great philosophical tradition of India had instructive love and respect for such a personal peace. At the same time he realized that personal peace is impossible to attain if we live in an atmosphere charged with violence and unrest. From the personal it moves to social level. We cannot attain personal peace without first attaining peace of others.

Peace at the interpersonal level is a state of freedom from hostility between persons. Freedom from hostility is the negative aspect of peace. Positive dimension of peace is friendliness. Gandhi always favoured positive peace. His emphasis was always on love and charity in the broadest sense. Gandhi always regarded even his so-called enemies, his possible friends. His search for peace was not only for freedom from hostility, but for the achievement of friendliness in interpersonal relations.

At group level peace is a negation of conflict between two racial, religious or ethnic groups. It is thus a state of harmony, and concord. To create such a state of harmony was Gandhi's life mission.

At social level peace is freedom from public disturbance and disorder. Gandhi created problems of law and order in his life time during freedom struggle of India. He justified his action on the ground that peace and justice are the two sides of the same coin. Instead of obeying an unjust law he disobeyed and defied it—not only personally, but also in a socially organized manner. This shows that in Gandhi's mind peace and justice coincided. At social level Gandhi gave more emphasis on justice. To him peace and justice must go together (Verma: 1978).

Gandhi derived that peace on earth is essentially attached to the moral conduct of human beings. And moral conducts should be the guidelines of our day-to-day life. Thus he observed, "Moral principles have no meaning unless they can be made to serve as guides of conduct in the daily affairs of men."

Peace does not imply any kind of cowardice to Gandhi. Peace of weak was not acceptable to him. According to him a strong will and ability to protect oneself is necessary for achieving and establishing peace.

Gandhi was of the opinion that strength did not come from physical capacity, it comes from indomitable will.

The fear, distrust and suspicion among people cause every discomfort in man's life. At the same time Gandhi recognized the differences among people and realized the need of maintaining them because they would enrich our culture. The main task is to remove fear and suspicion. But mere logic and cold assurance are poor weapons to fight these social evils. Instead, they can be removed only by faith and generosity. "Generosity is not only good morals, but is often good politics and sound expediency" (Madhilika: 1987).

In medical services a physician must have peace of mind to serve effectively the patients. His primary goal is to establish peace in the mind of patient and through it to the whole family of the patient. This is a noble service to the humanity. However, he can be distinguished from other public servants with regard to the environmental peace in the sense that he is always in the midst of sufferers, i.e. with the physically and mentally ailing people. Unlike the work environment in any other organization, the scene of suffering is the routine environment in any hospital (private or public), nursing home, dispensary etc. His profession does not permit the physician to have too much attachment to a particular patient or group of patients nor he is allowed to be emotional nor fearful. He is a strict regulator of all these passions through a strong mind. In other words, he must be a man of self-control. One can derive personal peace from self-knowledge and self-regulation. In the operation theatre a surgeon is to operate a patient not with the end of killing the patient but to save the patient's life. It is not his concern whether the patient is his enemy or friend, male or female, educated or uneducated, rural or urban etc. His only concern is the nature of disease and treatment of the patient. He is the saviour of patient's life. There he cannot be aggressive, but must be calm and peaceful. He cannot treat his enemy, who comes to him for treatment, as his enemy, but as patient. He prescribes medicine to a patient considering his or her nature of ailment and physical condition, not on the basis of his personal relationship. As Gandhi said personal peace can be derived thus from the peace of others. By saving the life of a patient or curing the diseases the physician gives peace and happiness not merely to the patient, but to a family and he receives well wishes as well from the patient's *atman.* This can be extended to the whole mankind as a very significant component of public service as saviour of man's life.

The search for peace is one of the most important problems faced by the mankind. Mahatma Gandhi has gone to the root cause of the strife in order to find a solution. The UNESCO has given only apt expression to Gandhian solution when it says, "since wars begin in the minds of men, it is there that the defense of peace must be laid."

Closely connected to the concept of Gandhi's peace is the 'means and end' concept. Gandhiji believed in the purity of means to attain any end. He was greatly opposed to the Machiavellian idea that ends justifies the means. To Gandhi ends and means cannot be separated from each other. Howsoever, pure the end may be, honest means has to be employed in order to attain that. Much of the strife, tensions and unrest in the world would disappear if nations employed the pure end and means to attain the end. In contemporary society there are instances of Machiavellian idea that end justifies the means. For example Kidney replacement is possible in medical sciences which gives a new birth to a patient. In order to save mother, brother, sister etc. it is alleged that in most cases the members of the family take shelter of fraud, deceit and cunningness to get the kidney of other people, human trafficking is another example where the motive of selling of the kidnapped people is found. The physicians may also be aware of it. Here is a confusion to average people either to accept or refuse what Gandhi said about this relationship. People who are involved in this kind of activity, especially the relatives or family members of the patient may go for it at a helpless condition considering it as a last resort.

The psychology, philosophy and activities of any human being are influenced and conditioned by his or her environment. Mahatma Gandhi was not an exception to it, said E.P. Menon in his article, *Gandhiji's Ashram Vows and their Relevance for Contemporary Social Situation.* One will have to agree with him when he said that very few people gain the capacity to look beyond and do think in such a way that their thoughts and actions create new environments and provide new directions to the future. Responding to the existing environment and being responsible to the creation of new environment were both equally important to him. During the three decades when Gandhi pervaded the entire Indian atmosphere like a colossus, he was fully conscious of all basic values and aspiration that Indian society stood for in its evolution through five thousand years. Therefore, he could easily assimilate the best that was latent in the indigenous culture and the best that was available from the modern technological and scientific civilization in new environment. (Menon: 1985) Let us now look into the Ashram Vows:

Ashram Vows: In 1915 in consultation with the inmates of the *ashram,* Gandhi drafted a list of vows to overcome the manifold temptation of daily life. However, Gandhiji observed, "the taking of a vow does not mean that we are able to observe it completely from the beginning; it does mean constant and honest effort in thought, word and deed with a view to the fulfillment. The following are some of the important vows:

1. Truth
2. *Ahimsa*
3. *Brahmacharya* or Celibacy
4. Control of the Palate
5. Non-stealing
6. Non-possession or poverty
7. *Swadeshi*
8. Fearlessness
9. Religious use of politics
10. Untouchables

Truth: Gandhi identified truth with God. One must speak the truth because it simplifies living and ensures correct path. It may be a bitter pill, but the follower of truth will gain immense strength and courage.

Ahimsa: *Ahimsa* literally means non-killing but Gandhiji broadened its measure by adding an important positive element. The followers of *Ahimsa* were bound not only not to hurt any living thing, but also to love everybody. (Gopalakrishnan: 1985) To Gandhi It is not a negative state of harmlessness, but a positive state of love, of doing good even to the evil doer. H.R.H., the Prince of Wales considered Gandhi as non-violent revolutionary person. Gandhi himself acknowledged it. He understood people and loved them as human beings, as could be seen from his campaign for the untouchables, and this became inescapably obvious to nearly all Indians and also to a great number of other people in and out of India (H.R.H: 1969).

Brahmacharya: To Gandhi *Brahmacharya* is the foundation of other vows. Though this vow is generally understood as regulation of sexual activity, Gandhiji felt the need of control of all senses, in thought, word and deed at all times and in all places. *Brahmacharya* helps self-discipline, self-control, self-purification, perfect control over all the senses and freedom from lust (Bharato: 1987).

Control of Palate: The control of palate is the outcome of many of Gandhiji's experiments for keeping the vow of *brahmacharya*. Six years of experiment showed that the *brahmachari's* ideal food is fresh fruit and nut. He firmly believed that food is taken essentially for sustenance and not for pleasure or to satisfy the palate. This *ashram* vow is related to *brahmacharya* and thereby it helps maintaining good health of an individual or it may be considered as a health security measure to be adopted by each individual. Gandhi said, "I found that complete control of the palate made the observance very easy, and so I now pursued my dietic experiments not merely from vegetarian's, but also from the *brahmachari*'s point of view. As a result of these experiments he saw that *brahmachari*'s food should be limited, simple, spiceless and, if possible, uncooked." (Autobiography: 1948) Gandhi's aims of this vow are:

1. To acquire control over the palate as a part of self-control in general;
2. To search for the simplest and the cheapest diet for identifying ourselves with the poor or the general masses;
3. To discover which diet is necessary for perfect health, as diet is the main source of health. (Iyer: 1986) Gandhi was aware of the evil consequences of over eating. Besides all other advantages control over palate may be considered as hygienic, economic and practical.

A doctor at the time of entry into service has to take an oath that he/she will not do any harm to the patient. This is nothing, but an oath of *ahimsa* as Gandhi thought of or every religion tells us. Gandhi administered the oath to all common men while medical oath is only for the medical service providers. In other services this kind of oath is not found in explicit terms. Since the medical services occupy a unique position by dealing with the problems relating to life and death of the patients this oath has a special meaning and very closely related to Gandhi's concept of non-violence and religious lessons. On the other hand, Gandhi made experiments with nature cure of diseases.

Khundrakpam Budhachandra Singh, while undertaking research for the degree of Doctor of Philosophy in Manipur University on *Gandhian Approach to Non-violence and Peace* has mentioned clearly about Gandhi's ideas on Food, Nature and Individuals. According to Gandhi, the nature cure implies that the treatment should be the cheapest and simplest possible. It must bring some reform to the life of an individual. It invites regulation of one's life in accordance with the laws of health. Gandhi's nature cure does not favour taking free medicine from hospital for the simple reason that free treatment from the hospital accepts charity. The man who does not take free treatment is free from charity and develops habit of self-help, which is one of the ways to enhance self-respect. He takes steps to cure himself by eliminating poisons from the system and adopts preventive measures against illness in future.

It is desirable to understand the use of the word 'health' in this context. Health here means body care. An individual has good health if his body is free from all diseases and carries on his normal activities without fatigue. The fundamental laws of health and hygiene are simple and one can easily learn them. "Promote the purest thoughts and banish all idle and impure thoughts; breadth the fresh air day and night; establish a balance between bodily and mental work; stand erect, sit erect and be neat and clean in everyone of your acts and let these be an expression of your inner condition. Balance and right food also play a significant role in good or healthy thinking of an individual. Because man becomes what he eats. He believes that the man who eats to live, who is a friend with five powers—earth, water, *akash*, sun and air and who is a servant of the God, the creator of all these, ought not to fall ill." (*Hind Swaraj:* 1.9.1946) Man's first deviation from the right path began when he started enjoying his right to use nature for his own convenience and exploitation of it without realizing his corresponding duties to it. Man should not forget that duty is the true source of right. Gandhi felt that man should desist himself not only from exploiting man, but also from exploiting nature and the natural resources. The accepted values of life should be truth and non-violence. Science has given us an unlimited mastership over nature, but has not taught us self-control. So, the individual in the present day society is swayed by greed, jealousy, anger, egoism etc. for the protection of mankind, minds of people should be inculcated by using self-propelled moral laws in our daily life. (Budhachandra Singh: 2011) A group of researchers in Washington also recently found that dieting intervention may be a promising approach for prevention of Hepatocellular Carcinoma (HCC) (*The Assam Tribune*: 8th Jan, 2014).

Non-stealing: Non-stealing is a vow automatically to be followed by anybody pursuing vows of truth and *ahimsa*. Need based requirements for immediate use when obtained through legitimate process ensured fulfillment of this vow. If any person takes anything which he does not need for immediate use and deprives another person of its use he is thieving, thought Gandhi. Man succumbs to accumulation of articles not needed immediately due to uncertainties of future and greed. Non-possession vow is a logical extension of non-stealing. Since simple living with minimum needs do not justify any property ownership, anyone pursuing the above two vows voluntarily reduces his personal wants. Gandhiji pointed out that material wealth increases at the cost of moral wealth and since the basic requirements of all individuals being common, greater attention has to be paid to moral wealth. Non-stealing has two meanings—negatively, it means non-exploitation and positively, it means selfless service and a feeling for welfare of all.

Swadeshi: The virtue of *Swadeshi* in thought and practice is one of the tenets of Gandhi's philosophy. The *ashram* members were to serve the motherland and immediate neighbourhood under the umbrella of *Swadeshi*. This allegiance should not be blind and static. On the contrary, institutions will have to be dynamic to adjust in a changing situation. (Umarani: 1985)

Gandhi's economic philosophy revolves round his concept of *Swadeshi*. Which literally means the mentality of returning to one's own country—to its culture and heritage, its own genius and tradition, its own ethos, its traditional customs and institutions after a proper re-appraisal of their survival value in the light of modern circumstances. Here Gandhi indicated mainly the revolutionary *Khadi* mentality. "It means a whole sale *Swadeshi* mentality, a determination to find all the necessities of life in India and that too through the labour and intellect of the village." (Tripathy: 1980)

The virtue of *Swadeshi* in thought and practice is one of the basic tenets of Gandhi. He defines *Swadeshi* as the spirit in us which restricts us to the use and service of our immediate surroundings, to the exclusion of the more remote. "Thus, as for religion, in order to satisfy the requirements of the definition, I must restrict myself to my ancestral religion, that is, the use of immediate religious surroundings. If I find it defective I should serve it by purging it of its defects. In the domain of politics I should make use of the indigenous institutions and serve them by curing them of their proved defects. In that economics, I should make use only the things that are produced by my immediate neighbours and serve those industries by making them efficient and complete where they might be found wanting. It is suggested that such *swadeshi*, if reduced to practice, will lead to the millennium." (*Young India*: 21.6.1919) Gandhi applied this principle in all walks of life and said, "*Swadeshi* in its purest form is the acme of universal service". By advocating the virtues of *Swadeshi*, Gandhi was against the exploitation of one nation by another, through multinational trade which necessitated the maintenance of large military force to protect the imperial economic interest. (Sethi: 1978)

A nation which has full strength based on non-violence can serve its neighbouring nations. In the '*Collective Works of Mahatma Gandhi*', it is mentioned that Gandhi wanted India to be strong enough so that she could offer willingly to sacrifice herself for the betterment of the world. Gandhi said, "The individual being pure, sacrifices for the family, the latter for the village, the village for the district, the district for the provinces, the province for the nation, the nation for all." (N.K. Bose: 42) Gandhi's law of *Swadeshi* is not a domestic law to be confined within the four walls of the nation, it embraces the global human society. Gandhi said, "*Swadeshi* is the only doctrine consistent with the law of humanity and love". (Government of India: 1964) In support of it R. Rolland said that the Gandhi's concept of laws of *swadeshi* has universal applicability. Because the concept of *swadeshi* based on love and service to motherland is not different in essence from our obligation to serve mankind. Our capacity to serve is conditioned by our knowledge of the world in which we live. It means that we can do best only to those who are immediately known to us and our neighbours and our country must be the first to receive our service. This in fact is nothing, but humanism or love of mankind. However, it is not narrow nationalism. (Rolland: 1969)

Traditional Medicine: The term "traditional medicine" refers to ways of protecting and restoring health that existed before the arrival of modern medicine. As the term implies, these approaches to health belong to the traditions of each country, and have been handed over down from generation to generation. Traditional systems generally have had to meet the needs of the local communities for many centuries. China and India, for example, have developed very sophisticated systems such as acupuncture and ayurvedic medicine. In practice, the term "traditional medicine" refers to the following components: acupuncture, mental healers and herbal medicine etc.

Over the years, the World Health Assembly has adopted a number of resolutions drawing attention to the fact that the most of the populations in various developing countries around the world depends on traditional medicine for primary healthcare, that the workforce represented by practitioners of traditional medicine is a potentially important resource for the healthcare and that medicinal plants are of importance to the health of individual communities.

Through the Traditional Medicine Programme, the World Health Organization supports Member States in their efforts to formulate national policies on traditional medicine including evaluation of practices and examination of the safety and efficacy of remedies, to upgrade the knowledge of traditional and modern health practitioners, as well as to educate and inform the general public about proven traditional health practices.

WHO is working closely with 19 collaborating Centers in ten countries: Belgium, China, Democratic Republic of Korea, Italy, Japan, Republic of Korea, Romania, Sudan, United States of America and Vietnam.

A genuine interest in various traditional practices now exists among practitioners of modern medicine and growing numbers of practitioners of traditional, indigenous or alternative systems are beginning to accept and use some of the modern technology. This will foster teamwork among all categories of health workers within the framework of primary healthcare. The reasons for inclusion of traditional healers in primary healthcare are manifold: the healers know the socio-cultural background of the people; they are highly respected and experienced in work; economic considerations; distances to be covered in some countries; the strength of traditional beliefs; the shortage of health professionals, particularly in rural areas, to name just a few.

A large proportion of the population in a number of developing countries still herbalists and bone-setters and on local medicinal plants to satisfy their primary healthcare needs. WHO estimates the traditional birth attendants assist in up to 95 per cent of all rural births and 70 per cent of urban births in developing countries.

Traditional medicine has maintained its popularity in a number of countries of Asia, such as China, India, Japan and Pakistan. In China, for example, traditional medicines (herbal preparations) account for 30 per cent to 50 per cent of the total medicinal consumption. In 1993, the total sales of herbal medicines amounted to more than US$ 2.5 billion. In Japan, from 1974 to 1989, there was a 15-fold increase in Kampoh ("Chinese method") medicinal preparations in comparison with only 2.6 fold increase in the sales of mainstream pharmaceutical products. The Japanese per capita consumption of herbal medicine appears to be the highest in the world.

During last decade, there has also been a growing interest in traditional and alternative systems of medicine in many developed countries. One-third of American adults have used alternative treatment and 60 per cent of the public in the Netherlands and Belgium, and 74 per cent in the United Kingdom are in favour of complementary medicine being available within the framework of the National Health Service. A survey among member states of the European Union in 1991, identified about 1400 herbal drugs used in the European Economic Community.

Medicinal plants are the oldest known healthcare products. Their importance is still growing although it varies depending on the ethnological, medical and historical background of each country.

Medicinal plants are also important for pharmacological research and drug development, not only when plant constituents are used directly as therapeutic agents, but also when they are used as basic materials for the synthesis of drugs or as models for pharmacologically active compounds.

Legislative controls in respect of medicinal plants have not evolved around a structured control model. There are different ways in which countries define medicinal plants or herbs. As a result, different approaches have been adopted with regard to licensing, dispensing, manufacturing and trading in order to ensure the safety, quality, and efficacy of medicinal plant preparations.

Herbal medicines are assuming greater importance in the primary healthcare of individuals and communities in many developing countries and there has been an increase in international trade in herbal medicines market is not adequately regulated, and the products are therefore unregistered and often not controlled by regulatory bodies. The establishment of regulation and registration procedures has become a major concern in both developed and developing countries.

WHO has compiled a list of medicinal plants which are widely used in primary healthcare. In July 1996, a WHO scientific group involving 100 experts from various countries around the world adopted the list which includes 28 monographs of 28 medicinal plants originally prepared by the WHO Collaborating Center for Traditional Medicine in Chicago, Illinois, United States of America. (*www.who.int/inf-fs/en/fact 134.html*)

Fearlessness: Fearlessness, said Gandhi, "connotes freedom from external fears—fear of diseases, bodily injury and death, of dispossession, of loosing one's dearest and nearest, of loosing reputation and like." As we are living under stress and strain all over, it is imperative that we cultivate deliberately an attitude of detachment and learn to take things pragmatically, or else there is every danger that we expose ourselves to several health related complications. (Umarani: 1985)

Fearlessness is one of the essential qualities of a good man and is included in the list of virtues of ancient India. In the *Upanishads*, *Vedanta* and *Gita* fearlessness has been appraised as one of the cardinal virtues. Therefore, Gandhi said that fearlessness occupied top position as it is indispensable for the growth of other noble qualities. (Gandhi, MK: 1983) The seeker of truth must overcome all these fears. He must be prepared to sacrifice everything just as *Harishchandra* did. For this faith in God is essential. (Yeravada: 1985)

Religious use of Politics: Since people and politics are inseparable it is imperative for people to carry forward their political activities on the same principles like non-violence, truth and morality. Similar is the case with regard to all the services to the people. (Umarani: 1985)

Gandhi rejected any religious doctrine that does not appeal to reason and is in conflict with morality. He said, "As soon as we lose the moral basis, we cease to be religious. There is no such thing as religion overriding morality. Man, for instance, cannot be untruthful, cruel and inconsistent and claim to have God on his side."

Gandhi was also convinced that morality by itself was not possible to be practiced unless strengthened by religion. So long as the seed of morality is not watered by religion, it cannot sprout. Without water it withers and ultimately perishes. Thus, it may be said that true or ideal morality ought to include true religion. To put the same thought differently, morality cannot be observed without religion. Morality should be observed as religion.

Gandhi related his concept of religion with its root meaning of the original Latin word "*religio*" (that which binds) and also with the Sanskrit word *Dharma*. Whatever is the terminology one uses, to Gandhi meaning is same:

"The root of religion is 'that which binds'. The root meaning of Sanskrit equivalent to *Dharma* is 'that which holds'. It sustains a person as nothing else does. It is rock-bottom of fundamental morality. When morality incarnates itself in a living man it becomes religion, because it binds, it holds, it sustains him in the hour of trial. In this way Gandhi defined religion in terms of morality, he held 'no man can live without religion'." (Pushparanjan: 1987)

T.S. Devadoss in his article, *Freedom, Equality and Peace—A Gandhian Perspective*, while discussing about a new social order in the Gandhian perspective has pointed out the ways for establishing peace as below:

"1. A conviction of the fundamental unity of the human family, and the equality and dignity of all human beings.
2. Vow regarding Untouchables.
3. A sense of the value of human dignity.
4. A realization that might is not right, that human power is not self-sufficient and absolute.
5. A belief that love, compassion, selflessness and the inner truthfulness and of the spirit have ultimately greater power than hate, enmity and self-interest.

6. A sense of obligation to stand on the side of the poor and the oppressed as against the rich and the oppressed.
7. A profound hope that good will ultimately prevail.
8. Man's spiritual and moral maturity must grow proportionately to his technical skill and power. It can be done if science and religion get together and work together in a harmonious relationship.
9. Commitment to violence cannot guarantee security, but universal commitment to practical non-violent alternatives can make us personally, nationally and globally much more secure.
10. 'Education for Peace' must be a subject for bringing forth creative human potential in the family, workplace and community.
11. No scheme of global peace can prove lasting unless it is linked to the creation of a new equitable world economic order. There can be no lasting peace unless the basic factors of exploitation and hegemony are removed.
12. The greatest need today more than ever before, is to educate the people and their Governments to have a greater understanding and awareness of the problems created by armaments race and of the need of disarmament." (Devadoss: 1987)

Untouchability: While giving a serious thought to the issue of untouchables Gandhi made a statement on 6th May, 1926 in *Young India* where he wrote regularly on it, as "If we are to make progress we must not repeat history, but make new history." He declared during *Vykom Satyagraha*, "Untouchability is a crime" and championed the cause of "the unapproachable and untouchables and the recognition of the most elementary human rights." By 1924 Gandhi had come to be known both in India and abroad as a revolutionary who had stirred 300 million people to revolt and who shook the foundation of British empire. In India Annie Besant said, "It is the queerest revolution that ever was.... and has had a queerest leader". If Gandhi condemned in most unmistakable terms the unjust rule of the Raj, he did not spare his countrymen of their inhuman treatment of the so-called untouchables: "I regard untouchability as the greatest blot on Hinduism.... We ought to purge ourselves of this pollution. We are not better than brutes until we have purged ourselves of the sins we have committed against our weaker brethren." When Vykom movement of *Satyagraha* began in the middle of 1924 he became involved in the movement. The movement was launched for one and half years on behalf of the untouchable of Travancore.

It is relevant to look the background of the community known as "untouchables" in India, which has been highlighted very specifically by Anima Bose in her article, *Gandhi's Satyagraha for Human Rights at Vykom,* 1924. In the early Vedic period, the *Shudra* population was not very considerable. It grew during later Vedic period. By the nineteenth century, their number had swollen to several millions. At the beginning of the twentieth century it is reported one-sixth of India's population consisted of the *Shudras*. In various parts of the country they came to be known by different names numbering more than four hundred. In the northern and central India they were known as "*chamars*", "*mochis*", "*mahars*", "*mahtars*", "*balmikis*", "*dome*", "*dhobis*", "*kahars*", "*kanjars*", "*khatiks*", "*tellis*" and "*tharus*". During the early stages, the *Shudras* did not suffer from disabilities. But during the later Vedic times, they progressively lost their rights and have since been deprived of elementary human rights continuously. They have been systematically subjected to negligence. They carried the stigma of untouchability, a hereditary stigma which nothing could remove, as Ambedkar said. Even their shadows were supposed to pollute the upper castes. They were segregated territorially, they were segregated from the society in every way. They denied the basic human and civic rights such as the use of public wells, schools, and temples. They had to take up all menial jobs. And yet the jobs that they performed were indispensable to society such as, agricultural labourers, artisans, barbers, washerman etc.

The first major movement for the removal of untouchability in no ambiguous term was the *Vykom Satyagraha* of 1924-25 in Kerala in the State of Travancore. Vykom is situated on the northern border of Travancore. The occasion arose when the priests of the temple at Vykom village assented that if the "Untouchables" walked on the roads round or converging to the sacred temple, the temple would be polluted. Human rights were being denied to a group for no other reason than that their birth and occupation. Gandhi said, "they do not want anything more than a recognition of the most elementary human rights."

The immediate goal of movement was the use of the road to the temple by the untouchables. But in essence the goal was to win the basic human rights of a section of the community who were subjected to injustice because of a blind tradition and ignorant custom docilely accepted by the Hindu society based on birth and occupation (Goyal: 1984).

Every vow of Gandhiji is good for individual and society. Gandhi realized that individual good is the stepping stone for social good. Individual morality is a preliminary step for social morality. To

Gandhi, good is a value laden term and he analyzed it in the context of morality.

Further, Ashram Vows of Gandhi has implied loyalty to truth, especially *Satyagraha* is nothing, but loyalty to truth. According to him, loyalty is the supreme virtue of morality. Loyalty is nothing but a devotion of a person to a cause. It demands a cause to which a man is loyal. Gandhi was conscious that loyalty is to be expressed in one's deeds. To Gandhiji loyalty is a supreme ethical principle. Gandhi was a loyal man and while being loyal he did not hinder loyalty of other people. His moral cause did not hamper the moral cause of others. In fact Gandhiji respected the loyalty in all men open heartedly. The first necessary condition for his loyalty was that he chose his cause according to his natural attitude. His loyalty was based on his *Swabhava* and *Swadharma*. Gandhiji's *Swadharma* was not his *Kuladharma* (observance of family rites as per one's own caste. His *Swadharma* was connected with one's *Swabhava* (One's own duty with one's nature or *Guna*). In fact Gandhi insisted on merit or capacity of a man to carryout certain duties.

Medical Services are highly influenced by the progress of science and technology. It has made service life comfortable and easy and less time consuming. But the man whose life made comfortable cannot be improved by it. Science is a progress towards while Ashram Vows is a progress within a man. It creates self-awareness and then self-realization. What is needed to-day is self-awareness along with the comfort given by science. (Gopalakrishnan: 1985)

Bread-labour: The most significant practical work which helps the individual to realize the ultimate values in their own lives, according to Gandhi is bread-labour. The bread-labour is described as 'the first moral law of life' in Gandhian social philosophy, as described by an authority on Gandhi. It would eliminate exploitation as well as more direct forms of violence. Through it an individual can enjoy the creative freedom and can avoid some external constraints. According to Gandhi, "Bread-labour is a veritable blessing to one who would observe non-violence". He went to the extent of saying that who performed bodily labour to earn bread had right to live, and that people engaged in intellectual pursuits were no exception. During Gandhi's time spinning was the ideal form of bread-labour. Today various forms of bread-labour have emerged. Even Government is providing various schemes of productive labour to be engaged by uneducated and rural people to earn bread for themselves. (Tripathy:1980)

John James Ruskin preached dignity of manual labour. His work on 'Unto This Last' was handed over to Gandhi by Henry S.L. Polak while he was on his train journey for twenty-four hours from Johannesburg to Durban in 1903. After going through the book Gandhi determined to change his life. He translated the book of Ruskin into Gujrati, his mother tongue and titled it, '*Sarvodaya*'.

Gandhi was especially influenced by three teachings of 'Unto This Last' as:

"1. That good of the individual is contained in the good of all.
2. That a lawyer's work has the same value as the barber's in as much as all have the same right of earning their livelihood from the work.
3. That a life of labour, i.e. the life of the tiller of the soil and the handicraftsman is worth living."

Count Leo Nickolaevich Tolstoy could also influence Gandhi. Tolstoy believed in the efficacy of manual labour for earning one's bread. He advocated performance of manual labour by everybody. It could serve the interest of the poor as well as of the rich.

To Gandhi God created man to work for his food and said that those who eat without work are thieves. The great nature has intended us to earn our bread in the sweat of our brow. Everyone, therefore, who idles away a single minute becomes to that extent a burden upon his neighbours and to do so is to commit a breach of the very first lesson of *ahimsa.*

The philosophy behind this is that every healthy individual must labour for his food and his intellectual faculties must be utilized in the service of mankind. The bread labour generates a sense of equality, eliminating distinction between rich and poor, touchables and untouchables. Thus, labour for Gandhi is a powerful unifying force and a great equalizer of persons. (Budhachandra Singh: 2011)

Human Rights: The concept of individual occupies a central position in Gandhi's thought. All individuals are born equals and have a right to equal opportunities. But all individuals do not have same capacity because of their differences in the degree of intelligence, colour, height etc. Further, while studying the problems of medical ethics as a researcher I have given a serious thought on this problem. Are all individuals born equals ? A social scientist may say, 'yes'. The parents and the social reformers may also say 'yes'. But can a medical scientist say 'yes' ? Inborn differentials cannot be denied by a medical scientist. For example, a baby who is dumb by birth, a baby, who is blind by birth, a baby who inherits physical deficiencies through the mechanism of birth cannot be ignored by a medical scientist. These people require special opportunities, depending upon the nature of their deficiencies for growth. The parents cannot deprive them from the love and affection as they are also their children. This kind of difference with the implication of inequality one has to take care while talking about human rights.

Freedom does not mean that individuals should be left alone to have their way in the society. For Gandhi, "there is no such thing as inherited or acquired superiority. I believe all men are born equal". Gandhi as humanist has this belief (Gandhi: 1924).

Qualities of the physicians: M. Ruthnaswamy, in his book titled, "*Principles and Practices of Public Administration*" discussed with interesting illustration of the qualities of the administrators which are applicable even to physicians. Truthfulness, honesty, trustworthiness, conformity to the moral standards of civilized society, physical soundness, a fair measure of education are required for every expert or professional:

Love for Knowledge: A physician must have knowledge of the facts. But he should not be mere slave of facts and this knowledge should not be acquired from books, official documents, learned reviews and newspapers and other printed works, but from conversation with patients and attendants. The study of the people, their way of life, their separate groupings, as physicians, their relationship with the colleagues, subordinates and superiors and others are necessary. Devotion to detail is another quality to be possessed by him.

Reason and Objectivity: The service of the state requires the physician to consider the family interest next to the state's interest which is possible through honest and efficient service to the patients. "Reason", said Richelieu, "ought to animate and cause the action of those that are in employment of public affairs." He wanted to exclude women of his time from public affairs solely for the cause that they allowed their conduct to be governed by emotion rather than by reason. Balance and matter-of-factness are aids to this objectivity.

Ability to anticipate events is another quality of the physician. He should not wait till things become dangerous or worst.

Mastery over the art of expression: Ability to write clearly, intelligently, precisely and economically is expected of everybody in office and in every profession. The outdoor workers are expected to write clear and intelligible reports. It is found that Lord Kitchener's failure as a War Minister in the First World War was due to his being tongue-tied in the

Cabinet while Winston Churchill and Lloyd George could always persuade their colleagues to accept their proposals.

Character: "There is greater need of character in administration than in war", said Napoleon.

Self-control: Self control is absolutely necessary to the physicians. Here mention may be made of Sir Ernest Shackleton, the great Antarctic explorer, who was most careful in the selection of men to accompany him on his voyages that he would not only test their general health and physique, but their temperament. On one of his voyages he went 2000 miles out of his way to land an officer who had revealed the possession of violent temper which he never tried to master.

Application: Application is more a moral than an intellectual quality. Not incessant work, but attachment to one's own in spirit, in thought, in affection was what Rechelieu meant by application. Pere Joseph, known in history as Grey Eminence, advised his master not to rely so much on his fortune and goodness but on his conduct and prudence. However, in certain services special qualities are required, for example, for police, courage, quickness of thought, an eye on detail and a reliable memory in addition to physical strength and agility are necessary (Ruthnaswamy: 1972).

Gandhi realized the differences in the individuals and pointed out that all individuals have not the same capacity because of their differences in the degree of intelligence. The highly talented individuals may earn more and a portion of earning by them may be spent for the welfare of the people. For this an individual must have the sense of sacrifice and love for the people.

Considering individual as the key to build-up a new social order in which each individual will be able to face his or her challenges to attain peace and happiness in life without disturbing others. While doing so one should not dishonour the social norms. Every individual has the right to pursue their moral objects and at the same time he or she has also the duty to allow others to do so. Here lies the need of individual freedom. Full development of personality of the individual is needed not only in the interest of the individual but in the greater interest of the society.

Another significant belief of Gandhi is that individual is the master of himself, of his thought, intentions, deeds and passions (Sharma: 1980). To Gandhi perfect social order must be free from all coercive authority and must be grounded in the free will of individuals (Tewari: 1983).

An individual is an agent of social transformation. For this, according to Gandhi, control of the self-interest of the individual is an essential prerequisite to transform the social relationships in terms of ultimate values. The values inculcated in the individual before they can find true social expression. He emphasized the need of a private moral effort on the part of the individual before he can qualify for social action (Tripathy: 1980).

Man has the duty to care for others. This is possible only through the development of moral qualities of an individual. A moral man always attempts to accommodate the interest of the society. (Mahatma: 1946) While recognizing mutual interdependence between individual and society Gandhi did not talk merely of functional-interdependence he embraced within it the value of harmony, integration of self with humanity also. The harmony between individual and society is a dynamic process. It evolves through clash of personality, interchange of opinion and exchange of ideas. Thus, the society is based on extended self of individuals, harmony, non-exploitation, equality and participation.

According to Gandhi 'inner voice' is the conscience of an individual. He also said the 'inner voice' of self-disciplined individual is not contrary to basic moral principles. Morality includes, as Gandhi said, nobleness of character, purity of soul and motive, the notions of truth, selfless service and goodness of means. A moral man always adopt moral principles for the solution of the problems—personal or social. We can have a dream of new human world when mutual relationship of the individuals depend on understanding of moral values of humanity. Full development of moral character can make a man perfect to the maximum level.

A peaceful disposition of the whole personality is indispensable for moral life. Because tranquility, calmness and mild temperament help development of morality. Gandhi said, "freedom from bad habits forms another element of morality." Habit is nothing, but capacity or tendency of an individual resulting from repetition of the same act. A man is considered as good or bad on the basis of his or her habits.

Every man has reasoning capacity. With this power an individual can decide what is right and what is wrong. An individual with good habit or moral habit will be guided in a positive and constructive way. This will help development of the concept of 'inner voice' within him. When individual becomes matured in thought and action based on moral and moral values, then he or she will be empowered by 'soul force' Once an individual becomes powerful with soul force he or she will be strong enough to be the seeker of truth and non-violent activist (Devi, Bimola: 2010).

Gandhi on Family: The family is a nucleus of the society. It is the primary and universal social institution in the world. Parents have the primary responsibility to take care of the children for full development of their personal qualities. They should create a congenial environment for the growth of the children and to educate them about the social norms and values.

The parents should develop high moral values and must be very strict disciplinarian. They should maintain cordial relationship with the children. According to Hindu *Shastra* a child should be lovingly taken care of up to five years, should be disciplined up to ten years with necessary instruction and persuasion. At the age of sixteen a friendly relationship should be maintained between parents and the children. After attaining the full adulthood the children will automatically develop self-respect. By playing this crucial role by the parents for the full development of personal qualities of their children they render great service to the nation.

Home is the first school and real education begins at home. According to Gandhi all parents should give prime importance to the formation of the character of their children. They must help the children to lead a simple life or to maintain economy in life.

Both father and mother should create an environment where peace, love, truth, kindness, sympathy and patience prevail. They must train the children in physical labour and avoid laziness. It is the duty of the parents to treat both sons and daughters equally. The children of broken families may create problems not only to the families but to the society as a whole. Here mention has been made of what Kumaran Assan, the famous Malayalam poet states, "Human life is a kind of pain in which good children are the medicines for the pains." A good child can give relief to unhappy parents.

Referring to the role of the mother in the process of formation of a good moral character it is noticed that she plays a crucial role in bringing up the children in a right direction. It is the mother who can help developing good conduct and behaviour of the children. Though both men and women are equals in life nobody can deny the differences between the two—their functions are also different. By educating her children she becomes the mother of the nation. One may think that by giving birth a woman can become a mother of the child, but by giving proper education for full development of personal qualities of the child she can become the mother of the nation.

In a family the father also has a significant role to play to create a congenial environment for the growth of the children. The father should himself be a strict disciplinarian, a religious person, to adopt rightful means to lead a truthful way of life. He may be considered as a promoter of peace in the family. Pointing out the qualities of a good father Gandhi said that he should not be a drunkard. Gandhi firmly believed that smoking and drinking will not only ruin his health and wealth, but the family will also be ruined. He was of the opinion that after completion of the age of seventeen sons should be treated by the father as his friends.

In a letter of 16th August, 1913, Gandhi advised his son Manilal, "You should be very much on your guard against laziness, see that you get-up not later than 4 O' clock in the morning, even if you have to force to yourself to do it. Make it a regular practice to complete the appointed work each day. Do everything after careful thinking and understanding. Always take pleasure and keen interest in being of service of others." In a letter of 26th 1914 he addressed to his son Manilal, "It is your duty not to take notice of my faults. A son should have devotion enough to his father, not to notice his shortcomings but to think of only of his virtues. I want to see your character pure, to see in you truthfulness, charity, straight-forwardness, tenderness, self-confidence, humility and goodness. But I want you to understand my deepest feelings and to attain true success in your life." (Government of India: Vol. XII: 1969).

As regards the duty of children, according to Gandhi, children are very important for the parents. Referring to his early life Gandhi said, "I believe whatever I achieved is due to my devotion to my parents and fruits of their blessings. When the parents have been given the place of a teacher and of God, they have been thought of as perfect beings, so that to their offsprings they are perfect. The children should not even entertain a doubt that what their parents say may be full of ignorance or error. However, the children have to be critical when parents issue an order which appear to them to be clearly *adharma*. At an early age the children may not decide what is to be done. But after attaining adulthood they become capable persons with high moral value and think for their duties.

One's respective *dharma* towards one's self, family, nation and the world cannot be divided into watertight compartments as Gandhi felt. One must sacrifice himself or herself in the interest of the family and the family must do so for the nation and the nation for the world. This sacrifice must be genuine and this genuineness emanates from self-purification. (Budhachandra Singh: 2011)

Gandhi learnt a lot from the members of the family. He learnt a significant lesson from Rambha, the old family nurse. He said, "There was fear in me of ghosts and spirits. Rambha suggested, as a remedy for this fear, the repletion of *Ramanama*. I had more faith in her than in her remedy, and so at a tender age I began repeating *Ramanama* to cure my fear of ghosts and spirits. This was of course shortlived, but the good seed sown in childhood was not sown in vain. I think it is due to that seed sown by that good woman Rambha that today *Ramanama* is an infallible remedy for me." The service to the ailing population is not an easy task. It requires patience, commitment to the profession, sacrifice and love for the humanity. These are the qualities the seeds of which have to be sown in the soil of family itself. Every member of the family, especially the children must cultivate them at the guidance and care of the parents.

Reading of *Ramayana* before his father left a deep impression on Gandhi. He said, "During his illness my father was in Porbandar. There every evening he used to listen to the *Ramayana*. The reader was a great devotee of *Rama*, Ladha Maharaja of Bileswar. That laid my deep devotion to the *Ramayana*. Today I regard the *Ramacharita Manasa* of Tulsidas as the greatest book in all devotional literature.

A few months after this we came to Rajkot. There was *Ramayana* reading. The *Bhagavata*, however, used to be read on every *Ekadashi* day (eleventh day of bright and the dark half of a lunar month). Sometimes, I attended the reading, but the recite was uninspiring. Today I see that the *Bhagavata* is a book which can evoke religious fervor. I have read it in Gujarati with intense interest, but when I heard portions of original read by Pandit Madan Mohan Malaviya during my twenty-one days fast, I wished I had heard it in my childhood from such a devotee as he is, so that I could have formed liking for it at an early age....

In Rajkot, however, I got early grounding in toleration for all branches of Hinduism and sister religions for my father and mother would visit the *Haveli* as also Shiva's and Rama's temples and take or send us youngsters there. Jain monks also would pay frequent visits to my father, and would even go out of their way to accept food from us—non-Jains. They would have talks with my father on subjects religious and mundane.

He had, besides, Musalman and Parsi friends, who would talk to him about their own faiths, and he would listen to them always with respect and often with interest. Being a nurse, I often had a chance to be present at these talks. These many things combined to inculcate in me a toleration for all faiths." (M.K. Gandhi: 1989)

He realized that the essence of all religions is morality.

Gandhi learnt the first lesson of *ahimsa* at the feet of his father. Once he committed theft along with his brother. Both of them chipped pieces from the brother's solid gold armlet in order to pay a debt they had. In remorse the young Gandhi decided to confess. He did this not by word of mouth, but in writing, a common practice of Gandhi. When he handed over the note to his father, the latter could not talk and his eyes were full of tears. He forgave Gandhi and was deeply impressed at his father's love. Later on he realized that this was nothing but *ahimsa.* When *ahimsa* becomes all-embracing, it becomes unlimited power. He concluded that a clean confession, combined with a promise never to commit the sin again, when offered before one who has the right to receive it, is the purest type of repentance. (Autobiography: 1959)

Gandhi's path of self-purification is three-fold:

1. One must be free from passions in thought, speech and action;
2. One must rise above the currents of love and hatred;
3. One must be free from attachment and repulsion. But it is a very difficult path to follow.

Gandhi also said that "to conquer the subtle passion seems to me to be harder than the physical conquest of the world by the force of arms."

Gandhi's mother, Putalibai was a woman of sharp intelligence and high common sense. The outstanding impression which left on Gandhi was that of saintliness. She was a religious lady and never took meals without offering prayers. The practice of self-restraint that Gandhiji observed through fasting and daily prayers had its roots in the influence of his mother on him. As regards his disciplinary observance he was deeply influenced by his mother. As a result he could keep his promise made to his mother while leaving for London in the face of all kinds of temptation. (Autobiography: 1957)

Another very significant contribution of Gandhi to the process of socialization is the food habit of the children. To him food should be taken as a matter of duty even as medicine to sustain the body, never for the satisfaction of the palate. Pleasurable feeling comes from satisfaction of real hunger. Therefore, it can be said that relish is dependent on hunger not on outside it. Because of our wrong habits and artificial way of living, very few people know what their systems requires. Our parents who bring us to this world do not, as a rule, have self-control. They forget that their way of living and habits influence the children very deeply. The mother's food during pregnancy is bound to affect the child. The mother tries to satisfy the child by offering all kinds of tasty food. She also offers the child little bit of whatever she herself eats and thus the child's digestive system gets a wrong training from time of its birth. Habits once formed difficult to shed. (Gandhi:1948)

Closely connected to above, the problem of intoxicants, Gandhi expressed his experience as below:

> "The intoxicants used in India might be taken as the following: alcohol, *bhang*, *ganja*, tobacco and opium. Alcohol or liquor includes the country made liquor and *arak*, besides the large quantity of liquor imported from foreign countries. All these should be strictly prohibited. Alcohol makes a man forget himself and while its effects last, he becomes utterly incapable of doing anything useful. Those who drink, ruin themselves and their people. They lose all sense of decency and propriety.
>
> There is school which favours limited and regulated consumption of alcohol and believe it to be useful. I have not found any weight in their argument. Even if we accept their view for a moment, we have still to face the fact that innumerable human beings cannot be kept under discipline. Therefore, it becomes our duty to prohibit alcoholic drinks even if it were only for the sake of this vast majority.
>
> Parsis have strongly supported the use of *tadi*. They say that although *tadi* is an intoxicant it is also a food and even helps to digest food stuff. I have carefully examined this argument and have read fair account of literature pertaining to this subject. But I have been a witness of the terrible straits to which *tadi* reduces the poor and therefore I have come to the conclusion that it can have no place in man's food.... None of the public workers have the same bitter experience of the evils of the drinking as I have had. In South Africa, most of the Indians going there as indentured labourers were addicted to drinking. The law there did not in my time permit Indians to take liquors to their houses except under a medical certificate. They could go to the drinking booths and drink as much as they liked. Even the women had fallen victims to this evil habit. I have seen them in the most pathetic condition. One who has seen those scenes near the public bars will never support drinking.
>
> African Negroes were not allowed to drink originally. Liquor may be said to have simply ruined them. Large number of Negro labourers are seen to waste all their earnings in drinking.
>
> And what about Englishmen? I have seen respectable Englishmen falling in the gutter under the effect of alcohol. There

> is no exaggeration in this statement. During the war many Englishmen had to leave the Transvaal. Some of them were taken to my home. One of them was an engineer and a good man in everyway, when not under the effects of alcohol. He was a theosophist. Unfortunately, he was addicted to drink, but as far as I know he never succeeded.
> On my return from South Africa to India I had similar painful experience of the evils of drink. Several Princes have been and are being ruined by liquor. What applies to them applies more or less to many rich youths...."

Today alcoholism and drug addiction are the serious ailments in the society affecting the youths very badly, causing domestic problems in the families and indiscipline in the services. The most serious aspect of it is that it affects the health of the people and becomes a challenge to the healthcare system of the country. (Gandhi: 1948)

To Gandhi addressing the needs of the most vulnerable persons is very important. Hungry, homeless, diseased persons require protection. Material progress beyond the requirement of the satisfaction of basic needs and comforts causes deterioration of moral values. The medical scientists deal with the ailing population of a country, who are vulnerable and who surrender themselves to the physician for getting relief of the disease.

***Sarvodaya*:** *Sarvodaya* is a composite term. It consists of two parts, "*Sarva*" and "*Udaya*". *Sarva* means 'all'. To Gandhi it is universal brotherhood, not only brotherhood of human beings, but all living beings. '*Udaya*' means rising or welfare. Therefore, *Sarvodaya* means welfare of entire humanity and all other creatures. It is related to the future generations and their legitimate right to our common heritage. The realization of this right requires integration of ethical-moral, social, economic and political life of man in a disciplined way. Therefore, it may be said that total development of an individual is possible through discipline and service. (Goyal: 1984)

Sarvodaya is based on truth and non-violence. To Gandhi the basis of *Sarvodaya* is all embracing love and non-violence; where no individual will be suppressed or exploited. N.K. Bose has pointed out that *Sarvodaya* is of universal applicability. It has its own worldview, view of life, social relationship, technology and values. Besides, *Sarvodaya* rests on the spiritual nature of human life, the essential unity of life, the existence of a benevolent law operating behind universal process.

Gandhi tried to translate his ideals into reality through his day to day life. Work was designed and worked out for full development of individual as well as society. Harmonious development, mutual trust and co-existence are the basic goals of *Sarvodaya*. Under *Sarvodaya* includes the concepts of decentralization, trusteeship, appropriate technology, *khadi* and village industries, *Swadeshi* and self-reliance, utilization of local resource and service to local people, face to face communities depending on nature. Gandhi formulated constructive programme to bring about social reform and upliftment of the society. It was a programme to build the nation from the bottom.

Gandhi's constructive programme includes certain specific activities, such as 1. Communal unity, 2. Removal of untouchability, 3. Prohibition, 4. *Khadi*, 5. Other village industries, 6. Village sanitation, 7. Basic education, 8. Adult education, 9. Upliftment of women, 10. Education in health and hygiene, 11. Provincial language, 12. Propagation of *Rashtra-bhasha*, 13. Promotion of economic equality etc. (Budhachandra: 2011)

Brother A.T. Ariyaratne, leader of the Sri Lanka *Sarvodaya* Movement said, "*Sarvodaya* also means the harnessing of the goodness of all the awakening or the liberation of all." *Sarvodaya* recognizes the oneness of all mankind, and thus attempts to transcend all man-made barriers of caste, colour, race, religion and nationality in the realization of its aims and objectives. The objectives of *Sarvodaya* are:

> "The liberation of the individual from all inner defilements of greed, hatred, ignorance and other oppressive elements that have enslaved him; the liberation of the rural and urban communities from poverty, ill-health, ignorance and dependency from conditions existing within the communities as well as the economic and political subjugation and exploitation carried out by outside agencies and bureaucracies.
>
> The liberation of the world family of man from distrust, enmity, hatred, wars and ills such as environmental pollution, attendance on technological advancement".

In striving towards the realization of these objectives, *Sarvodaya* aspirants seek to practice eight traditional virtues in their individual as well as their community life. Four of these principles are for personal development: Loving kindness towards all, or reverence for all life compassionate action or helping people to overcome suffering; altruistic joy or experiencing happiness when fellow human beings are happy; and learning to maintain mental balance or equanimity at times of loss as well as gain, fame or blame. The four salient principles of healthy social life are: sharing, pleasant speech, constructive activity and equality.

Kampadoo quoted from Arusha Declaration, in which President Nyere of Tanzania states so eloquently in consonance with United Nations Declaration of Human Rights:

> "The opportunity, of full development—physical, moral and spiritual, should be assured to every member of the community—man, woman and child. The development of man's full personality should not be hampered by unjust conditions, or crushed by economic pressure."

In the introduction of Vinoba Bhave's book "The Third Power", the late Jayprakash Narayan states: "The power of coercion and of the law have both failed to solve the basic problems of human society. Some third power is needed. It is this power which Mahavira, Buddha, and Jesus have set before us in such masterly fashion—the power of love, non-violence and compassion." Service and humanity are the keys to create the culture of *Sarvodaya* and medical service is one which is equipped with both of them (Kampdoo: 1986)

In the perspective of peace, Gandhi's revolutionary mode of action for transforming individual and society, adopted the challenging goal of *Sarvodaya,* welfare of all accompanied by potential constructive programme for democracy and development of the society. Peace can be experienced as it is a state of mind only. (Government of India: 1966)

Any development strategy must provide for all-aided flourishing of human potential and not just economic growth. Development, in the words of Phil Karp, "is the process, by which an environment is attained in which all members of a society are given an opportunity to reach their full potential as human beings." A viable strategy for development should lay emphasis on eradication of poverty, full employment; elimination of social and economic inequalities with the entire rural sector as well as between town and village; and participation of entire population in the development process. To achieve these goals there has to be a high degree of decentralization and technological improvements which increase the requirement of labour, maximizes the production of scanty resources, and aims primarily at raising human welfare rather than merely stepping up economic growth. A strategy for tackling these problems revolves round self-supporting agriculture; labour-intensive public works; labour intensive light industry, social service programmes for family planning, education, healthcare and nutrition; self-reliance and self-help; institutional, organizational and administrative reform and rural-urban coordination. (S.K. Sharma: 1979)

While looking to the different approaches to economic development one may classify these approaches into two groups—narrower approach and wider approach. The narrower approach relates to economic development maximizing the aggregates of economy: increasing national income, output, per capita income and raising the standard of living. These are some of the different objectives of such approach. Efforts to accumulate more and more of wealth, to consume and to live luxurious life and to produce for earning a high profit in a free and competitive society guided by the market forces are the essence of such approach to economic development. Against this, the other approach to economic development which is broader, does not see that the mere increase in income and production should be the target of economic development. This approach is concerned with the type of development which is to ensure the structural changes in the social and economic systems of the country so as to provide the basic needs of the people. Professor Myrdal, Professor J. Tinbergen and many others are of the opinion that mere increase in national and per capita income and production might create different social and economic problems. Social justice, distributive justice are more important for meaningful economic development.

Gandhian approach to economic development comes within the purview of broader approach. It deals basically with human problems concerned not only with social and economic ends, but essentially with attainment of highest satisfaction of life—the realization of inner self through containment of and liberation from material wants. It means that the people everywhere act more purposefully to improve their living conditions and thus also change their community in such a way as to make these striving more possible and effective. To Professor Mehta, Gandhian approach calls for "quality of life" in place of "quality of living" and "standard of life" in place of "standard of living".

In the present approach it is found that all that come across in terms of trade, commerce, financial arrangements and human attitudes are attempts to continue with the past practices of short term gains of limited groups or communities. These attitudes, structures and arrangements do not provide long term solution to the problems of mankind.

The Gandhian approach to economic development is the real solution to the problems with which the world economy is concerned. The relevance of Gandhian ideas becomes more and more important in the sense that his ideas provide a key to the dilemma of the growth of the contemporary world economy (Tripathi: 1979).

Gandhi also maintained that a non-violent social order will have to be constructed on the basis of economic equality. By equality he meant guarantee of a minimum standard of consumption to all. He argued that everyone must have a balanced diet, a decent house to live in, facilities for the education of one's own children, and adequate medical care. True individual freedom—the opportunity for the moral and spiritual development of human beings—is possible only when the individual is free from hunger and unemployment. His ability and willingness to question his superiors and their decisions and thereby gain a measure of self-control over his life and environment and make his preferences count in the final determination of social policy depend upon his freedom from hunger. The provision of adequate food and education, medical care, employment, housing, and other basic requirements for human development is essential.

Gandhi accepted the fact that there will be inequalities of skill, industry, intelligence, and opportunity. He recognized that people with talent will earn more. But he wanted them to take what was required for their legitimate needs and to leave the rest to be used for the society. Ideally he preached the doctrine of non-possession, as he believed that real happiness and contentment comes not from self-indulgence and multiplication of wants, but from deliberate and voluntary reduction of wants. He wanted the rich and the elite to take initiative in dispossession with a view to a universal diffusion of the spirit of contentment. As a practical matter, he was willing to accept, in the transitional phase, income differentials that are considered fair by the society. He proposed to fix a decent minimum living wage and a ceiling for the maximum income that can be allowed to a person in society. The difference between such minimum and maximum income should be reasonable and equitable and variable from time to time, so that we can move towards the obliteration of the difference. (Desai:1981)

Freedom and Democracy: The President of America Abraham Lincoln who is considered as the father of democratic thought tried to preserve individual rights and liberty. He defined Democracy as, "Government of people, by the people and for the people". This concept, however, was not developed at that time to embrace social justice and economic freedom.

The freedom movement in India under the leadership of Gandhiji may be called as a process of democratization because he tried to humanize the whole concept of democracy through the movement. He realized that every human institution is prone to danger. Therefore, the people must be alert and sensitive to humanize it by putting it in the right direction. To quote Gandhi:

> "There is no human institution that has not its dangers. The greater the institution, the greater chances of abuse. Democracy is an institution and therefore it is liable to be greatly abused. The remedy, therefore, is not avoidance of Democracy but reduction of possibility of abuse to a minimum." (*Young India*: 7.5.1931).

Gandhi's mission was to liberate the poor and oppressed classes. The poor must enjoy equal opportunity as the rich and for that *Swaraj* must be achieved. Again, *Swaraj* is possible only through democratic way of life. Gandhi said, "India is trying to evolve true democracy, i.e. without violence. Our weapons are those of *Satyagraha* expressed through *Charakha*, village industries, removal of untouchability, communal harmony and non-violent organization of labour as in Ahmedabad. These mean mass effort and mass education." (*Harijan*, 18.5.1940)

Gandhi accepted democracy as a way of life. He was anxious to establish democratic values. Preservation of such values can only bring about a new social order where "all for one and one for all" can truly function. It is a vast programme of mass education. But the democratic educators must also display the democratic values in their way of life. Mass is never attracted through simple prophecy not can he be taught. Mass follows the examples and practices of the individuals. According to Gandhiji, the essence of democratic way of life is that individuals must have mutual respect and sympathy for each other. Each individual shall keep his fellow man ahead of him in respect of enjoying social responsibilities. This retrospective desire to stand for each other's cause will create an atmosphere of social responsibilities. To Gandhi social justice and individual freedom do not stand in contrary to each other. Their aims and objectives are same. Discipline and restraint in the life of individual will only help him to achieve the social well-being. In the words of Gandhiji:

> "A born democrat is a born disciplinarian. Democracy comes naturally to him who is habituated normally to yield willing obedience to all laws, human or divine....let those who are

ambitious to serve democracy qualify themselves first the acid test of democracy. Moreover, a democrat must be utterly selfless. He must think or dream not in terms of self or party, but only of democracy.... I value individual freedom, but you must not forget that man is essentially a social being. He has risen to his present status by learning to adjust his individualism to the requirement of the social progress. Willing submission to social restraint for the sake of the whole society enriches both the individual and the society of which one is a member." (*Harijan* 27.5.1939)

Pandya said that never before in human history as we know it, have fundamental moral values such as truth, justice, brotherhood of man and non-violence, been applied so effectively in man's relations in the political field and especially in the mutual dealings of organized groups and nations, as during Gandhi's time under his own leadership. By insisting on such basic qualities to be a part of the process of social training directed towards collective struggles in the interest of larger objectives, Gandhi introduced a new sense of responsibility in the mind of the individual. Such a training and commitment to moral values indirectly helped the economic animal in man to be less aggressive when it came to the realm of partaking the economic gains of collective labour. This factor can be traced in his philosophy of "bread labour" which was a compulsory component in the personal life-style of these social revolutionaries. (Pandya: 1980)

Jagadish Prakash and Nageswar Rao in their paper, *Gandhian Persepective to Socialism* stated that the method of attaining socialism differ from country to country. Socialism must be evolved out of the traditions and cultures of its own people which will be able to produce desired results. Thus what may be food for one country can easily be poison for another. Acharya Narendra Deva in his presidential address at second National Conference of Praja Socialist Party on 26th December, 1955 at Gaya advocated the same and pointed out that there is no classic straight line. The masses are to be set in motion only along that road that fits each country and the prevailing circumstances, which is usually a round about road.

Gandhi's concept of socialism is nothing, but democratic socialism which emphasizes the equality by noble means. Gandhiji also made a distinction between possession and possessiveness. In his view, the evil lies not in possession as such, but in the attitude of possessiveness. This has been confirmed with a narration of an incident—a multimillionaire friend of Gandhiji went to him to seek his blessings and to renounce, his wealth as well as business activities. Gandhiji told him that he did not want the renouncement either of his wealth or of his business activities, but what he wanted was their application for the services of the poor and the oppressed. He desired the capitalists to become trustees of the nation by running their business with integrity and efficiency and for the welfare of the people. (Prakash and Rao: 1980)

Buddhadeva Bhattacharya, in his writing, *Gandhian Socialism and Its relevance to India Today* has said that the socialists should have that was most precious in Gandhi's psyche, namely his seminal humanism, his unbounded love for humanity, his readiness to suffer and make the supreme sacrifice for the liberation of the people. Secondly, his message of fearlessness and courage is a legacy that will inspire mankind forever. Thirdly, the Gandhian technique of dealing with large numbers of human beings *en masse*, his method of evoking self-confidence and a creative response in them, of building up their initiative step and then hurling them into action in a disciplined manner at the crucial historical moment. As has been correctly pointed out by an eminent Marxist theoretician that it should be the endeavour of any socialist in the phase struggle against poverty, exploitation and inequality, to learn and imbibe as much as may be possible or necessary of that humanism and mass approach which made Gandhi the leader of suffering humanity for all time." (Bhattacharya: 1980)

Referring to the economic aspect of man's life Gandhi said, "economics is untrue which ignores and disregard moral values. The extension of the laws of non-violence in the domain of economics means nothing less than the introduction of moral values as a factor to be considered in regulating international trade."

The Gandhian views on the relation between economics and ethics were borrowed from the ancient Indian writings on *Varta* and *Arthashastra* underlying the supremacy of ethics (*dharma*). For instance, Kautilya says: "whenever in any matter there is a conflict between administrative law on the one hand and traditional code (sacred law) on the other, the matter must be settled in accordance with *Dharma*, sacred laws". According to Yajnavalkya, "When two *smritis* conflict with each other the question should be solved with the help of the principles laid down by the old usage. The rule is when economics comes into conflict with the sacred law "*Dharma Sutra*" the latter is more forceful." The same principle was propounded by Narada: "When the rules of sacred science and *Arthashastra* are variance, the king ought to discard the dictates of economics and follow the precepts of ethics." (Kurien and Sivaraman: 1976).

A rigid economic equality in the social structure imposed from above is a dead equality. Man is a social discerning and intelligent being is and ought to be, capable of voluntarily sharing his possessions among his fellow-beings, which way alone ensures his development to the full.

The trusteeship idea implies the benevolent use of the superfluous wealth possessed by the rich for the benefit of the society. It asked the possessors to enjoy their wealth by renouncing it in the interest of humanity. "Earn your crores by all means. But understand that your wealth is not yours; it belongs to the people. Take what you need for your legitimate needs, and use the remainder for society" (Tewari: 1976). Saul Karsz has correctly stated that economics and ethics cannot be divorced for the simple reason that "there does not exist an economics in general and an ethics in general". Always we find economic system related to a particular ethical system (Choudhuri: 1976).

Human Nature: In Gandhi's thinking human nature was changed primarily through conscious self-efforts of individuals, inspired as it may be by examples of love and suffering for others. It was a subjective, purifying process with the aid of prayers, fasting, sacrifice, suffering etc. Social forms had little to do with it. The soul force operated every second of the day and had great impact on man.

With the death of Gandhi it was as if a great restraining influence had been murdered and his message began to die away as did the embers of his funeral pyre. Today violent methods seem to be taken for granted in many organizations. The excuse is frequently that all else has failed and that institutional violence must be met with a similar response.

The Prince of Wales said that violent techniques are used in demonstrations on behalf of worthy causes and causes that may require fighting for, but that fighting should be directed with perseverance against people's minds rather than bodies and possessions. The Prince said, "I personally can see no point whatsoever in using unnecessary and utterly barbaric force. All it does is to set people's minds more firmly against the perpetrators. Gandhi, by his fast and disobedience campaigns engendered sympathy throughout India and indeed world. There are many causes at the moment for which people feel, rightly or wrongly, desperately anxious. I myself have discovered in a small way that it is perseverance that counts, even if you are frustrated 10 or 20 times over. In the course of your persistence you probably touch human susceptibilities of sympathy and appreciation, and if uncalled for violence is met with a passive resistance that sympathy will increase by leaps and bounds.

Those against whom you are persevering are after all only human and eventually something will crack. The consequent sense of achievement is overwhelming and it is far easier to justify something obtained legitimately and peacefully than brutally and senselessly.

The only trouble about this is that it requires effort, will power and self-discipline. Some would have us believe these are out-of-date concepts, but as long as man has an ounce of humanity left, remembers the example of Gandhi they will survive." (H.R.H: 1969)

Organizational Constraints: Administration of an organization is not an easy task. It faces several limitations and problems, both internally and externally.

Among the internal problems are lack of adequate number of workers with proper motivation and understanding. To a large number of workers this is just a job, and they leave organization as soon as better opportunities are available. This not only prevents the organization from taking up certain programmes they may wish to but also disrupts the continuance of the existing programmes, maintenance of proper records and dates, and the efforts to have social and historical analysis of the situation.

These workers when they come for jobs fail to perceive the basic element of the voluntary efforts, i.e. people's involvement. Their whole attitude is very casual and, as such they fail to inspire people and instill in them a sense of confidence in the organization. Coupled with this is the failure to develop an efficient leadership.

While all the organizations believe in the totality of development efforts, very few give equal emphasis to all aspects of it. There is a tendency to compartmentalize without realizing that one sustains the other. For example, emphasis on economic programmes, without an adequate stress on the social efforts, even limits the achievement of the economic programmes.

The external factors which have also limited the functioning of the organizations are many. Resistance from vested groups is a major hurdle. When any voluntary effort meets some success, it also meets opposition from those who wield some power as they feel that their own power base is being eroded. They make efforts, by spreading false rumours about the programmes and activities to create a situation, in which the poor may get alienated from the organization and in extreme cases, even become apprehensive about them.

Another problem which the organizations are facing is with regard to human nature. As is the case with human nature, when some one gets some authority and power, he feels that he should centralize the entire authority to himself.

Another limitation which the organizations have to face is the apathetic attitude or lack of cooperation from the officers concerned with development. However, these limitations cannot deter the organizations from working towards achieving their goals. The achievements may be possible through certain strategies, such as, First, it is necessary to create greater confidence in the minds of the people about the organizations by involving them in all aspects of activities. Secondly, organizations should try to improve the quality of the existing workers through training and orientation. This would aim at changing the attitude of workers and also in developing skills in the management. Thirdly, due attention should be given to improve the quality of functioning through periodical analysis of the strengths and weaknesses. Finally, efforts have to be made in sharing each other's experiences and maintaining continuous dialogue between them, so that, an environment of mutual trust and goodwill is created and the whole attempt of organizations develop into a great movement with proper vision. (Study Report:1981)

The 2nd October, 2014 is a memorable day for the people of India. Because for the first time in the political history of independent India a nationwide attempt has been made by the Government of India under the leadership Narendra Modi as Prime Minister to translate the Gandhi's dream of neat and clean India into reality. The nation took an oath (Swachchhta Pledge) as:

> "Mahatma Gandhi dreamt of an India which was not only free, but also clean and developed. Mahatma Gandhi secured freedom for Mother India. Now, it is our duty to serve Mother India by keeping the country neat and clean. I take this pledge that I will remain committed towards cleanliness and devote time for this. I will devote 100 hours per year that is two hours per week to voluntary work for cleanliness. I will neither litter nor let others litter. I will initiate the quest for cleanliness with myself, my family, my locality, my village and my workplace. I believe that the countries of the world that appear clean are so because their citizens don't indulge in littering nor do they allow it to happen. With this firm belief, I will propagate the message of Swachchh Bharat Mission in villages and towns. I will encourage 100 other persons to take this pledge which I am taking today. I will endeavour to make them devote their 100 hours for cleanliness.

> I am confident that every step I take towards cleanliness will help in making my country clean." (The Government of India: 2014)

Gandhi's devotion to service was mirrored in his application to the nursing service of the wounded soldiers in South Africa, his nursing and sheltering a leper at home till his hospitalization, his overseeing cleanliness of *Harijans*' abodes during the Bombay plague (1896) and so on. His manual labour in his farms bore ample testimony to his belief in dignity of labour. (Hasan: 2.10.2014)

Village sanitation was the primary consideration in Gandhi's scheme of rural reconstruction. He recommended simple, inexpensive and effective remedies for tackling the problem of village insanitation. These aimed at not only keeping the surroundings clean but also sought to convert the dirt into a source of wealth. So he suggested, "lanes and streets have to be cleansed of all rubbish, which should be classified. There are portions which can be turned into manure, portions which have simply to be buried and portions which can be directly turned into wealth. Every bone picked-up is valuable raw material from which useful articles can be made or which can be crushed into rich manure. Rags and waste paper can be turned into paper, and excrete picked-up are golden manure for the village field."

Again, he said, "But the chief thing to remember is not necessity of burying all the refuse for the double purpose of promoting the villagers' health and their material condition, through the better yield of their crops which the manure must produce. Attention to hygiene is undoubtedly the first step to village reconstruction."

He looked upon supply of pure water to villages as of glorious service fraught with incalculable benefit to the suffering humanity of India, since its neglect was responsible for many of the diseases suffered by the villages. To him sanitation is the most effective way for dealing with disease, since, for him nature is the first physician, which is continuously repairing what man has damaged.

He believed that where the rules of personnel, domestic and public sanitation are strictly observed and due care is taken in the matter of diet and exercise, there should be no occasion for illness and disease.

Nature cure was a part of his plan of self-reliant society, for this kind of system of fighting disease depends on self-help and seeks to procure everything in the village. It relies on right and balanced diet. So to produce enough vegetables, fruits and milk in the villages is essential part of nature cure. It is most suitable for villages because it does not depend upon costly equipment. "My nature cure", Gandhi argued, "is designed solely for villagers and villages. Therefore, there is no place in it for microscope, X-rays and similar things. Nor is there room in nature cure for medicine, such as quinine, emetine and penicillin. Personal hygiene and healthy living are of primary importance.... All that can possibly be had from the five agencies of nature must be taken and used. They are earth, water, ether, fire and wind.... If necessary, curative herbs that grow locally, may be used." (Malhotra & Sharma: 1977)

The high standard of material living is prone to disintegration in society. There is every possibility of creating suspicion and jealousy in the minds of men because it stands as a hindrance in the way to human touch in social relationships. Without mutual trust and fellow feeling social life is not at all possible. The trust plays a significant role in human relations. Most of the administrative and professional constraints can be removed by this mutual trust. It is more true in medical sciences, especially in the relationship between physician and patient and other personnel in the service system. Today the Multinational Companies have started business practices in many countries. The internet expedites discussion and understanding among practitioners. With the increase of these facilities there arises wide scope for their misuse by the modern man as well as mechanization of human relationship. In developing countries, it may appear as a threat to the nation as well as to those who misuse them. It works as a factor of corruption embracing the largest section of the society in India.

The dangerous aspect of it in a developing country is that the family has become a strong source of corruption or the tacit supporter of it. Family is an informal and very powerful school to shape the character of a child. Gandhi talked of '*Swadeshi*' and 'Self-Rule' so that, human security and self-discipline with moral power can be achieved.

Education has always been a lifelong and comprehensive affair. The purpose of education is to give people enhanced awareness, greater openness, the courage to question and perseverance in searching solution. The objective of initial education is to equip one with basic minimum levels of knowledge, attitude, values etc. to begin with one's own life journey. [Chiranjivi J. Nirmal (ed.) 1999]

Independence must begin at the bottom, said Gandhi, just as peace originates in the mind of a man. One can go a step further and say that independence must begin in the individual's thought mirrored in his way of life. Every village has to be self-sustained and capable of managing its affairs even to the extent of defending itself against all kinds of odds. (*Harijan*, 28th July, 1948) During the freedom movement, it was often conceived that Panchayats would serve as substitute to bureaucratic authoritarianism. Gandhi explaining the *Swadeshi* movement advocated that Village Panchayats should be a living force which can be utilized basically for three purposes: 1. To restrict us to use and service of our immediate surroundings; 2. To correspond between representatives and represented; and 3. To develop self-government according to the need. (Khan: 1969) But unfortunately, it became a subject of debate resulting refusal of constitutional status to the grassroots level democracy. During the general discussions, the Draft Constitution was largely criticized for not incorporating the Village Panchayats in the Constitution. But B.R. Ambedkar, Chairman of the Drafting Committee opposed it by saying that, a village was nothing, but a "... a den of ignorance, narrow-mindedness, and communalism". (CAD: 1966) However, Dr Ambedkar's apprehension was developed not in vacuum. The rural communities were constrained by various ailments during that period, like caste system, untouchability, domination by the traditionally privileged class etc. and Dr. Ambedkar fought for the cause of untouchables. (Palmer: 1973). However, leaders like K. Santhanam, Professor N.G. Ranga, Alladi Krishnaswami, Begum Aizaz Rasul, H.V. Kamath, Renuka Ray, V.I. Muniswami Pillai, Pandit Thakur Das Bhargava, Professor Shibanlal Saksena and many others commented on the statement of Dr. Ambedkar and discussion took place on the issue. Ultimately, on 22nd November, 1948, K. Santhanam moved an amendment for the adoption of a new article as Directive Principle and after a debate for a short time the article 40 of the Constitution was incorporated with the provision for it in the Constitution of India. (CAD: 1966) Today again the importance of grassroot democracy was realized by the Government of India and by 73rd and 74th (Constitution) Amendment Acts have provided the constitutional status to them. The Panchayat system has embraced *Gram Sabha* also in which all the adults whose names are incorporated in the Voters' list are the members with the freedom to participate in the administration of the village. The next to *Gram Sabha* there remains family as an informal social organization. The family's role is very significant in inculcating in the members the values of human dignity, accountability, responsibility and responsiveness. The environment in the village depends on the environment of the families, which again influences the members of the higher stratus of administration. Burke also contributed to the view that the dignity of human being came through socialization. Men obey social norms because they saw themselves as an integral part of it. (Mukherjee) The impact of family on administration may be said direct and effective. Each family can be converted to a source of moral strength in administration.

The village Panchayats can play a significant role in extending help to the healthcare system of the country by adopting simple measures like maintaining cleanliness, good sanitation system, making the villagers aware of the preventive measures, protecting the life from diseases caused by water, polluted environment, providing effective administration of locally available dispensaries and making provision for easy access to the dispensaries and other healthcare facilities to the villagers. It will provide economy in healthcare system to the rural masses and help educating them about the preliminary measures for maintaining good health of the people. Indian traditional societies depended mainly on indigenous medicines administered by the local experts and on locally available medicinal plants. This indigenous system may be modified to adjust it with the modern system of healthcare services. What is needed is the personnel involved in the process must be able to command confidence of the local people through their efficiency, honesty and sympathetic approach while rendering service to the rural people.

The ancient Indian traditions always remind us our human duties. The Vedic literature discusses the subject matter of man's duty profusely. Vedic attitude is all pervasive. *Rig Veda* lays stress on pure and virtuous duty. Violence does not mean to kill.

The proclamation of *Mahabharata* tells us that labour is the only means to attain desired ideals. Labour may be righteous and unrighteous. Desired ideals gained through unrighteous labour may make a man but it is transitory and insignificant. Righteous labour is the harbinger of eternal grandeur, dignity and eternity. (Sinha: 2002)

Traditions are not established in a day. Indian traditions are ever flowing right from the dawn of civilization till today. They have shown the path of humanity not to India but to the entire world. They are the path finders. They are the beckoning light and have imparted vitality and wisdom to the world over.

The tradition of giving priority to duties has been handed over to us right from the time of Manu. Indian traditions have peeped into rights and duties very minutely. Relation between the two has been given thorough pondering and discussion. From the point of view of etymology, the subject matter of action, comes under the ambit of duty. Duty predicates action. So, the word 'duty' is used comprehensively. Gandhi simply brought to light Indian tradition and with the help of it he tried to unite people together to fight against foreign rule.

A human being is not inclined to do any work devoid of some motive or interest. Right is the reward and duty is its cause or means. There can be no work without motive or purpose. Means invokes no interest if there is no desire of fruit. There is interdependence between right and duty. Right is the result and duty is the means. He who sows the seeds will have the right to harvest the crops. It is ridiculous and ironical if a person exerts his right to harvest the crops though he has never been to the fields. Today we are confronting a very strange phenomenon. To gain our right we pay little heed to our duty. We are making effort to enjoy our rights without doing our genuine duty through strike and demand. If we cut the very branch on which we are sitting our fall is sure. We will be like Kalidasa who used to cut the branch of a tree on which he was sitting. Duty done never goes fruitless. If we do our duty honestly and efficiently the right will follow naturally. (Jha: 2002) This is the lesson which has universal value. Indian civilization, like any other human civilization is based on ancient traditions and values. Looking to the history of human civilization from its dawn one finds its dynamic nature. Man's life itself is changeable. From the cave man to the democratic man he has to travel a long way struggling at every step of the journey. Natural calamities and attack of wild animals forced the cave man to search for some shelter for protection and then the question of survival made them mobile in search of water and foodgrain and in course of time they settled down on the banks of the river. Thus, human security and survival were the two major factors for dynamic character of human civilization. Then man's creative capacity helped him to invent new things contributing to human progress and today man reaches a stage where he can exercise authority to utilize nature for his own progress. In the whole process of change human security, survival of man, progress of human civilization etc. have become serious challenges to a nation. In independent India on the line of '*Sarvodaya*' Community Development Programme was introduced but it could not work well. After that also the Government of India adopted several rural oriented schemes. Unfortunately, these schemes could not be implemented effectively due to various reasons—like lack of coordination among different government departments, failure to motivate the villagers to participate in the programmes, inability of the representatives of the people to realize the importance of the schemes etc.

Now, under the leadership of Narendra Modi, as Prime Minister, the Government of India launched "Swachchh Bharat" Scheme which may be said as public health oriented movement on 2nd October, 2014 nothing but a reminder of Gandhi's scheme for improvement of sanitation condition in the villages involving each villager. Then on birth anniversary day of Lok Nayak Jayprakash Narayan, the social reformer introduced "Sansad Adarsh Gram Yojana" (Member of Parliament Ideal Village Scheme). Under this scheme every Member of Lok Sabha has to take the responsibility, during his or her tenure, of building three ideal villages in his or her own constituency. Similarly, each Member Rajya Sabha has to build-up three villages in his or her own state. This is a scientific way of entrusting responsibility in specific term. It helps self-evaluation of the activities of the MPs. The people will also have the opportunity to see the progress of the villages. The most significant point is that it will induce the villagers to participate directly and specifically in the administration of the country. The participation brings involvement, involvement will inculcate the sense of responsibility and accountability at the village level itself. These qualities of a man cannot be imposed from the top, these have to be cultivated at the bottom by each and every member. Development is a dynamic process with upward trend and it can be sustained if every individual equipped with these qualities. This effort of the Government is rooted in the Gandhi's scheme of self-purification through self-analysis and self-knowledge for achieving self-discipline. A self-discipline individual is an asset in the medical services handling the basic issues of human security.

Further, since the development is a process with innovation and change in every service (whether public or private) it becomes extremely easy to carry out corrupt practices without being detected and even if they are detected defense measures are so circuitous and sophistic in nature that it is not possible for common men to understand the problem to find out the ground reality. On many occasions people not only tolerate corruption, but also adopt corrupt practices in certain compulsive situations. For example, a person from a remote area having some official work in connection with his profession at the country's headquarter or at the headquarter of his state is generally compelled to get things done on payment of "Speed Money" on the frequent refusal to take action on his request without bribe by the concerned person in the office. It is not possible for him to visit the office very frequently by leaving his official duty and family responsibility. Further he may not be in a position to do so due to financial constraints. Under these circumstances, he will certainly make calculation in terms of money, time constraint, travelling difficulties etc. Ultimately, he prefers to pay bribe in the form of speed money to get the work done. Similarly, a patient depend upon the physician's advice and guidance. In addition, in the case of medical sciences most notable point is that patient who approaches physician never tells lie of his suffering, though we cannot root out the possibility of mistakes to be committed by the patient. The patient may commit mistake out of ignorance, lack of misunderstanding, fear complex etc. In return to the truth telling the patient, the physician must provide efficient or expert services necessary for cure. In such a situation when blackmailing, cheating, exploitation, inhuman treatment like human trafficking for selling and buying of human organs, providing inefficient service to the patient take place, the position of the service providers is reduced to that of a betrayer. It demands flourishing of human qualities in the medical service providers. The mischievous people may deceive both the patient and service providers by motivating them in different ways. In this situation, the physicians at the crossroad and it is with human power they have to take the decision. Mere expertness without human approach the very Oath of rendering service to humanity may be a farce.

The World Bank has identified corruption as the single greatest obstacle to economic and social development. Corruption undermines development by distorting the Rule of Law and weakening the institutional foundation on which nations' security and progress depend. (Treadwell: 2005)

The concept of *Ahimsa* is not new. It is mirrored in the writings of great thinkers of the world. It is also rooted in ancient Hindu and other religious writings. It occurred in *Upanishad* itself, where it was listed as one of five ethical virtues. Indian *Rishis* and Saints and even Kings practiced it. They had faith on 'Soul Force'. Gandhi as a symbol of Indian culture attracted by the Tolstoy's writings and thus strengthened his belief on 'Soul Force'. His concept of non-violence has a humanitarian approach. This came to light during his stay in South Africa. His human feelings were sharpened by the inhuman conduct against Non-Europeans in South Africa. As his life and ideas were highly influenced by Indian culture, Gandhi did not adopt any violent attitude towards those who were involved in inhuman conduct in that country. In South Africa, though Gandhi was in the midst of political activities, he was active as a humanitarian to vindicate human rights (Jhunjhunwala: 2002).

While addressing in UN in September 2014 Modi, Prime Minister of India referred ancient tradition of our country and said, "Let us work towards adopting an International Yoga Day." Noting that Yoga is "an invaluable gift of our ancient tradition", he said, "it is not about exercise, but to discover the sense of oneness with yourself, the world and the nature." Yoga is the 5,000 year-old Indian physical, mental and spiritual practice that aim to transform body and mind. "Yoga embodies unity of mind and body; thought and action; restraint and fulfillment; harmony between man and nature; a holistic approach to health and well-being" he said. (http://times of india.india times.com/india/At-UN-general-assembly-PM-Narendra-Modi-rebukes-Pakistan-for-its-Kashmir-obsession/articleshow/436523)

Dr. Bhim Rao Ambedkar was one of the social reformers in India who made a sincere effort to eradicate weaknesses of Hindu social system by building it on the basis of freedom, equality and social justice. He fought against untouchability. Swami Vivekananda also said that even for self-perfection an individual requires freedom. The health of the human society is possible only when its members are morally strong.

Each religion is flooded with rich moral values and has inward looking orientation. While realizing the need of knowledge of the moral principles associated with religion, devotion to them is also essential to remove moral vacuum in the human society. This devotion may be called religion in a wider perspective. The spirit of oneness is a significant aspect of each religion. This aspect of religion was flourished in the culture of the ancient society. In every family a child is first introduced to the members of the family to which it is born. It is also taught the way it should behave towards each other. Thus, the process of socialization begins immediately after the birth of a child. These norms or behavioural patterns constituted the foundation of group or social life uniting people together. Religion as mentioned above had its roots in the ancient human society, which was simple and where the members had personal or face to face relationship. Gradually with the increase of population, spread of education and progress of science and technology, the society is becoming complex day-by-day. While moving from traditional society to modern one, the members fail to carry with them the human or social values and ethical principles to the complex modern society. The situation in modern society also apparently creates an impression that old traditional human values originated in the ancient, simple and naïve communities are not relevant as we are entering into the world of expert knowledge and competition in every walk of life. Improved Information and Communication Technology comprising of television, radio, internet, mobile in addition to newspapers, books, journals etc. is enough to construct modern human civilization. As a result it is noticed that the modern society is abstract and sophisticated in nature where everything is mechanized and institutionalized. Man has become a part of this mechanism. Even the charity is not excluded from being institutionalized. In short, we are now almost in a depersonalized society. Somehow we fail to realize the depth and pervasiveness of religion's power. I have high appreciation of the statement of Malvin Rader, "The impulse of the higher religions is to extend the community-mindedness of the close, intimate, concrete group to the wider sphere of the immense, impersonal, abstract society. Religion begins with the immediate ties of love and to take the love that is cultivated in the most intimate circles and to extend it to the widest circle that the human imagination can trace." Further, it is also stated that the need for communion and self-transcendence is the result of solitariness. Religion is return from solitariness to community. It is man's endeavour, by an inward personal adjustment to feel at home in the world. Mere rituals cannot help us in this effort, what is needed to-day is the understanding of core principles and devotion to them if we want to strengthen the ailing Indian society of to-day.

The religious leaders belonged to the societies which were simple, compact and ancient in nature. With the movement of the societies from traditional to modernity some changes are taking place—such as simplicity to complexity, face-to-face relationship to indirect relationship, from informal to formal relationship. Today we are reaching a stage where the process of dehumanization of human society has become active.

M.N. Roy, while appreciating the progress of science as a significant factor to energize man's creative capacity and in helping him to realize the negative consequences of superstition, has pointed out that a confraternity of morally and spiritually liberated individuals is the fundamental requirement for the realization of a better and healthier society. Tagore, Aurobinda, Roy etc. also contributed to this view.

The religions which were a significant component of Indian philosophy and social life to integrate people through their assertion on human values and *ahimsa* are overshadowed by excessive ritualism. It is noticed specifically in the case of performance of *pujas* of several Hindu Gods and Goddesses. Another change is found in the process of education which is giving a serious blow to it. To-day competition is how to secure more marks than how to acquire more knowledge resulting disintegrating the whole education process from midst of social life or social relationship based on love, affection, mutual respect for human dignity and ethical principles which are sustaining the continuity of human civilization.

In the public services merit of the candidates is judged on the basis of money power not on the qualities and efficiency of the candidates. To be very simple, it may be said selling of jobs and selling of seats in the professional educational institutions including medical colleges has become open secret practice, though it is most unwelcome practice in a democracy. One must understand incompleteness of human beings and their interdependence in the society and the need of full development of personality as a member of the society through education for the very existence and development of human society. These are very well treasured in the Gandhi's philosophy.

It is no denying a fact that the evolution of societal forms of living throughout the animal world has been an innate response to the compulsions of self-preservation. However, unlike rest of the animal world, the human attribute of reason has permitted our species to break the biological barriers and subjugate, to some extent, nature to human will. This has opened up several dimensions for societal development within the human species far beyond those found in the rest of the animal world. Even to-day self-preservation is the basis of social living. Dr. R.P. Sapru has indicated two major components of self-preservation—security and sound health. Education helps development of inherent powers of men. Through education a man can develop his capacities to control the personalities his environment and fulfill his aspiration. In short, education brings all-round and harmonious development of the personalities of the individual such as physical, intellectual, esthetic, social, economic, religious, cultural and realization of social needs. (Sapru: 1986)

Life is changeable. Human mind is always prone to change. New ideas and knowledge widen our mental horizon and create conflict in the mind provoking our thought. In this situation man's capacity to search and accept the right way to move is needed. Every change cannot lead us to human progress. Indian society is facing a serious challenge of change in life. In some areas impact of change is very slow and not perceptible. On many occasions people realize it when the negative impact of it is irreversible and serious damage has already done to the society or the nation. B. Ramesh Babu, in his address on *Legitimate Globalisation: Towards New Universal Norms and Values* pointed out that the most crucial change needed, however, is in our attitude towards change. Humanity's greatest challenge does not lie in coming up with new ideas. It lies in escaping from old ones. Mere material advancement, without any redeeming humane values or spirituality, will not or cannot lead to real progress.

Today every society whether 'open' or 'traditional' is constrained by its own peculiar problems. The traditional society in India is moving towards modernization through the process of transition. In a transitional society, the members always suffer from the problems like indecisiveness, confusion, imitation of superficial things, disliking of long standing social customs and traditions, unhealthy competitions amongst families. The traditional society is experiencing several serious problems—buying and selling of jobs at all levels of administration, demand for speed money to expedite the administrative process including transfer and promotion of public servants, bribery in the process of admission in the professional colleges, buying and selling of votes at the time of election to the legislature, illegal transaction of landed and other permanent property, misuse of money, time and energy by the youths, lack of parental control on the children, violation of human rights etc. The healthy traditions of the social life are distorted in the name of being modern. For example, community work, family tie, social relationship etc. are fast deteriorating. Mutual trust has been replaced by mutual suspicion, elderly members of the family are neglected, the children are heavily engaged in internet/ television etc. In short, the earlier process of socialization of the children with human values and ethical principles has disappeared both in family and school. Naturally, the fruits of it are reflected in each and every field of public service. With the increase of responsibilities of the state and change of role of service providers due to globalization and privatization and commercialization and increasing awareness of the people of their rights whole administration is at the crossroad.

In the educational institutions students are more trained to be fitted in the competition of job market than to maintain a balance to educate or inculcate in them human qualities along with it. The academic competition and human power must go hand in hand. This aspect of man's life is neglected to a great extent by the modern India builders. The students are not educated along with the natural way of human life in the society so that while returning to it after completion of their education they have to earn money by serving a human society which he or she missed at the preparatory stage. Human society is to be served with human touch. The experience in India shows that the human gap which is maintained at the process of education or preparation for the future life of a child remains as a big gap in his service life also. Human society is to be served by a human being with expert knowledge. Otherwise we are heading towards dehumanization of the human society. Accumulation of a huge amount of money and property which remain unused and causes tension to the accumulators, the undesirable comfort provided to the children as part of socialization or taking care of the children etc. require a fresh look in India.

Another significant aspect of man's life in India is religion. The existing scenario reaffirms that religion is an inalienable component of individual and social life in India. Religious festivals are found in rural as well as in urban areas on equal footing. The youths are attracted by the celebration of religious occasions in different temples. However, the negative aspect of it is the emphasis on the rituals only setting aside core principles of religions. Attempt has to be made to de-emphasize the rituals. Human aspect of religion should be given more emphasis instead of emphasis on rituals. (B. Ramesh Babu)

The then Prime Minister of Japan, Mr. Masayoshi Ohira, in January, 1979 initiated several Study Groups in Japan with certain interesting terms of reference. They were 'The Garden City State Concept Study group', 'The Age of Culture Study Group', 'The Study Group on Economic Performance in the Cultural Age', 'The Historical Evolution of Science and Technology Study Group', etc. the reports of these groups are published by the 'Foundation of Advanced Information and Research, Japan'. The reports recognize that rapid industrialization had produced what were referred to as the 'advanced nation's diseases', in the societal structure. One of such is 'the growth of individualization.' They create neurotic individualistic possessive tendencies characteristic of an acquisitive society. These tendencies, the reports predicted, produce a conflict with the growing consensus for evolving a cultural society and fostering of interdependence. The report on the Historical Evolution of Science and Technology says:

"In the highly industrialized society isolated and alienated individuals have created the main cause of 'illness' of civilized countries which has reduced significantly the vitality of the society. It may be interpreted as an expansion of the living space of mankind being limited by the barrier of 'finiteness of the globe'.

Speaking on the 'Economic Management in the Age of Cultural Priorities' it is found that according to the report:

"In order to secure existence with honour and vitality in the coming twentyfirst century, what harmony should be realized between people, culture and economic principle and how should economic management be undertaken? The following five basic philosophies may be sought after in economic management in the age of cultural priorities:

1. Respect for Humanity

2. Respect for Independence
3. Respect for Creativity
4. Respect for Regionality
5. Respect for Internationality

Without the development of the inner culture of man all our worldly possessions become the means of his own destruction, science and technology, if recognized as ethic neutral, will surely destroy our great civilization. Without a perception of the morality of the means and ends intellect becomes a self-stultifying instrument. The scornful impatience of the egoist wrecks his mission."

The Government of India is also making efforts to make an appeal to each one of us for being accountable and responsible for our activities, to be human to our people to begin with the family members, especially the parents and elderly members, to put an end to violence in the family through the Right to Information Act, the Domestic Violence Act, Maintenance of Parent and Old People Act in the beginning of the twentyfirst century itself. These have direct appeal to human heart.

Coming to medical services, it is found that unprecedented development of medical knowledge and scientific skill is not confining a physician to the care of the disease of a patient only. His social responsibility is increasing beyond expectation. For example, contraception, abortion, sterilization, sex change, cosmetic operations, organ transplantation etc. are very complex issues. A physician's responsibility is extended through these issues to non-patients also. These situations require a physician to make a moral choice. Today with the assertion of individual's right to freedom earlier paternalistic authority of the physician has become to some extent eroded. The only purpose for which power can be rightfully exercised over any member of a civilized community against his will, is to prevent harm to other. (*en.wikipedia.org/wiki/paternalism*)

We can conceptualize one facet of the right to health as a "human right to healthcare". Notably, it encompasses both patient and service provider's rights in the delivery of healthcare services, the latter being similarly open to frequent abuse by the state. The patient right in healthcare delivery includes the right to privacy, life and quality care, as well as freedom from discrimination, torture and cruel, inhumane or degrading treatment. Service provider's right includes the right to quality standards of working conditions, the right to associate freely and the right to refuse to perform a procedure etc. It is found that in developing countries with weak rule of law, healthcare providers are often forced to perform procedures which negate their morals, deny marginalized groups the best possible standards of care, breach patient confidentiality and conceal crimes against humanity and torture. (*en.wikipedia.org/wiki/right to health*)

Gandhi always insisted on the concept of "integration". What he talked of is the Integration of word, work and thought of a man. All the three must make a concerted effort towards a particular goal by which both the individual and the society will be benefitted. It helps cure of several social diseases, like hypocrisy, mutual distrust, feeling of alienation, fear etc. and at the administrative level it contributes significantly for strengthening morale in the organization. If we look it from the wider perspective it is found that our social life demands both horizontal as well as vertical integration from the ancient to the present and in the present life integration with environment and changes which take place every moment. In the life of an individual also one cannot delink his or her birth and death and the developments that take place in the journey from birth to death. Life exists in between the two. All these constitute the totality of a man's life.

In the similar way if we analyze the state of medical services to an individual, the service providers take care of past life of the patient and also the family background in the context of particular diseases. The development of modern medicine and technology in the medical world cannot do away the significance of the traditional medicine, which is also known as indigenous or folk medicine. It comprises knowledge systems that developed over generations within various societies before the era of modern medicine. The World Health Organization defines traditional medicine as, "the health practices, approaches, knowledge and beliefs incorporating plant, animal and mineral-based medicines, spiritual therapies, manual techniques and exercises, applied singularly or in combination to treat, diagnose and prevent illness or maintain well-being."

In some Asian and African countries, up to 80 per cent of the population relies on traditional medicine for their primary healthcare needs. When adopted outside of its traditional culture, traditional medicine is often called complementary and alternative medicine.

The WHO also notes, though, that "inappropriate use of traditional medicines or practices can have negative or dangerous effects" and that "further research is needed to ascertain the efficacy and safety" of several practices and medicinal plants used by traditional medicine systems.

In the written record, the study of herbs dates back 5,000 years to the ancient Sumerians, who described well-established medicinal uses for plants. Ancient Egyptian medicine of 1000 BC are known to have used various herbs.

Many herbs and minerals used in Ayurveda were described by ancient Indian herbalists such as Charaka and Sushruta during the 1st millennium BC. The first Chinese herbal book was the *Shennong Bencao Jing*, compiled during the Han Dynasty, but dating back to a much earlier date, which was later augmented as the *Yaoxing Lun* (Treatise on the Nature of Medicinal Herbs) during the Tang Dynasty. Early recognized Greek compilers of existing and current herbal knowledge include Pythagoreanism, Hippocrates, Aristotle, Theophrastus, Dioscorides and Galen.

Indigenous medicine is generally transmitted orally through a community, family and individuals until "collected". Within a given culture, elements of indigenous medicine knowledge may be diffusely known by many, or may be gathered and applied by those in a specific role of healer such as a shaman or midwife. Three factors legitimize the role of the healer—their own beliefs, the success of their actions and the beliefs of the community. When the claims of indigenous medicine become rejected by a culture, generally three types of adherents till use it—those who born and socialized in it who become permanent believers, temporary believers who turn to it in crisis times, and those who only believe in specific aspects, not in all of it. (*en.wikipedia.org/wiki/Traditional medicine.*)

Now, the present Government with Narendra Modi as the Prime Minister is aiming to integrate Ayurveda with modern medicine. The Government is planning to set-up an exclusive drug control department to facilitate research and development, monitor quality control and standardize the manufacturing of medicinal products of Ayurveda and other traditional Indian treatment systems. The chief objective of the mission is to encourage integration of Ayush with modern medicine and create a healthcare system that can be emulated globally and which will achieve the universal goal of health for all. There is growing accessibility for Ayurveda globally and several nations have shown interest in partnering India to popularize it locally.

"Under newly created AYUSH (Ayurveda, Yoga and Naturopathy, Unani, Siddha and Homoeopathy) Mission, the Centre would provide funding support to states wanting to set-up manufacturing facilities and create manpower for the traditional medicine industry." It is said by the Health Minister, Harsh Vardhan at the inauguration of the Arogya Expo organized alongside the 6th World Ayurveda Congress. Nilanjan Sanyal, Secretary, AYUSH noted that one-third of the World's population lacks access to healthcare. Ayurveda and other traditional systems have great potential to address this health lacuna since they already meet the healthcare requirements of 80 per cent of the rural population in India. However, these traditional medicinal products have to be validated scientifically for the practitioners to have credibility and patients to have confidence. (*The Assam Tribune*, 7th November, 2014)

The religions are also full of guidelines for taking care of health of the people. The Hindu religion, for example provides enough scope to learn various tips for maintaining good health through diet, meditation, religious customs etc. Here let me also mention about Buddha's teachings as pointed out by Dr. Lalit Shyam in a daily local English newspaper of Assam. While discussing the Buddha's teachings for a peaceful world Dr. Shyam said, "Buddha was rightly described as the king of physicians……The Buddha was a great psychologist too who gave immense importance on mind." According to the teachings of the Buddha, the mind is the forerunner of all events and happiness. *Dhammapada* opens with a clear assertion that the mind is the forerunner of all that we are, the maker of our character, the creator of our destiny. It is from the mind there arises happiness or sorrow and suffering. If an individual does an act of righteousness, there arises happiness. If he does an immoral activity, the mind produces sorrow and suffering to the individual. These activities proceed from the volition of the mind. If the mind is controlled and cultured and trained to do only the moral acts, there shall arise only happiness to the individual. Our restless mind is the source of great suffering. There is no suffering if the mind is peaceful and happy.

By mind the world is led, by mind the world is moved. And all good and bad things exist in the world because of the mind. The practice of meditation is the only way by which an individual can control his mind and culture it for perfection and spiritual attainments.

Samatha or calmness meditation and *Vipassana* or Insight medication rediscovered by the Buddha over 2557 years ago is the effective means by which we can learn in depth to reach the real life centre, and understand what life is all about, how suffering ceases after it occurs, how life-quality development can be done, and how real peace can be achieved by human beings. This is the method of practice followed by Gautam Buddha leading to his enlightenment over 2557 years ago. These two meditation techniques are non-sectarian and practised by all without any distinction of race, caste, religion and nationality. The techniques teach how to develop the mind go hand in hand with material development so that life will be truly peaceful. Spiritual development is meditation leading to peaceful mind. When the mind is peaceful, spiritual insight or wisdom is achieved. When we have meditation and wisdom, all other virtues will come about. The essence of meditation in Buddhist philosophy is pure calmness of mind together with equanimity by wisdom without prejudice. Besides, the purpose of meditation is not merely to cure physical diseases, but as the by-product of mental purification, many psychosomatic diseases get eradicated. The highest achievement will be the attainment of *Nirvana*, the cessation of all sufferings and realization of perfect bliss. Meditation practice is the way to lasting peace.

At this critical juncture the Buddha's methods of meditation practice to the modern world has great relevance as it is the only way by which people can control their mind. Buddhism has spread without fire or sword, spread its doctrines of tolerance, peace and compassion to a world in turmoil and sufferings. (*The Assam Tribune*, 26th May, 2013)

Shriman Narayan talked about moral values envisaged by Mahatma Gandhi as, "During last two decades, our country has doubtless, achieved notable results in various sectors of national development, and it would be improper to underestimate, much less denounce, our own achievements. Nevertheless, the fact remains that we have not paid adequate attention towards strengthening the ethical principles of our people. Gandhiji always stressed the imperative need for raising the moral stature of the human beings, while attempting to raise the standard of material living. He repeatedly reminded us that a nation did not become great merely by erecting huge buildings, establishing giant factories and multiplying wealth for economic prosperity." (Narayan, Shriman: 2005) Modern technology has to be applied for the survival of human society.

References

Autobiography of Gandhi: The Story of My Experiments with Truth, Beacon Press, Boston, 1957.

An Autobiography by Gandhi: Navajeevan Publishing House, Ahmedabad, 1959.

Babu, B. Ramesh: His address on *Legitimate Globalisation: Towards New Universal Norms and Values: Man in India*: 90 (1-2): 309-409.

Bharato, K.S. and Mani: *The Foundations of Gandhian Thought*, Bharati, 1987.

Bhattacharya, Buddhadeva: Gandhian Socialism and Its Relevance in India Today; *Journal of Gandhian Studies*: Institute of Gandhian Thought and

Peace Studies, Gandhi Bhawan, University of Allahabad, Allahabad, Vol. 7, No. 27, Jan-Apl. 1980.

Bose, N.K.: *Selection from Gandhi*, Navajivan Publishing House, Ahmedabad, 1957.

Budhachandra Singh, Khundrakpam, Gandhian Approach to Non-Violence and Peace: an unpublished Ph.D. thesis submitted to the Department of Political Science, Manipur University, 2011.

Chiranjivi J. Nirmal (ed.) 1999: *Human Rights in India*, Oxford University Press; 1999.

Choudhuri, Dr. Keshab: A Limited-frame reference to Gandhian relevance: *Journal of Gandhian Studies*; April-July, 1976, Vol. No. 10-11.

Devadoss, Dr. T.S. *Freedom, Equality and Peace—A Gandhian Perspective*: *Journal of Gandhian Studies:* Institute of Gandhian Thought and Peace Studies, Gandhi Bhawan, University of Allahabad, Allahabad, Vol. 14, Nos. 54-55, Jan-April, 1987.

Desai, Suresh A., The Role or Price System in Gandhian Economics: Gandhi Marg, *Journal of the Gandhi Peace Foundation*; No. 24, Vol. 2, Number 12, March 1981.

Devi, Ksh. Bimola: Relevance of Gandhian Thought in the Present Day Society; *Manipur Today*, Republic Day, Dept. of Information and Public Relations, 26.12.2010, Vol. XXXI, No. I.

Dogra, Km. Sandhaya Deep: Mahatma Gandhiji's Social Philosophy: *Journal of Gandhian Studies*: Institute of Gandhian Thought and Peace Studies, Gandhi Bhawan, University of Allahabad, Allahabad, Vol. 7, No. 28, July 1980.

Gandhi: *Young India*; 13th November, 1924.

Gandhi, 1948, *Key to Health*, this book was written by M.K. Gandhi in Gujarati language and translated in English by Sushila Nayar, first published in October 1948, Navajivan Publishing House, Ahmedabad-380 014.

Gandhi, M.K.: *From Yeravda Mandir, Ashram Observance in Action*, Sage Publication, New Delhi, 1985.

Ghosh, Dr. Raghunath: *The Gandhian Concept of Truth: In the Light of Advaita Vedanta and its Relevance in Modern Society*: *Journal of Gandhian Studies:* Institute of Gandhian Thought and Peace Studies, Gandhi Bhawan, University of Allahabad, Allahabad, Vol. 12, Nos. 47-48, April/ July 1985.

Gopalakrishnan, Dr. R.: Gandhiji's Asharam Vows and their Relevance for the Contemporary Social Situation: *Journal of Gandhian Studies*: Institute of Gandhian Thought and Peace Studies, Gandhi Bhawan, University of Allahabad, Allahabad, Vol. 12, Nos. 47-48, April/July 1985.

Guha, Ramchandra: *Gandhi Before India*, Penguin Book, 2013.

Government of India (Ministry of Information and Broadcasting), New Delhi: *Collected Works of Mahatma Gandhi*, 1969, Vol. 22.

Ibid., Vol. XII, 1969.

Ibid., Vol. XIII, 1964.

Goyal, O.P., *Studies in Modern Indian Political Thought*, Kitab Mahal, Allahabad, 1984.

Grover, Dr. D.C., *Satyagraha: As Answer to International Conflict*; Institute of Gandhian Thought and Peace Studies, Gandhi Bhawan, University of Allahabad, Allahabad, Vol. 4, No. 16, July 1977.

Hasan, Nawab Md. Dilwar: The Saint we know as Gandhi, *The Assam Tribune*, 2nd October, 2014.

HRH, the Prince of Wales: *Text of Speech at the Royal Albert Hall*, London, 1969.

Iyer, Raghavan: *The Moral and Political Writings of Mahatma Gandhi*, Oxford, 1986.

Jhunjhunwala, Bharat Ed. *Governance and Human Rights*, by Kalpaz Publications, Delhi-110052, 2002.

Jha, Vidyananda: *Priority Given to Human Rights in Ancient Indian Tradition:* Published in the book; *Governance and Human Rights*, edited by Bharat Jhunjhunwala, Kalpaz Publications; Delhi, 2002.

Kampadoo, Peter Lakhsmanen: Way Five: The Sarvodaya Way: *Journal of Gandhian Studies*: Vol. 14, No. 53, October 1986, Institute of Gandhian Thought and Peace Studies, Gandhi Bhawan, University of Allahabad, Allahabad.

Khan, Zia Uddin, Mathur and Iqbal Narain Ed: *Panchayati Raj, Planning and Democracy*, Asia, 1969.

Kurien, K. Mathew and Mythily Sivaraman: *Gandhian Approach to Property and Relations and Class Comflict*: 1986, Institute of Gandhian Thought and Peace Studies, Gandhi Bhawan, University of Allahabad, Allahabad, Vol. 3, Apl-July 1976, No. 11-12.

Madhilika, Smt.: Gandhiji and Contemporary Ideologies Regarding Freedom, Peace and Equality. *Journal of Gandhian Studies*: Institute of Gandhian Thought and Peace Studies, Gandhi Bhawan, University of Allahabad, Allahabad, Vol. 14, Nos. 54-55, Jan-April 1987.

Mahatma: *Harijan*, 5th May, 1946.

Malhotra, Dr. S.L. and Dr. S.K. Sharma: *Towards Village Swaraj, Research Monograph*; Department of Gandhian Studies, Punjab University, January 1977, Chandigarh.

M.K. Gandhi: An Autobiograhy Or the Story of My Experiments with Truth, Navajivan Publishing House, Ahmedabad, 1989.

Mukherjee, Subrata and Sushila Ramswamy: *A History of Political Thought (Plato to Marx)*: Prentice Hall of India; New Delhi.

Narayan, Shriman: *Gandhi: The Man and His Thought:* Publication Division, Government of India, New Delhi, 2005.

Palmer, N.D. *The Indian Political System*, Houghton Mifflin Co., Boston, 1973.

Pandya, V.D.: *Gandhian Perspective to Democracy and Socialism*: Institute of Gandhian Thought and Peace Studies, Gandhi Bhawan, University of Allahabad, Allahabad, Vol. 14, Nos. 54-55, Jan-April, 1987.

Prabhu, R.K. and U.R. Rau: *The Mind of Mahatma Gandhi*, Oxford University Press, London, 1945.

Prakash, Dr. Jagadish and Nageswar Rao: *Gandhian Perspectve to Socialism*: Institute of Gandhian Thought and Peace Studies, Gandhi Bhawan, University of Allahabad, Allahabad, Vol. 7, No. 27, November 1, 1980.

Pushparanjan, A.: Are Religions One ? *Journal of Gandhian Studies*: Institute of Gandhian Thought and Peace Studies, Gandhi Bhawan, University of Allahabad, Allahabad, Vol. 7, No. 27, November 1, 1980.

Quartey, Francis Ofosu: *Gandhian Concept of Non-violence*: Published in Journal of Gandhian Studies, Vol. 7, No. 28, July 1980, Gandhi Bhawan, University of Allahabad, Allahabad.

Rolland, R.: *Mahatma Gandhi: The man who become one with the Universal being*. Translated by Catherine D. Groth, New Delhi, Publication Division, Government of India, 1969 (referred in Budhachandra's unpublished Ph.D. thesis, titled Gandhian Approach to Non-Violence and Peace).

Robinson, Joan: *Freedom and Necessity: An Introduction to the Study of Society*: George Allen & Unwin Ltd., 1970.

Ruthnaswamy, M., *Principles and Practice of Public Administration,* Fifth edition; Central Book Depot, Allahabad, 1972.

Sapru, Dr. R.P., *The Conflict of Ethics and Social Justice in Developing Countries*; Dr. R.P. Sapru was an Associate Professor, Dept. of Cardiology, Postgraduate Institute of Medical Education and Research, Chandigarh. Published under the auspices of Indian Council of Medical Research the Conference papers. The International Conference was held in New Delhi 1986. The topic was *Health Policy: Ethics and Human Values*. It was held in collaboration with the Council of International Organization of Medical Sciences (Geneva). Compiled by Dr. P.C. Bhatta, Secretariat, IMA House, May, New Delhi.

Sethi, J.D: *Gandhi Today*: Viikas Publishing House; Delhi, 1978.

Sharma, Dr. S.K.: *Gandhi's Objectives and Development Styles*; Institute of Gandhian Thought and Peace Studies, Gandhi Bhawan, University of Allahabad, Allahabad, Vol. 7, October, 1979, No. 25.

Sharma, M.L.: *Gandhi as a Socialist*; Deep & Deep Publications, New Delhi, 1980.

Sinari, Dr. Ramakant: *The Culture of Peace and Gandhi's Commitment*: *Journal of Gandhian Studies,* Vol. 5, No. 21, Oct. 1978.

Sinha, Anil Kumar: *Human Rights in Mahabharata*: Governance and Human Rights, edited by Bharat Jhunjhunwala, Kalpaz Publications; Delhi, 2002.

Study Report: A Study Report on Voluntary Efforts: Their Contribution and the Methodologies of People's Participation, sponsored by the Department of Rural Reconstruction, Ministry of Agriculture, Government of India in 1978. Referred in Gandhi Marg, *Journal of the Gandhi Peace Foundation*, 24 March, 1981.

Tewari, A.P.: *Gandhian Approach to Class Conflict and Property Relations,*

Institute of Gandhian Thought and Peace Studies, Gandhi Bhawan, University of Allahabad, Allahabad, Vol. 3, Apl-July, 1976, Nos. 11-12.

Tewari, A.P.: *Gandhiji's Concept of an Ideal State*; Institute of Gandhian Thought and Peace Studies, Gandhi Bhawan, University of Allahabad, Allahabad, Vol. IV, July, 1983, No. 40.

Treadwell, Donald and Jill B. Treadwell: 2005; Public Relations Writing; second edition; Response Books, A Division of Sage Publications, New Delhi.

The Assam Tribune, 8th October, 2014: Note (Eating white meat, fish may lower liver cancer risk: Washington: 7th October - eating lots of white meat such as poultry or fish may reduce the risk of developing liver cancer, scientists say.

Ibid., 8th Apr., 2014.

Ibid., 7th Nov., 2014.

Ibid., 28th Nov., 2013.

Researchers studied the relationship between meat intake and the risk of hepatocellular carcinoma (HCC).

They analyzed studies published between 1956 and 2013 and found that eating white meat or fish may reduce the risk of developing liver cancer by 31 per cent and 22 per cent respectively. Consuming red meat, processed meat, or total meat was not associated with the liver cancer risk.

"The present mega-analysis indicates that a high level of white meat or fish consumption can reduce the risk of HCC significantly, while intake of red meat, processed meat or total meat is not associated with HCC risk," researchers wrote in the study published in the *Journal of Alimentary Pharmacology and Therapeutics*.

"Our findings suggest that dietary intervention may be a promising approach for prevention of HCC, which still need to be confirmed by further well-designed prospective studies and experimental research." PTI

The Government of India: Swachchh Bharat Mission; Ministry of Urban Development, Ministry of Drinking Water & Sanitation, Ministry of Panchayati Raj; appeared in *The Assam Tribune*, 2nd October, 2014.

Tripathi, Anil: *Gandhiji's Social Philosophy*: Published in *Journal of Gandhian Studies*, Vol. 7, No. 28, July 1980, Gandhi Bhawan, University of Allahabad, Allahabad.

Tripathi, B.K., *Gandhian Approach to Economic Development*, Institute of Gandhian Thought and Peace Studies, Gandhi Bhawan, University of Allahabad, Allahabad, Vol. 7, No. 25, October 1979.

Umarani, R.I.: *Gandhiji's Ashram Vows and their Relevance for Contemporary Social Situation*: *Journal of Gandhian Studies*, Institute of Gandhian Thought and Peace Studies, Gandhi Bhawan, University of Allahabad, Allahabad, Vol. 12, Nos. 47-48, April-July, 1985.

Verma, Dr. Surendra: *Modern Search for Peace*: *Journal of Gandhian Studies*: Vol. 5, No. 21, Oct., 1978.

Wilson, Harold: *Text of Speech by the British Prime Minister, the Rt. Hon. Harold Wilson*, M.P. at the Royal Albert Hall, London, 1969.

FOUR
Human Rights
Means and End of Medical Sciences

The concept of human rights is a great contribution of human thought to the culture and civilization of every nation. It is flourishing at every stage of the progress of human civilization embracing new areas of man's interest. Gradually, human rights are developing in different dimensions. (Baxi: 1994). The dynamic nature of the concept of human rights is reflected in the definition offered by Harold J. Laski in his book, *Grammar of Politics* when he said, "rights are those conditions of social life without which no man can seek to be himself". It indicates wide meaning and evolutionary character of the concept. Similar is the case when Professor Hobhouse put it as, "rights are what we expect from others and others from us and all genuine rights are conditions of social welfare". Here addition has been made of the relationship between the rights and duties. Gandhi also asserted that the true source of right is duty. The rights are required not only for development of personality of an individual, but also to fulfill the social responsibilities of an individual. (Sharma: 1998)

Any discussion on human rights cannot be divorced from its normative aspect of connotation. Social Sciences are normative sciences and as a part of social sciences human rights set certain norms or ideals for establishing a peaceful society. At the same time these rights have support of the norms of the society. These are nothing but moral principles that set out certain standards of human behaviour and regularly protected as legal rights in national and international law. They are commonly understood as inalienable Fundamental Rights to which a person is inherently entitled simply because she or he is human being.

(en.wikipedia.org/wiki/Human Rights)

From the above, it is found that human rights are inherent to all human beings whatever their nationality, place of residence, sex, national or ethnic origin, colour, religion, language, or any other status. All are equally entitled to their human rights without discrimination. These rights are all interrelated, interdependent and indivisible.

(www.ohchr.org/en/issues/pages/whatarehuman rights.aspx)

Human rights are the claims of an individual for the realization of human qualities, which the nature has bestowed on him or her as human being. (Naseema: 2002)

The concept of human rights is closely connected to human dignity. The principles of human rights constitute a strong device to ensure protection of dignity of each and every individual in the society. This also invites equal respect and development of human qualities, such as, intelligence, talent and conscience and satisfaction of spiritual needs.

Dignity provides a sense of value. The human rights and their observance may be considered as an indicator of awareness of an individual of the dignity of others and thus adherence of human values. Self-realization is not possible in isolation of social life because it is a part of common humanity. (Sharma: 1998)

Human rights entail both rights and obligations. In the modern democracy, States assume obligations and duties under international law to respect, to protect and to fulfill human rights. The obligation to respect means that states must refrain from interfering with or curtailing the enjoyment of human rights. The obligation to protect requires states to protect individuals and groups against human rights abuses. The obligation to fulfill means that states must take positive action to facilitate the enjoyment of basic human rights. At the individual level, when we are entitled to our human rights, we should respect the human rights of others.

(www.ohchr.org/en/issues/pages/whatarehuman rights.aspx)

The above discussion reflects the universal character of the doctrine of human rights. However, the universal character of human rights cannot do away with the diversity that exists in the global human society. Canely and Jones stated clearly that the universality of these rights has to be safeguarded in a world characterized by diversity—a world in which people live in different circumstances, bear different cultures, profess different religions, and pursue different ways of life. Further, human individuals exhibit different physical and personal characteristics. They also exhibit differences as members of different societies and professions. These differences do not stand as a hindrance to accept the universal character of human rights. Simple reason for it is that in spite of these differences, the truth is that all are human beings. The social values, customs and traditions differ from country to country and in the same country amongst different communities. India had the experience of the diversity in beliefs and values adhered by different ethnic groups which have affected the human rights of individuals. For a long time the doctrine of human rights, was not asserted by certain sections of the Indians, especially in the rural and hill areas who gave priority to the social customs and traditions to human rights. (Canely and Jones: 1945) Without respect for human rights social life is not possible because it requires mutual respect for each other, fellow feeling, co-existence of differences of opinion etc.

The doctrine of natural rights was translated into practical reality when King John was made to acknowledge that there were certain rights of the subject which could not be violated even by a Sovereign in whom all power was legally vested. It is said that king John's barons forced him to grant Magna Carta, the Charter of Liberties that placed the English king under the law. It is a Charter agreed by king John of England at Runnymede, near Windsor, on fifteenth June, 1215 and was confirmed in definitive form by Henry III in 1225. It is a crucial document for England's history, likely best known of all documents surviving from medieval England. Its attempt to impose the law's limitations on a ruler is summarized in chapter 39:

> No freeman shall be taken or imprisoned, or dispossessed or outlawed or exiled or in any way ruined, nor will we go or send against him except by the lawful judgement of his peers by the law of land.

The document, essentially a peace treaty between king John and Barons guaranteed that the king would respect feudal rights and privileges, uphold the freedom of the Church, and maintain the nation's laws. Although more a reactionary than a progressive document in its day, the Magna Carta was seen as a cornerstone in the development of democratic England by the later generations.

(https://en.wikipedia.org/wiki/Magna - Carta accessed on 28.6.2015)

The doctrine of natural rights, is itself, an offshoot of the doctrine of natural law. Since the natural law consists of rules founded on the primary instincts of man as modified by his inborn perception of what is right or wrong, it would follow that natural rights would constitute the primary rights and obligations of men towards each other's as soon as they begin to live in a society.

Just as natural law stands above the law of the land, so natural rights are supposed to be of a higher sanctity than legal rights. They exist independent of the law of land. The philosophers, in spite of their controversial views on the origin of rights they agree on the point that there are certain basic and inalienable rights which are inherent in free and civilized human beings. A political society is necessary not to create them but to secure them. (Basu: 2007)

One of the oldest records of Human Rights is the Statute of Kalisz (1264) giving privileges to the Jewish minority in the Kingdom of Poland such as protection from discrimination and 'hate speech.' *en.wikipedia.org/wiki/human rights, accessed on 19.5.2014*

The movement continued through the repeated confirmation of the Magna Carta and the Petition of Right, 1628 and culminated in the Bill of Rights, 1689, which enacted in a parliamentary statute the declaration which the people made the Prince and Princess of Orange to subscribe at their accession in 1688.

The doctrine of natural rights received further impetus at the hands of the great protagonists of the Social Contract in the seventeenth and eighteenth centuries, particularly, Locke and Rousseau, who sought to trace the genesis of political society and Government in an agreement into which individuals entered to form a collective society to ensure their general interests and objects, but at the same time without interfering with their 'natural rights' which already belonged to them as human beings (Basu: 2007).

The earliest conceptualization of human rights is credited to ideas about natural rights emanating from natural law. In particular, the issue of universal rights was introduced by the examination of extending rights to indigenous peoples by Spanish Clerics. In Britain in 1689, the English Bill of Rights and the Scottish Claim of Right, each made illegal a range of oppressive governmental actions. Two major resolutions occurred in eighteenth century in the United States (1776) and in France (1789), leading to the adoption of the United States Declaration of Independence and the French Declaration of the Rights of Man and of the Citizen respectively, of which established certain legal rights. Additionally, the Virginia Declaration of Rights of 1776 encoded into law a number of fundamental civil rights and civil freedoms.

en.wikipedia.org/wiki/human rights, accessed on 19.5.2014

The emergence of humanitarian ideas during the eighteenth and nineteenth centuries in Europe and other countries contributed to a clear understanding of human rights. An example of humanitarian intervention was the military action agreed in 1827 by Great Britain, France and Russia against the Ottoman Empire, reportedly to bring to an end the sufferings of the Greek population under Turkish rule. (Sunanda Raj: 1999)

These were followed by developments in philosophy of human rights by philosophers such as Thomas Paine, John Stuart Mill and G.W.F Hegel during the eighteenth and nineteenth centuries. The term human rights came into use sometime between the Paine's the *Rights of Man* and William Lloyd Garrison's 1831 writings in *The Liberator*, in which he stated that he was trying to enlist his readers in "the great cause of human rights".

en.wikipedia.org/wiki/human rights, accessed on 19.5.2014

In the nineteenth century human rights became a central concern over the issue of slavery. Slavery in Europe and the slave trade in Africa and Asia occupied whole of nineteenth century. The prohibition of slave trade had been the main objective of international concern. Various treaties and agreements were concluded throughout the century towards the end. (Sunanda Raj: 1999)

A number of reformers, such as William Wilberforce in Britain, worked for the abolition of slavery. This was achieved in the British Empire by The Slave Trade Act, 1807 and the Slavery Abolition Act, 1833. In the United States, all the northern States had abolished the institution of Slavery between 1777 and 1804.

The movements for rights and efforts of several social leaders were successful in bringing significant social changes over the course of the twentieth century in the name of human rights. In Europe and North America, labour unions brought about laws granting workers the right to strike, establishing minimum work conditions and forbidding or regulating child labour. The women's right movement succeeded in gaining for women the right to vote. National Liberation Movement in many countries succeeded in driving out colonial powers. One of the most influential was Mahatma Gandhi's Movement to the native India from British rule.

en.wikipedia.org/wiki/human rights, accessed on 19.5.2014

What is Natural law? Natural law is mixed up with a number of high ideals—such as morality, justice, ethics, right, reason, good conduct, equality, liberty, freedom, social justice, democracy etc. To Earnest Barker natural law is a "way of looking at things—a spirit of human interpretation in the mind of the judge and jurist."

According to Plato (427-347), the doctrine that natural law meant natural justice that is, justice is harmony of man's inner life and harmony is the quality of justice and it is achieved by reason and wisdom over desires. Plato is of the view that it is the intelligent man—the philosopher who should be the king. Aristotle expounded the theory of natural law and positive law in clear terms. He said, "The purpose of state, community and law is to enable man to realize good life that is living according to virtue." (Dias, R.W.M: 1994)

The importance that Aristotle attaches to the individual will always carry universal appeal. It is because of it Aristotle may be regarded as the father of modern individualism. His ideas on family and property as natural and necessary institutions for the development of individuality, received wide support. His statement that "state comes into existence for the sake of life, but continues to exist for good life" was a very significant declaration supporting the cause of the individual and indicating the duties of the state. Although he admitted that a man has personal value only as a member of the state, the state is not an end in itself. Because the fullest development of man's personality is not possible through a complete control of man by the state. The state has to allow individual to lead a complete life through exercise of freedom. (Ebenstein, W.)

The Stoics represented another school of thought who came into existence after the death of Aristotle. The Stoic philosophy also emphasized individualism. To them good was virtue and evil was vice. Virtue and vice consisted respectively in right and wrong disposition of will. The will was under the control of the individual. Therefore, they held that the attainment of good is wholly within the power of each individual. A life in accordance with nature meant to them two things—firstly, he would justifiably seek the fulfilment of his simple, natural instincts; secondly, because the mankind was naturally one family, he would seek to serve his fellowmen. The Stoics interpreted nature as reason. They had immense faith on the rationality of men. A life according to nature meant co-operation with all forces of good. (Sabine: 1949)

The contribution made by Cicero toward development of human rights is of great importance. He said '*Res-Public is Res-Populi*', which means the affairs of the state is the affairs of the people. State exists for the enforcement of law for common good. Based on such a law, the state is to be regarded as an ethical community. If state deviates from moral laws it will lose justification for its existence. To Cicero, the state is an association of human beings who are united together by a common agreement about law and right and by the desire to participate in mutual advantages. Explaining the reason of its coming together is not weakness, rather a sort of natural affinity for each other, because they are endowed with the instinct of gregariousness which is inborn.

Cicero devoted very heavily to the discussion on justice. Justice, according to him consists of acting according to the law of nature, which is the dictate of reason. (Singh, S.: 1966)

The concept of natural rights as being derived from natural law may be traced from the Stoic philosopher Cicero who in his *De Legibus*, said, "....we are born for justice, and....right is founded not in opinion, but in nature. There is indeed a true law, right reason, agreeing with nature and diffused among all, unchanging and everlasting". (Basu: 2007).

After the end of Roman civilization chaos and conflicts had swept Europe. The authority of church became supreme. The church fathers were interested in maintenance of law and order in the society. With this end in view the natural law was given religious flavour. The Christian fathers like Ambrose, Austin and Gregory postulated the supremacy of divine law over all other laws by making the divine law the ultimate criteria of divine reason. (Singh, S.: 1966)

The natural law of the modern era was in essence different in form and spirit from that of medieval age, which was dominated by church, priests and holy Christian saints. After renaissance and reformation in the fourteenth and fifteenth centuries natural law ceased to exist to be associated with Church or Divine God.

The natural law of modern classical era was marked by its two distinctive features, first, it was more secularized, political and non-religious in form and content. The new natural law philosophy moved away from its theological or divine origin and founded it once again on human reason exclusively. Second, the medieval thinkers had made individual as mainly the object having many duties and obligations towards Pope and the Emperor. The emerging natural law in the modern era became a theory of natural right of man and state, which dominated the British, the French and American revolutions in the seventeenth and the eighteenth centuries. (Singh, Dr. Deepa: 2002)

Each state has had its own different history in relation to human rights. For example, in England, human rights are traced back to the days of King John and Magna Carta of 1215 AD. This was followed by Petition of Rights of 1627 AD and the Bill of Rights of 1688. The Declaration of Rights of Man adopted in 1789 by the French National Assembly gave recognition to the fundamental human rights which became the basic general principles of the "Constitutional Law of Civilized States." In nineteenth century human rights became a part of the law of nearly all European States and in the national constitutions of the liberated colonies which became the developing states of the Third World. Thus, formal national laws is well established almost all-over the world with varying degrees of enforceability. Thus, both international charters and national constitutions framed after Second World War have shown an increasing realization of the truth that peace within and among the nations can be lasting only if it is based on human rights and socio-economic justice. (Nagendra Singh: 1981)

Rex Martin, in his article titled, *Are Human Rights Universal*? answered in negative to this question. He referred to the distinction between natural rights and human rights on the ground that the natural rights was a doctrine of universal rights, at least of those basic moral rights that were thought to hold good in a state of nature. The United Nations of Organization accepted the Universal Declaration of Human Rights on 10th December, 1948 with the view that these were founded on morality and universal in character.

Since the later part of nineteenth century the notion of natural rights have become fragile. Martin indicated that after Second World War universal rights made a return to the center stage, first in the United Nations Charter, 1945, then in the Universal Declaration of Human Rights, 1948 followed by various international covenants and treaties. But this return is not towards old notion of natural rights. The return is a deviation from the old concept of natural rights.

Natural rights have nothing to do with the society, as they are held by a man simply because he is a human being. These rights have the orientation of good of the people irrespective of time and place. But the notion of human rights is rooted in the concept of the society. Human rights represent fundamental interests of such persons, such as personal autonomy, participation in the social institutions, practices of self-governance, security, dignity, health and well-being. It is true that the distinction between the natural rights and the human rights exists if one looks them from the social background. The idea of natural rights was conceived during pre-societal period or in the early stage of the process of evolution. Gradually, with the improvement or strengthening of the social life the contemporary notion of human rights emerged from the crude nature of natural rights. In course of time human rights are expanding with the changes of social life or the progress of human civilization.

However, it may be admitted that universalization of moral grounds or norms for human rights is difficult. While it may be possible in the case of some areas, there are several areas which remain outside the notion of universalization. It is not merely because of diversity in culture, tradition, geographical location, religion, language, education etc., it is also due to the growth of an individual from childhood to adulthood or the mental maturity of an individual which he or she gains during the span of life.

Martin argued that there is no single argument or justification for universal human rights that would be accepted as normatively sound by each one of us everywhere. His assumption is that at the initial stage the authors and the supporters of Universal Declaration believed that the rights incorporated in the UDHR had moral background, however, they identified no single moral ground or justification in support of the universal nature of these rights. Rather, the founders believed that a variety of recognized moral systems and conventional moralities would justify and support these rights either in the sense that they would overlap or converge on the UDHR set of rights or in the sense that each constituent moral system, taken on its own, or most of them would morally endorse and support the UDHR set of rights or most of them. But in any country having diversity in culture, religion, customs and traditions can provide undisputable normative ground for these rights. The concept of norm is dynamic and the members of an organized or modern society try to adjust or modify the norms according to their convenience or situation. However, it has to be admitted that the assertion on these rights by the civil society is noteworthy in the significant/fundamental human interests. Therefore, it is difficult to deny the moral authority behind the human rights incorporated in the UDHR. (Martin: 2013)

The original meaning of civil society was linked to the concept of civility. It emerged during the seventeenth and eighteenth centuries at a time when earlier ties of blood, kinship and religion were breaking down. The growth of states and the establishment of a rule of law gradually eliminated private and often violent methods of settling disputes and created the conditions for new forms of social interaction based on commonly accepted means of communication.

Civil society meant respect for individual autonomy, based on security and trust among people. It required regularity of behaviour, rules of conduct, respect for law and control of violence. It is a society in which the strangers act in a civilized way towards each other, treating each other with mutual respect, tolerance and confidence.

The theorist of civil society faced with the problem how to reconcile individual autonomy with society, how to distinguish private concerns from public realm. The answer for eighteenth century thinkers was that society was held together by moral sentiments and natural affections. Civil society was an ethical arena, a realm of public morality, based on individual conscience. Later, as secular morality came to supplant religious injunction, this public realm was understood to be held together by the nature, the natural tendency for affection, sympathy and friendship, and experience, the notion that natural behaviour is learned, and that through experience men come to understand that altruism behaviour sustains the public realm which is required for individual autonomy. (Kapoor: 2001)

However, the phrase 'civil society' has a range of meanings in contemporary usage. It is sometimes considered to include the family and the private sphere, and referred to as the 'third sector' of society distinct from Government and business.

The civil society concept goes back to Aristotle's phrase, "*koinonia politke*" appeared in his "Politics" where it means, a "community", commensurate with the Greek city-state (polis) characterized by a shared norms and ethos, in which free citizens on an equal footing lived under the rule of law. The end of civil society was common well-being.

The literature on relations between civil society and democratic political society have their roots in early classical liberal writings like those of Alexis de Tocqueville. However, they were developed in a significant way by twentieth century theorists like Gabriel Almond and Sidney Verba, who identified the role of political culture in a democratic order as vital.

More recently, Robert D. Putnam has argued that even non-political organizations are vital in Democracy, this is because they build social capital, trust and shared values which are transferred into political sphere and help to hold society together facilitating understanding of interconnectedness of society and interests in it.

(en.wikipedia.org/wiki.civil_society)

Relationship between Ethics and Human Rights: The interdependence of human rights and ethical principles is an undeniable fact. The ethical principles constitute a strong device to safeguard human rights while laws of a country can create an environment for generating inner power to realize the strength and significance of these principles in the global human family. The tragic events, worst and violent situations faced by different nations in the path of progress of human civilization create confusion in the minds of the people making them frustrated and indecisive to confirm their faith on the human power and to adopt ethical or moral principles in his way of life. The progress of science and technology helps the indecisive man to move from the stage of indecisiveness towards acquiring decision making power to stabilize his shaky mind and he tries to confirm his belief on the irrelevance of moral or ethical principles in the modern civilization or his modern way of life. But we must remember that unless the use of scientific products are directed by human power for the service to humanity the safeguard of human rights will remain as a slogan only causing severe damage to humanity itself. Human rights may also be considered as a very strong thread to unite different nations in the world, different communities in a nation, different families in a community and different members within the same family passing through different multicolour social cultures.

The World Medical Association has pointed out that in the recent times medical ethics has been generally influenced by the development of human rights. In a pluralistic and multicultural world, with many different moral traditions, the major international human rights agreements can provide a foundation for medical ethics that is acceptable across national and cultural boundaries. Kofi Annan said, "In the twentyfirst century I believe that the mission of the United Nations will be defined by a new, more profound awareness of the sanctity and dignity of every human life, regardless of race or religion. This will require us to look beyond the framework of states and beneath the surface of nations and communities. We must focus, as never before, on improving the conditions of the individual men and women who give the state or nation its richness and character" (Kofi Annan: 2002).

Shirin Abadi, the winner of Nobel Peace prize also said, "People are different, and so are their cultures; people live in different ways, and civilizations also differ; people speak in a variety of languages; people are guided by different religions; people are born with different colours, and many traditions influence their lives with varying colours and shades; people dress differently and adapt to their environment in different ways; people express themselves differently. Music, literature and art reflect different styles as well; But despite these differences, all people have one single common attribute: they are all human beings—nothing more, nothing less. And however different they may be all cultures embrace certain common principles. No culture tolerates the exploitation of human beings. No religion allows the killing of the innocent. No civilization accepts violence or terror. Torture is abhorrent to the human conscience. Brutality and cruelty are appalling in every tradition.

In short, these common principles, which are shared by all civilizations, reflect our fundamental human rights. These rights are treasured by everyone, everywhere.

So, cultural relativity should never be used as a pretext to violate human rights, since these rights embody most fundamental values of human civilizations. The Universal Declaration of Human Rights is needed universally, applicable to both East and West. It is compatible with every faith and religion. Failing to respect our human rights only undermines our humanity. Let us not destroy this fundamental truth; if we do, the weak will have nowhere to turn." (Shirin Abadi: 2002)

Evolution of Human Rights: As stated above the concept of human rights is rooted in the beginning of human civilization. In the journey of human civilization people acquired rights and responsibilities through their membership in a group—a family, indigenous nation, religion, class, community, or state. The Hindu *Vedas*, the Babylonian Code of Hammurabi, the Bible, the Quran, and the Analects of Confucius are five of the oldest written sources which address questions of people's duties, rights and responsibilities. In addition, the Inca and Aztec Codes of conduct and justice and an Iroquois Constitution were Naïve American sources that existed well before the eighteenth century. In fact all societies, whether in oral or written tradition, have had systems of propriety and justice as well as ways of tending to the health and welfare of their members.

Precursors of Twentieth Century Human Rights Documents: Documents asserting individual rights, such as the Magna Carta (1215), the English Bill of Rights (1689), the French Declaration of the Rights of Man and Citizen (1789), and the US Constitution and Bill of Rights (1791) are the written precursors to many of today's human rights documents. Yet many of these documents, when originally translated into policy, excluded women, people of colour and members of certain social, religious, economic, and political groups. Nevertheless, oppressed people throughout the world have drawn on the principles these documents express to support revolutions that assert the right to self-determination.

Contemporary international human rights law and the establishment of the United Nations (UN) have important historical antecedents. Efforts in the nineteenth century to prohibit the slave trade and to limit the horrors of war are prime examples. In 1919, countries established the International Labour Organization (ILO) to oversee treaties protecting workers with respect to their rights, including their health and safety. Concern over the protection of certain minority groups was raised by the League of Nations at the end of the First World War. However, this organization for international peace and cooperation, created by the victorious European allies, never achieved its goals. The League floundered because the United States refused to join, failure of the League to prevent Japan's invasion of China and Manchuria (1931) and Italy's attack on Ethiopia (1935).

Ultimately with the outbreak of the Second World War League disappeared.

The idea of human rights emerged stronger after Second World War. The extermination by Nazi Germany of over six million Jews, Sinti and Romani (gypsies), homosexuals and persons with disabilities horrified the world. Trials were held in Nuremburg and Tokyo after Second World War and officials from defeated countries were punished for committing war crimes.

United Nations of Organization and Human Rights: The First World War of 1914-1919 resulted human tragedy which was never occurred before in the history of human civilization. A.C. Roy has given an account of the major loss caused by the war as, "the loss of life involved in the war had been twice the number of the total number of deaths involved in the previous wars occurred during the period between 1790-1913. The war of 1914 and 1918 had involved a mobilization of 65 million men of whom 13 million had died in actual war or of injuries and 7 million were crippled and disabled, the destruction on both sides were so extensive that distinction between the combatants and non-combatants was completely vanished. Two-thirds of the world population were affected by this war. It has not yet been possible to ascertain definitely the exact loss of property. The death rate of the civilian was much greater than that of the military personnel and that was due to famine, epidemics, raids and indiscriminate attacks of both belligerents. In a word, in its scope and intensity, in the scale of destruction and in the involvement of every national interest, the First World War was certainly unprecedented" (Roy: 1991).

The violent nature of the First World War was a serious threat to the nations of the world. Untold miseries of the people compelled the world community to give a serious thought to explore ways of establishing peace and cooperation amongst nations (Anand: 2001).

In the beginning of 1919, the representatives of large number of nations of the world assembled at Paris to finalize the Peace Treaty. But the right of representation to the conference was closed to Germany, Austria, Hungary, Turkey and Bulgaria. Among the representatives who were present in the Conference were President Woodrow Wilson of America, the British Prime Minister Lloyd George, the French Foreign Minister George Clemenceau and the Italian Prime Minister Vitoria Orlando, an ex-Professor of Political Philosophy at Princeton, a brilliant orator, an idealist and a man of rigid convictions, Woodrow Wilson assumed a significant role in the conference. In spite of several constraints, such as lack of well-defined principles, conflicting interests of different states, ideological differences among the leaders etc. the League of Nations was formed on the basis of the last point of the fourteen points of US President Woodrow Wilson in January 1920.

On 8th January, 1918, Wilson analyzed his "Fourteen Points" as the basis of world peace in the US Congress. His last point was, "an international organization shall be established affording mutual guarantees of political sovereignty and territorial integrity of all powers and strong or weak." In conclusion Wilson said, "An evident principle runs through the whole programme I have outlined. It is the principle of justice to all people and nationalities and their right to live on equal terms of liberty and safety with one another, whether strong or weak". But The League of Nations failed due to aggressive attitude of Japan, Italy and Germany and non-involvement of other nations resulting break-up of Second World War in 1939. (Roy: 1991)

Attempts to establish an international organization for establishing peace and security in the world began even before the end of the Second World War. As early as in 1941, attempts were made to form an international organization. The London Declaration of 12th June, 1941 may be identified as the first formal attempt to establish such an organization when all the nations fighting against Hitler expressed their willingness to create a world free of wars and based on social and economic equality. This was followed by the Atlantic Charter of 14th August, 1941 with the aim of establishing peace and security through an international organization. On 1st January, 1942 the Axis – Coalition of twenty six countries assembled in Washington and endorsed the decision of the Atlantic Charter and there US President Franklin Roosevelt coined the term "United Nations" to indicate the unity of allied powers with an aim of fighting against common enemy. It also emphasized the need to move towards world peace.

On 30th October, 1943, Britain, United States, and Soviet Union expressed in Moscow the need of creating an international organization based on the principle of equality of all peace loving states. On 1st December, 1943, the Tehran Conference was held with the purpose of securing cooperation and active participation of all nations. A significant step was taken when a Great Power Conference was held in 1944 at Dumbarton Oaks near Washington at the initiative of United States. The conference took place for three months from August to October. It prepared a draft of the Charter of the United Nations. After several rounds of discussion and conferences the draft Charter was signed by fifty one

States on 26th June, 1945 in San Francisco, USA and it was ratified by States' Parliaments and ultimately on 24th October, 1945, the United Nations of Organization was created with the aim of establishing peace and security in the world.

The Charter of UN promised to "reaffirm faith in fundamental human rights, in the dignity and worth of the human person, in the equal rights of men and women and of nations large and small.....and to promote social progress and better standards of life in larger freedom." (Chatterjee: 2010) In fact, the United Nations of Organization's basic objective is to establish an international commitment to protect human rights of the members of the global human family. This enthused the United Nations to adopt the Declaration of Human Rights on 10th December, 1948 as below:

Universal Declaration of Human Rights, 1948

Preamble: Whereas recognition of the inherent dignity and of the equal and inalienable rights of all members of the human family is the foundation of freedom, justice and peace in the world;

Whereas disregard and contempt for human rights have resulted in barbarous acts which have outraged the conscience of mankind, and the advent of a world in which human beings shall enjoy freedom of speech and belief and freedom from fear and want has been proclaimed as the highest aspiration of the common people;

Whereas it is essential, if man is not to be compelled to have recourse, as a last resort, to rebellion against tyranny and oppression, that human rights should be protected by the rule of law;

Whereas it is essential to promote the development of friendly relationship between nations;

Whereas the peoples of the United Nations have in the Charter reaffirmed their faith in fundamental human rights, in the dignity and worth of the human person and in the equal rights of men and women and have determined to promote social progress and better standards of life in large freedom;

Whereas Member States have pledged themselves to achieve, in cooperation with the United Nations, the promotion of universal respect for and observance of human rights and fundamental freedoms;

Whereas a common understanding of these rights and freedoms is of the greatest importance for the full realization of this pledge;

Now, therefore,

The General Assembly,

Proclaims the Universal Declaration of Human Rights as a common standard of achievement for all peoples and all nations, to the end that every individual and every organ of society, keeping this Declaration constantly in mind, shall strive by teaching and education to promote respect for these rights and freedoms and by progressive measures, national and international, to secure their universal and effective recognition and observance, both among the peoples of member states themselves and among the peoples of territories under their jurisdiction.

ARTICLE 1:

All human beings are born free and equal in dignity and rights. They are endowed with reasons and conscience and should act towards one another in a spirit of brotherhood.

ARTICLE 2:

Everyone is entitled to all the rights and freedoms set forth in this Declaration, without distinct of any kind, such as race, colour, sex, language, religion, political or other opinion, national or social origin, property, birth or other status.

Furthermore, no distinction shall be made on the basis of the political, jurisdictional or international status of the country or territory to which a person belongs, whether it be independent, trust, non-self-governing or under any other limitation of sovereignty.

ARTICLE 3:

Everyone has the right to life, liberty and security of person.

ARTICLE 4:

No one shall be held in slavery or servitude; slavery and the slave trade shall be prohibited in all their forms.

ARTICLE 5:

No one shall be subjected to torture or to cruel, inhuman or degrading treatment or punishment.

ARTICLE 6:

Everyone has the right to recognition everywhere as a person before the law.

ARTICLE 7:

All are equal before the law and are entitled without any discrimination to equal protection of the law. All are entitled to equal protection against any discrimination in violation of this Declaration and against any incitement to such discrimination.

ARTICLE 8:

Everyone has the right to an effective remedy by the competent national tribunals for acts violating the fundamental rights granted him by the constitution or by law.

ARTICLE 9:

No one shall be subjected to arbitrary arrest, detention or exile.

ARTICLE 10:

Everyone is entitled in full equality to a fair and public hearing by an independent and impartial tribunal, in the determination of his rights and obligations and of any criminal charge against him.

ARTICLE 11:

1. Everyone charged with a penal offence has the right to be presumed innocent until proved guilty according to law in a public trial at which he has had all the guarantees necessary for his defence.
2. No one shall be held guilty of any penal offence on account of any act or omission which did not constitute a penal offence, under national or international law, at the time when it was committed. Nor shall a heavier penalty be imposed than the one that was applicable and at the time the penal offence was committed.

ARTICLE 12:

No one should be subjected to arbitrary interference with his privacy, family, home or correspondence, nor to attack upon his honour and reputation. Everyone has the right to the protection of the law against such interference or attacks.

ARTICLE 13:

1. Everyone has the right to freedom of movement and residence with the border of each state.
2. Everyone has the right to leave any country, including his own, and to return to his country.

ARTICLE 14:

1. Everyone has the right to seek and to enjoy in other countries asylum from prosecution.
2. This right may be invoked in the case of prosecution genuinely arising from non-political crimes or from acts contrary to the purpose and principles of the United Nations.

ARTICLE 15:

1. Everyone has the right to a nationality.

2. No one shall be arbitrarily deprived of his nationality nor denied the rights to change his nationality.

ARTICLE 16:

1. Men and women of full age, without any limitation of race, nationality or religion, have the right to marry and to found a family. They are entitled to equal rights as to marriage, during marriage and at its dissolution.
2. Marriage shall be entered into only with the free and full consent of the intending spouses.
3. The family is the natural and fundamental group unit of the society and is entitled to protection by society and the State.

ARTICLE 17:

1. Everyone has the right to own property alone as well as in association with others.
2. No one shall be arbitrarily deprived of his property.

ARTICLE 18:

Everyone has the right to freedom of thought, conscience and religion; this right includes freedom to change his religion or belief, and freedom, either alone or in community with others and in-public or private, to manifest his religion or belief in teaching, practice, worship and observance.

ARTICLE 19:

Everyone has the right to freedom of opinion and expression; this right includes freedom to hold opinions without interference and to seek, receive and impart information and ideas through any media and regardless of frontiers.

ARTICLE 20:

1. Everyone has the right to freedom of peaceful assembly and association.
2. No one may be compelled to belong to an association.

ARTICLE 21:

1. Everyone has the right to take part in the government of his country, directly or freely chosen representatives.
2. Everyone has the right to equal access to public service in his country.
3. The will of the people shall be the basis of the authority of government; this will shall be expressed in periodic and genuine elections which shall be by universal and equal suffrage and shall be held by secret vote or by equivalent free voting procedures.

ARTICLE 22:

Everyone, as a member of the society, has the right to social security and is entitled to realization, through national efforts and international cooperation and in accordance with the organization and resources of each State, of the economic, social and cultural rights indispensable for its dignity and the free development of his personality.

ARTICLE 23:

1. Everyone has the right to work, to free choice of employment, to just and favourable condition of work and protection against unemployment.
2. Everyone, without any discrimination, has the right to equal pay for equal work.
3. Everyone, who works has the right to just and favourable remuneration ensuring for himself and his family an existence worthy of human dignity, and supplemented, if necessary by other means of social protection.
4. Everyone has the right to form and to join trade unions for the protection of his interests.

ARTICLE 24:

Everyone has the right to rest and leisure, including reasonable limitation or working hours and periodic holidays with pay.

ARTICLE 25:

1. Everyone has the right to standard of living adequate for the health and well-being of himself and his family, including food, clothing, housing, and medical care and necessary social service, and the right to security in the event of unemployment, sickness, disability, widowhood, old age or other lack of livelihood in circumstance beyond his control.
2. Motherhood and childhood are entitled to special care and assistance. All children, whether born in or out of wedlock, shall enjoy the same social protection.

ARTICLE 26:

1. Everyone has the right to education. Education shall be free, at least in the elementary and fundamental stages. Elementary education shall be compulsory. Technical and professional education shall be made generally available and higher education shall be equally accessible to all the basis of merit.
2. Education shall be directed to the full development of the

human personality and to the strengthening of respect for human rights and fundamental freedoms. It shall promote understanding, tolerance and friendship among all nations, racial or religious groups, and shall further the activities of the United Nations for the maintenance of peace.

3. Parents have a prior right to choose the kind of education that shall be given to their children.

ARTICLE 27:

1. Everyone has the right freely to participate in the cultural life of the community, to enjoy the arts and to share in scientific advancement and its benefits.
2. Everyone has the right to the protection of the moral and material interest resulting from any scientific, literary or artistic production of which he is the author.

ARTICLE 28:

Everyone is entitled to a social and international order in which the rights and freedoms set forth in this Declaration can be fully realized.

ARTICLE 29:

1. Everyone has duties to the community in which alone the free and full development of his personality in possible.
2. In the exercise of his rights and freedoms, everyone shall be subject only to such limitations as are determined by law solely for the purpose of securing due recognition and respects for the rights and freedom of others and of meeting the just requirement of morality, public order and the general welfare in a democratic society.
3. These rights and freedom may in no case be exercised contrary to the purpose and principles of the United Nations.

ARTICLE 30:

Nothing in this Declaration may be interpreted as implying for any State, group of person any right to engage in any activity or to perform any act aimed at the destruction of any of the rights and freedoms set forth herein.

Thus, it is found that the process of internationalization of human rights is rooted in the formation of League of Nations at the end of First World War. The second step was taken by the world community before the end of Second World War by forming the United Nations of Organization. The specific declaration on human rights was found with the adoption of Universal Declaration of Human Rights, which was drafted by Nobel Peace Prize Winner Rene Cassin on 10th December, 1948. This Declaration may be said as the guarantor of human dignity to develop and use of human qualities, intelligence, talents, social, and spiritual needs of individuals.

The International Conference on Human Rights held at Tehran in 1968 may be considered as a significant stepping stone for promotion of human rights. The conference was a call on all states to ensure that "all means of education" should be used in stimulating interest in the safeguard of human rights in the wave of changes in the world. The United Nations in the same year appealed to the member states to introduce and encourage the principles of the UN Declaration of Human Rights and other Declarations. Thus, UN has taken steps in fostering its global efforts for promotion of social justice and human rights.

UNESCO in its recommendations relating to human rights underlined the need of understanding and respect for all peoples culture, civilization, values and ways of the life and strengthening of struggles against all forms of racialism, fascism and apartheid.

On 19th December, 2011, UN General Assembly adopted Declaration on Human Rights Education and Training in New York. This landmark document recognizes the right of every one of the planet's seven billion people to have access to human rights education, a lifelong process involving all ages, all parts of society, and every kind of education, formal and informal.

The Declaration satisfies not simply what one should learn about human rights, but also how ("through human rights, which includes learning and teaching in that respects the rights of both educators and the learners") and also why ("for human rights, which includes empowering persons to enjoy and exercise their rights and to respect and uphold the rights of others.").

The adoption of this new Declaration also offers educators and policy makers an occasion to reassess national policies and priorities in the light of international standards. If as the Declaration states, "human rights education and training is essential for the promotion of universal respect for and observance of all human rights and fundamental freedoms for all", then human rights education is not only the entitlement of every human being, but also a necessity for responsible global citizenship."

(http:/www.hrea.org/index.php?doc_id=1808, 6.12.2014)

In June 1993, when UN World Conference on Human Rights was held in Vienna (Austria), there was unprecedented gathering of participants—about 7000 participants representing 171 states and many national, international bodies and NGOs. It had a very wide perspective while making recommendations on human rights and fundamental freedom. It appealed to all states and institutions to include human rights, humanitarian laws, democracy and rule of law to the curricula of all learning institutions in formal and non-formal settings. Human rights education must include peace, democracy, development and social justice. (Vij: 2000)

The World Conference on Human Rights in the Vienna Declaration and Programme of Action (1993) stated that human rights education, training and public information were essential for the promotion and achievement of stable and harmonious relations among communities and for fostering mutual understanding, tolerance and peace. The Conference recommended that States should strive to eradicate illiteracy and should direct education towards the full development of human personality and the strengthening of respect for human rights, humanitarian law, democracy and rule of law as subjects in the curricula of all learning institutions in formal and non-formal settings.

It was followed by the Proclamation of UN Decade for Human Rights Education on 23rd December, 1994. The proclamation of the General Assembly goes as:

> Guided by the fundamental and universal principles enshrined in the Charter of the United Nations and the Universal Declaration of Human Rights;
> Reaffirming article 26 of the Universal Declaration of Human Rights, according to which "education shall be directed to the full development of the human personality and to the strengthening of respect for human rights and fundamental freedoms";
> Recalling the provisions of other international human rights instruments, such as those of article 13 of the International Covenant on Economic, Social and Cultural Rights and article 28 of the Convention on the Rights of the child, that reflect the aims of the aforementioned article;
> Taking into account Commission on Human Rights Resolution;

Resolution 1993/56 of 9th March, 1993, in which the Commission recommended that knowledge of human rights, both in its theoretical dimension and in its practical application, should be established as a priority in education policies;

Considering Commission on Human Rights Resolution 1994/51 of 4th March, in which the Commission encouraged the United Nations High Commissioner for Human Rights to include among his specific objectives a plan of action for the United Nations decade for human rights education and invited the Secretary-General to submit to the General Assembly at its forty-ninth session, through the Economic and Social Council, a plan of action for a decade for human rights education;

Convinced that human rights education should involve more than the provision of information and should constitute a comprehensive life-long process by which people at all levels in development and in all strata of society learn respect for the dignity of others and the means and methods of ensuring that respect in all societies;

Convinced also that human rights education contributes to a concept of development consistent with the dignity of women and men of all ages that takes into account diverse segments of society, such as children, indigenous peoples, minorities and disabled persons;

Taking into account the efforts to promote human rights education made by educators and non-governmental organizations in all parts of the world, as well as by intergovernmental organizations, including the United Nations Educational, Scientific and Cultural Organization, the International Labour Organization and the United Nations Children's Fund;

Convinced that each woman, man and child, to realize their full human potential, must be made aware of all their human rights—civil, cultural, economic, political and social:

> Believing that human rights education constitutes an important vehicle for the elimination of gender-based discrimination and ensuring equal opportunities through the promotion and protection of the human rights of women;
>
> Considering the World Plan of Action on Education for Human Rights and Democracy convened by the United Nations Educational, Scientific and Cultural Organization at Montreal from 8th to 11th March, 1993, according to which education for human rights and democracy is itself a human right and prerequisite for the realization of human rights, democracy and social justice;
>
> Recalling that it is the responsibility of the United Nations High

Commissioner for Human Rights to coordinate relevant United Nations Education and Public Information programmes in the field of human rights;

Taking note of the report of the United Nations High Commissioner for Human Rights, in paragraph 94 of which he declared that human rights education is essential for the encouragement of harmonious inter-community relations for mutual tolerance and understanding and finally for peace;

Aware of the experience in human rights education of United Nations peace-building operations, including the United Nations Observer Mission in El Salvador and the United Nations Transitional Authority in Cambodia;

Bearing in mind the Vienna Declaration and the Programme of Action, adopted by the World Conference on Human Rights on 25th June, 1993, in particular section II, paragraphs 78 to 82 thereof:

- Takes note with appreciation of the report of the Secretary General on human rights education, submitted in accordance with the request contained in the General Assembly resolution 48.127 of 20th December, 1993;
- Proclaims the ten-year period beginning on 1st January, 1995, the United Nations Decade for Human Rights Education;
- Welcomes the Plan of Action for the United Nations Decade for Human Rights Education, 1995-2005, as contained in the report of the Secretary General, and invites Governments to submit comments, with a view to supplementing the Plan of Action;
- Invites the Secretary General to submit proposals, taking into account the views expressed by Governments, for the purpose indicated in paragraph 3;
- Appeals to all Governments to contribute to the implementation of the Plan of Action and to step up their efforts to eradicate illiteracy and to direct education towards the full development of the human personality and to the strengthening of respect for human rights and fundamental freedoms;
- Urges governmental and non-governmental educational agencies to intensify their efforts to establish and implement programmes of human rights education, as recommended in the Plan of Action, in particular by preparing and implementing national plans for human rights education;
- Requests the United Nations High Commissioner for Human

Rights to coordinate the implementation of the Plan of Action;

- Requests the Centre for Human Rights of the Secretariat and the Commission on Human Rights, in cooperation with member states, human rights treaty-monitoring bodies, other appropriate bodies and competent non-governmental organizations, to support efforts of the United Nations High Commissioner for Human Rights to coordinate the Plan of Action;
- Requests the Secretary General to consider establishing a voluntary fund for human rights education, with special provision for the support of the human rights education activities of non-governmental organizations, to be administered by the Centre for Human Rights;
- Invites the specialized agencies and United Nations programmes to contribute, within their respective spheres of competence, to the implementation of the Plan of Action;
- Requests the Secretary General to bring the present resolution to the attention of all members of the international community and to intergovernmental and non-governmental organizations concerned with human rights and education;
- Calls upon international, regional and national non-governmental organizations, in particular those concerned with women, labour, development and the environment, as well as all other social justice groups, human rights advocates, educators, religious organizations and the media, to increase their cooperation with the Centre for Human Rights in implementing the United Nations Decade for Human Rights Education;
- Requests the existing human rights monitoring bodies to place emphasis on the implementation by member states of their international obligation to promote human rights education; Decides to consider this matter at its fiftieth session under the item entitled, "Human Rights Education".

(http:/www.un.org/documents/ga/res/49/a49r184.htm 6.12.2014)

On 19th December, 2011, UN General Assembly adopted Declaration on Human Rights Education and Training in New York. "This landmark document recognizes the right of everyone of the planet's seven billion people to have access to human rights education, a lifelong process involving all ages, all parts of society, and every kind of education, formal and informal.

The Declaration satisfies not simply what one should learn about human rights, but also how and why.

The adoption of this new Declaration also offers educators and policy makers an occasion to reassess national policies and priorities in the light of international standards. If as the Declaration states, "human rights education and training is essential for the promotion of universal respect for and observance of all human rights and fundamental freedoms for all, then human rights education is not only the entitlement of every human being, but also a necessity for responsible global citizenship."

(http:/www.hrea.org/index.php?doc_id=1808, 6.12.2014).

The institutional development in human rights took place with the beginning of international multilateral treaty regime with appropriate monitoring mechanisms. Before the World Conference on Human Rights which was held at Teheran no human rights treaty body existed. By the time of the World Conference at Vienna, several treaty bodies had come up under seven treaties, such as—The International Covenant on Civil and Political Rights, 1977; The International Covenant on Economic, Social and Cultural Rights, 1966; The Convention on the Elimination of all Forms of Racial Discrimination, 1966; The Convention on the Suppression and Punishment of the Crime of Apartheid, 1973; The Convention on the Elimination of Discrimination against Torture, and the Convention on the Rights of the Child, 1989.

These are Universal treaties, the sense that they are open to all States. At the center stands the International Covenant on Civil and Political Rights, with its detailed provisions and rather substantive monitoring procedures. The Covenant on Economic, Social and Cultural Rights has also developed monitoring procedures—in part modeled on the committee under the Civil and Political Covenant, and in part fashioned for their own separate needs. (Bakshi: 2004)

With the goal of establishing mechanisms for enforcing the UDHR, the UN Commission on human rights proceeded to draft two treaties: The International Covenant on Civil and Political Rights (ICCPR) and its Optional Protocol and the International Covenant on Economic, Social and Cultural Rights (ICESCR). Together with the Universal Declaration, they are commonly referred to as the International Bill of Human Rights. The ICCPR focuses on such issues as the right to life, freedom of speech, religion and voting. The ECESCR focuses on such issues as food, education, health and shelter.

In addition to the Covenants in the International Bill of Human Rights, the United Nations has adopted more than 20 principal treaties further elaborating human rights. These include conventions to prevent and

prohibit specific abuses like torture and genocide and to protect especially vulnerable populations, such as refugees, women etc.
(http:www1.umn.edu/humanrts/edumat/hreduseries/hereandnow/Part-1/short-history.htm, 27.8.2004)

It is found that the concept of human rights originated in different backgrounds and orientations. In western countries, it had right orientation while in the east it had duty orientation. In the ancient world the people had bitter experience of social life. Each city-state consisted of more slaves than free persons. In the east it had duty orientation.

Evolution of Human Rights in India: Since Indus Valley Civilization, the Indian culture has been the product of syntheses of diverse cultures and religions that came into the contact with enormous Indian sub-continent over time (Nehru: 1946).

Indian culture perceives the individual, the society and the universe as an organic whole; everyone is the child of God, and all fellow-beings are related to one another, belonging to a universal family. Religious prayers would ask of God to make all peoples of the world happy. An ancient text runs thus: "I seek no Kingdom, nor Heaven nor rebirth, but I wish that all living beings be spared of the manifold pains and distress."

"In fact, the Buddha doctrine of non-violence in deed and thought" says Nagendra Singh, "is a humanitarian doctrine par excellence, dating back to the third century B.C." According to the *Gita*, "he who has no ill will to any being, who is friendly and compassionate, free from egoism and self-sense, even-minded in pain and pleasure and patient" is dear to God. It also says that the divinity in humans is represented by the qualities of "non-violence, truth, freedom from anger, renunciation, aversion to fault finding, compassion to living beings, freedom from covetousness, gentleness, modesty and steadiness, that a good human being ought to have."

Nagendra Singh believes that the individual in ancient India existed as a citizen of the state and in that capacity he had both rights and obligations. These rights and duties have largely been expressed in terms of duties (*Dharma*)—duties to oneself, to a family, to other fellowmen, to the society and the world at large. The *Karmayoga* chapter in the *Gita* expounds the necessity for the performance of work without selfish attachment to results, with a view to securing the welfare of the world. If inter-individuals and social relations are expressed in terms of comprehensive web of duties, rights cease to be privileges to be specifically claimed, but a condition that would promote human, and hence social welfare. Hence Kautilya prescribed not powers, but "duties of a

King". One of the King's duties was: "when in court he shall never cause his petitioners to wait at the door." One of the ground rules for the King was: "In the happiness of his subjects lies his happiness; in their welfare, his welfare; whatever pleases himself he shall not consider as good, but whatever pleases his subjects he shall consider as good" (IWCOHR: 1997).

Rekha Bhardwaj, in her article, *Significance of Scriptures in Highlighting Human Rights*, pointed out that the *Vedas* constitute a unique document of the religious consciousness of the human race, urging it to contain ideals, principles and teachings for the welfare of humanity. The *Upanishads* are known as the *Vedantas* or the end of the Vedas because they represent the culmination of *Vedic* teachings, i.e. to imbibe ourselves with the feeling of brotherhood (Bhardwaj: 2000).

Referring to the existence of caste system in India, it is said in the study report of IWCOHR that it arose from the principle of division of labour as method of social organization. The caste system encompassed *Brahmins* (the priestly or teacher class), *Kshatriyas* (ruling class or nobles), *Vaishyas* (the tradesmen, agriculturists) and *shudras* (unskilled workers). As the *Gita* says, "the fourfold order was created by Me according to the divisions of quality and work". Radhakrishnan points out, "The emphasis is on *Guna* (aptitude) and *Karma* (function) and not on *Jati* (birth). The *Varna* or the order to which we belong is independent of sex, birth or breeding. A caste determined by temperament and vocation is not a caste determined by birth and hereditary. According to *Mahabharata,* the whole world was originally one class but later it became divided into four divisions on account of the specific duties.

The historical responses came from Buddhism and Jainism both of which emphasized on the principles of equality, non-violence and denial of materialistic pleasures. The advent of the Muslim rulers from the north brought with them teachings of Islam. This historical process of synthesis aided by enlightened reformers, and great Kings like Asoka and Akbar, now forms the foundation of the Indian culture. On it stands the coexistence and mutual respect for diverse religious and philosophical beliefs. (ICWOHR: 1997)

The Indian National Congress which was formed under the leadership of A.O. Hume in December 1885 hoped that the British Government would create an environment in which the Congress would be able to improve the social, economic and political conditions of India. In the beginning of the twentieth century, the freedom fighter, Lokmanya Bal Gangadhar Tilak declared "*Swaraj*" (self-rule) is my birth right and I will have it." During the First World War though the Indians helped the British Government to a grreat extent it was not reciprocated by the British with due recognition. Therefore, when President Woodrow Wilson of America enunciated his famous right of self-determination for the oppressed nationalities, Lokamanya Tilak took the opportunity and submitted a memorandum to the Paris Peace Conference in 1919 demanding the right to self-determination for the people of India because under the foreign rule no Fundamental rights could be enjoyed. This act of Tilak inspired Mahatma Gandhi to prepare a programme of Non-Cooperation in 1920.

Motilal Nehru, the leader of the *Swaraj* Party in the Central Legislative Assembly constantly demanded formation of a Constituent Assembly to draft a Constitution of India. The Indian thought was also influenced by the Constitution of the Irish Free State framed in 1921 which incorporated a Bill of Rights.

The Commonwealth of India Bill, drafted by the National Convention under the inspiration of Annie Besant in 1925 embodied a declaration of rights almost similar to the provisions of the Irish Constitution. Within two years of the publication of the Commonwealth of India Bill came the announcement of the appointment of the Indian Statutory (Simon) Commission. In the forty-third session of Indian National Congress, a resolution was taken to set-up a Committee to draft a *Swaraj* Constitution for India on the basis of the declaration of rights.Accordingly a committee was constituted with Motilal Nehru as its Chairman. Jawaharlal Nehru was its Secretary. There were nine other members in the committee. The committee submitted a report to Simon Commission signed by Motilal Nehru, Ali Iman, Tej Bahadur Sapru, M.S. Aney, Mangal Singh, S. Qureshi, Shubhas Ch. Bose and G.R. Pradhan. The committee demanded in the report the right of Indians to draft their own constitution. It forwarded two arguments in support of its report—the conditions in Ireland before the treaty were almost close to that of India, as the country's first concern was to secure fundamental rights to the people of the country which had been denied to them. Secondly, to inculcate the sense of security amongst the minorities.

But, the British Government did not honour the demand of the Indian people. The Simon Commission observed, "Abstract declarations are useless unless there exists the will and the means to make them effective."

The Joint Parliamentary Committee on the Government of India Bill, 1935 endorsed the observations of the Simon Commission on the demand for a constitutional guarantee of Fundamental Rights to subjects of British India. The rulers of Indian States did not agree to grant any functional rights to the people of their States. The Committee, however, conceded that the there were some legally recognized principles which could be included in the new Constitution. Accordingly, the Government of India

Act, 1935 conferred certain rights and forms of protection on British subjects in India.

In 1939, the Second World War broke out and in 1942 the Indian National Congress under the inspiration of Mahatma Gandhi launched the Quit India Movement. With the end of Second World War the issue of granting Independence to India and conferring certain Fundamental Rights was reopened.

The Cabinet Mission Plan conceded the demand for the Constituent Assembly as well as the need for a written guarantee of fundamental rights in the Constitution of India. It recommended the appointment of an Advisory Committee on the Rights of Citizens, Minorities and Tribal and Excluded Areas, containing the interests affected, which would prepare a list of fundamental rights. It also recommended the constitution of an Advisory Committee. The subject of fundamental rights and its incorporation in the Constitution of India was discussed in detail by the Sapru Committee under the chairmanship of Tej Bahadur Sapru in 1945.

The Objectives Resolution moved by Pandit Jawaharlal Nehru was adopted by the Constituent Assembly on 22nd January, 1947. Two days after adoption of the Objectives Resolution introduced by Jawaharlal Nehru, the Constituent Assembly elected an Advisory Committee for reporting on fundamental rights and other matters. The Advisory Committee was constituted on 12th February, 1947 with 54 members and Sardar Vallabhbhai Patel was its Chairman. (Agarwal: 1986)

The first meeting of the Advisory Committee of the Constituent Assembly on fundamental rights, rights of minorities was held on 27th February, 1947. Vallabhbhai Patel was unanimously elected chairman of the committee. The Committee appointed five subcommittees including one on fundamental rights. After examining various drafts on fundamental rights placed before it the committee prepared its report (Shiva Rao).

The Constitution of India has provided for fundamental rights of the citizens of India and the Directive Principles of State Policy. The Constitution of India included two chapters—Chapter III and Chapter IV dealing with the Fundamental Rights and the Directive Principles of State Policy. The Constitution (Forty Second Amendment) Act, 1976 inserted Duties, a new Chapter, Part IV A containing Fundamental Duties which are covered by Article 51 A.

Fundamental Rights are as follows:

The Right to Equality
The Right to Freedom

The Right against Exploitation
The Right to Freedom of Religion
Cultural and Educational Rights
Right to Constitutional Remedies. (Kapur: 1989)

Fundamental Duties are:

- To abide by the Constitution of and respect its ideals and institutions, the National Flag and the National Anthem.
- To cherish and follow the noble ideals which inspired our national struggle for freedom.
- To uphold and protect the sovereignty, unity and integrity of India.
- To defend the country and render national service when called upon to do so.
- To promote harmony and the spirit of common brotherhood amongst all the people of India transcending religions, linguistic and regional or sectional diversities, to renounce practices derogatory to the dignity of women.
- To value and preserve the rich heritage of our composite culture.
- To protect and improve the natural environment including forests, lakes, rivers and wildlife, and to have compassion for living creatures.
- To develop the scientific temper, humanism and the spirit of inquiry and reform.
- To safeguard public property and to abjure violence and
- To strive towards excellence in all spheres of individual and collective activity so that the nation constantly rises to higher levels of endeavour and achievement (Bakshi: 2004).

The Government of India passed the Protection of Human Rights Act in 1994 to provide for the constitution of a National Human Rights Commission, State Human Rights Commissions and Human Rights Courts for better protection of human rights and for matters connected therewith or incidental thereto. The functions of the National Human Rights Commission are:

- Inquire, *suo motu* or on a petition presented to it by a victim or any other person on his behalf, into complaints of—(i) violation of human rights or document thereof or (ii) negligence in prevention of such violation, by a public servant;

- Intervene in any proceeding involving any allegation of violation of human rights pending before a court with the approval of such court;
- Visit, under intimation of to the state government, any jail or any other institution under the control of the state government, where persons are detained or lodged for purposes of treatment, reformation or protection to study the living conditions of inmates and make recommendations thereon;
- Review the safeguards provided by or under the constitution or any law for the time being in force for the protection of human rights and recommended measures for their effective implementation;
- Review the factors, including acts of terrorism that inhibit the enjoyment of human rights and recommend appropriate remedial measures;
- Study treaties and other international instruments on human rights and make recommendation for their effective implementation;
- Undertake and promote research in the field of human rights;
- Spread human rights literacy among various sections of the society and promote awareness of the safeguards available for the protection of these rights through publications, media, seminars and other available means;
- Encourage the efforts of non-governmental organizations and institutions working in the field of human rights;
- Such other functions as it may consider necessary for the promotion of human rights. (Nirmal: 1999)

Rights may also be considered as limits on man's activism. His movement, activities and social relations are guided by social norms and country's laws. Whenever he crosses the limits or goes beyond his rights to act social disorder begins and people starts revolting. For example, the case of *Mahabharata* may be cited. *Kauravas* trespassed their limits and tries to deprive *Pandavas* of their rights. *Pandavas*, especially Arjuna expressed the unwillingness before Lord Krishna to fight against their relatives and *Gurus*. Krishna persuaded him to ahead to fight as it was a *Dharma Yudh* to regain rights. Krishna said, "If you will not carry on this righteous warfare, then casting away your own duty and thine honour, thou will incur sin." Today in India trespass of rights and exploration of ways to limit the duties in every field, public or private have become the routine affairs. Further, greed for money and power has dethrone love for human being from the heart of service providers. Indian culture gives importance to money and wealth for comfortable life. But it should never be acquired through unfair means, unethical deeds and unrighteous methods. Today India is experiencing all these evils compelling the common people to come out to the street for safeguarding their rights. (Jhunjhunwala ed: 2002): The tradition of giving priority to duties has been handed over to us right from the time of Manu. Indian traditions have peeped into rights and duties very minutely. Relation between the two has been given thorough pondering and discussion. From the point of view of etymology, the subject matter of action, comes under the ambit of duty. Duty predicates action. So, the word duty is used comprehensively.

A human being is not inclined to do any work devoid of some motive or interest. Right is the reward and duty is its cause or means. There can be no work without motive or purpose. Means invokes no interest if there is no desire of fruit. There is interdependence between right and duty. Right is the result and duty is the means. He who sows the seeds will have the right to harvest the crops. It is ridiculous and ironical if a person exerts his right to harvest the crops though he has never been to the fields. Today we are confronting a very strange phenomenon. To gain our right we pay little heed to our duty. We see it in the shape of strikes. If we cut the very branch on which we are sitting our fall is sure. Duty done never goes fruitless. To fight squarely for right is not essential. Do your duty and the right follows naturally.

The *Vedas*, the *Puranas* and *Smritis* make us acquainted with the ancient Indian traditions. Root or source of the *Puranas* and the *Smritis* is the *Vedas*. Vedic literature discusses the subject matter of man's duty profusely. Vedic attitude is universal and all pervasive. Personal, household, social, national and worldly duties are stressed in the *Vedas*. *Rig Veda* lays stress on pure and virtuous duty. Violence does not mean only to kill. Violence is done even when we torture, rebuke and violate the human dignity through our mind, speech and body. Greed of wealth other than your own is not your duty. It is sin rather. (Jha: 2002)

In ancient India also rights of men were not absolute. Restrictions were imposed on the rights on the basis of virtue and vice. For example reference may be made of *Atharvaveda*. In one verse of it man prays to God to bestow wealth on him in plenty because it is the means to keep the worldly activities in motion. In reality even *dharma* cannot be performed without money. Therefore, it is found that the Indian culture attaches importance to money. But at the same time it also said that wealth should not be acquired through foul means, unjust deeds and unrighteous methods. Unscrupulous ways had no place in the Indian tradition (Misra: 2002).

Part IV of the Constitution of India contains the Directive Principles of State Policy. The object of these Principles is to embody the concept of a welfare state. However, the Directive Principles do not confer any enforceable rights and their alleged breach does not invalidate a law, nor does it entitle a citizen to complain of its violation by the state so as to seek mandatory relief. The positive aspect of these principles is that these have been held to supplement fundamental rights in achieving a welfare state. These principles may also been described as the forerunners of the U.N. Convention on Right to development as an inalienable human right.

Directive Principles of State Policy incorporated in the Constitution of India are classified into three categories—

First Category

(a) Provision for adequate means of livelihood;
(b) Removal of monopolization of material resources;
(c) Non-concentration of wealth in the hands of few;
(d) Equal pay for equal work to both men and women;
(e) Securing employment for men, women and children so that their health is not undermined;
(f) Safeguarding the children and young men against exploitation and moral degradation;
(g) Taking steps to provide for work, education and public assistance in cases of unemployment, old age, sickness and disablement;
(h) Improving the conditions of work and providing material relief;
(i) Securing for all workers reasonable wages and a decent standard of life, reasonable leisure and cultural opportunities;
(j) Free and compulsory education for all children up to the age of 14 years; and
(k) To raise the standard of living and to improve public health.

Second Category

- State shall take steps to organize village Panchayats and make them powerful enough to work as units of self-government;

- To encourage cottage industries on an individual or cooperative basis in the villages;
- State shall work for the uplift of the Scheduled Castes and Scheduled Tribes by educating them and protecting their economic interests;
- State shall consider it primary duty to stop the use of intoxicating drinks and drugs except for medical purpose;
- Improvement of breeds of cattle and stop the slaughter of cows and calves;
- State shall protect the monuments and place of historic interest from destruction and disfigurement;
- The state shall take steps to separate judiciary from executive.

Third Category

- To secure international peace and security;
- To maintain good and honourable relations between nations;
- To foster respect for international law and treaty obligations;
- To encourage settlement of international disputes by arbitration and other peaceful means.

Here mention may be made of the following articles:

Article 38 provides the state to secure a social order for the promotion of welfare of the people as:

> Article 38 (i): The state shall strive to promote the welfare of the people by securing and protecting as effectively as it may a social order in which justice, social, economic and political, shall inform all the institutions of the national life.
> Article 38 (2): The state shall, in particular, strive to minimize the inequalities in income and endeavour to eliminate inequalities in status, facilities and opportunities, not only amongst the individuals but also amongst groups of people residing in different areas or engaged in different vocations.

Article 39 relates to certain principles of Policy to be followed by the state: The state shall, in particular, direct its policy towards securing:

- That the citizens, men and women equally, have the right to an adequate means of livelihood;
- That the ownership and control of the material resources of the community are so distributed as best to subserve the common good;
- The operation of economic system does not result in the concentration of wealth and means of production to the common detriment;
- That there is equal pay for equal work for both men and women;
- That the health and strength of workers, men and women, and the tender age of children are not abused and that citizens are not forced by economic necessity to enter avocations unsuited to their age and strength; and
- that children are given opportunities and facilities to develop in a healthy manner and in conditions of freedom and dignity and that childhood and youth are protected against exploitation and against moral and material abandonment.

Article 41 is related to right to work, to education and public assistance in certain cases—"The state shall within the limits of its economic capacity and development, make effective provisions for securing the right to work, to education and to public assistance in cases of unemployment, old age, sickness and disablement and other cases of undeserved want".

Article 42: "The state shall make provision for securing just and human conditions of work and for their maternity relief."

Article 47: "Impose a duty on the state to raise the level of nutrition and the standard of living and to improve public health." (Bakshi: 2002)

In the Constituent Assembly Dr. Bhim Rao Ambedkar, the Chairman of the Drafting Committee emphasized in his final speech as:

> "We must begin by acknowledging the fact that there is complete absence of two things in Indian society. One of these is equality. On the social plane, we have in India a society based on the principle of graded inequality which means elevation for some and degradation for others. On the economic plane we have a society in which there are some who have immense wealth as against many who live in abject poverty. On the 26th January, 1950, we are going to enter into a life of contradictions. In politics

> we will have equality and in social and economic life we will have inequality. In politics we will be recognizing the principle of one man one vote and one man one value. In our social and economic life, we shall, by reason of our social and economic structure, continue to deny the principle of one man one value. How long we shall continue to live this life of contradictions? How long shall we continue to deny equality in social and economic life? If we continue to deny it for long, we will do so by putting our political democracy in peril. We must remove this contradiction at the earliest possible moment or else those who suffer from inequality will blow up the structure of political democracy which this Assembly has so laboriously built up."

What is required to implement the constitution in the best interest of the nation as dreamt by the members of the Constituent Assembly is nothing, but efficient and dedicated workers with moral leadership. In this context, a very significant statement of Dr. Ambedkar may be referred as:

> "However good a constitution may be, it is sure to turn out bad because those who are called to work it, happen to be a bad lot. However bad a constitution may be, it may turn out to be good if those who are called to work it, happen to be a good lot. The working of a constitution does not depend wholly upon the nature of the constitution. The constitution can provide only the organs of State, such as the legislature, the executive and the judiciary. The factors on which the working of those organs depends are the people and the political parties they will set up as the instruments to carry out their wishes and their politics. Who can say how the people of India and their parties will behave?" (Krishna Iyer: 1995).

What was the apprehension of Dr. Ambedkar has become true. India is facing acute dearth of honest and dedicated manpower in today's India. Almost every service is crying for moral leadership. Ethical principles have been thrown out, well established Indian tradition has been distorted in the name of modernization. Bribery which is the common form of corruption is appearing as a deadly weapon to destroy India's age old human tradition. Gaps and flows of the Constitution have become convenient devices to satisfy the selfish interests of the service providers. Commitment to the cause of the nation and the goals of the Constitution of India is neither honoured nor adhered by the people. Under this situation, human rights of the people are not safe. Best way to cultivate human culture in the existing situation is to sensitize the significance of human rights education through both formal and informal ways of group life.

The aims of human rights education are:

- To strengthen respect for human rights and fundamental freedoms;
- To develop fully the human personality and the sense of human dignity;
- To promote understanding and tolerance among diverse national, ethnic, religious and linguistic groups; and
- To empower people to participate actively in social activities.

The aims of human rights education are reflected in a definition adopted by UNESCO's International Congress on Education of Human Rights and Democracy in 1993 as "Human rights education is a human right, a precondition for sustainable development, the civil, social and democracy." It was also accepted that "human rights education provide protection from discrimination, unfair treatment, undemocratic attitude, deterioration of cultural values, exploitation, bondage, human rights illiteracy, abuses of human rights at any level."

(Human Rights teaching, file:/A/Node002/network%209f amyo/ human%20Rights%20t Teaching htm.26.5.2005)

Right to Health: The Free encyclopaedia says that the right to health is the economic, social and cultural right to a universal minimum standard of health to which all individuals are entitled. The concept of a right to health has been enumerated in international agreements. The significant of them are the *Universal Declaration of Human Rights*, *International Covenant on Economic, Social and Cultural Rights* and the *Convention on the Rights of Persons with Disabilities*. However, there remains conflicting areas in the interpretation and application of the right to health due to considerations such as how to define health, what minimum entitlements are encompassed in a right to health, and which institutions are responsible for ensuring a right to health.

The Preamble of the 1946 World Health Organization (WHO) Constitution defines health broadly as "a state of complete physical, mental and social well-being and not merely the absence of disease or infirmity."

The Constitution defines the right to health as "the enjoyment of the highest attainable standard of health", and enumerates some principles of this right to health as healthy child development; equitable dissemination of medical knowledge and its benefits; and Government provided social measures to ensure adequate health.

Frank P. Grad credits the WHO Constitution as "claiming ....the full area of contemporary international public health", establishing the right to health as a "fundamental, inalienable human right" and governments cannot abridge, and are rather obliged to protect and uphold. The WHO Constitution, notably, marks the first formal demarcation of a right to health in international law.

Article 25 of the UN's Universal Declaration of Human Rights, 1948 states that "everyone has the right to a standard of living adequate for the health and well-being of himself and of his family, including food, clothing, housing and medical care and necessary social services." The Universal Declaration makes additional accommodations for security in case of physical debilitation or disability, and makes special mention of care given to those in motherhood or childhood.

The Universal Declaration of Human Rights is noted as the first international declaration of fundamental human rights, both freedoms and entitlements alike. United Nations High Commissioner for Human Rights, Navanethem Pillay writes that the Universal Declaration of Human Rights "enshrines a vision and organic whole, taking all human rights—civil, political, economic, social, or cultural—as an indivisible and organic whole, inseparable and interdependent."

Health is also briefly addressed in the United Nations International Convention on the Elimination of All Forms of Racial Discrimination, which was adopted in 1965 and entered into effect in 1969. The Convention calls upon States to "prohibit and to eliminate racial discrimination in all forms and to guarantee the right of everyone, without distinction as to race, colour, or national or ethnic origin, to equality before law", and references under this provision "the right to public health, medical care, social security and social services."

The United Nations further defines the right to health in article 12 of the 1966 International Economic, Social and Cultural Rights, which states: "The States Parties to the present Covenant recognize the right of everyone to the enjoyment of the highest attainable standard of physical and mental health. The steps to be taken by the States Parties to the present Covenant to achieve the full realization of his right shall include those necessary for:

- The reduction of the stillbirth-rate and of infant mortality and for the healthy development of the child;
- The improvement of all aspects of environmental and industrial hygiene;
- The prevention, treatment and control of epidemic, endemic, occupational and other diseases;
- The creation of conditions which would assure to all medical service and medical attention in the event of sickness.

(http://en.wikipedia.org/wiki/Right_to_health_equity 8.12.2014)

The Human Right to Health is also protected by several international conventions and declarations such as:

- Article 25 of the Universal Declaration of Human Rights.
- Article 12 of the International Covenant on Economic, Social and Cultural Rights.
- Article 24 of the Convention on the Rights of the Child.
- Article 5 of the Convention on the Elimination of All Forms of Discrimination.
- Articles 12 and 14 of the Convention on the Elimination of All Forms of Racial Discrimination against Women.
- Article 25 of the Convention on the Rights of Persons with Disabilities.

(https:/www.nesri.org/programs/what-is-the-human-right-to-health-and-health-care)

The analysis of the human right to healthcare shows that everyone has the right to the highest attainable standard of physical and mental health which includes access to all medical services, sanitation, adequate food, descent housing, healthy working conditions and a clean environment. It may be stated in brief as below:

- The human right to health guarantees a system of health protection for all.
- Everyone has the right to the healthcare they need and to living conditions that enable us to be healthy, such as adequate food, housing and a healthy environment.
- Healthcare must be provided as a public good for all, financed publicly and equitably.
- It also means that hospitals, clinics, medicines and doctors' services must be accessible, available, acceptable and of good

quality for everyone, on an equitable basis, where and when needed.

The healthcare system must be guided by the following key human rights:

Universal Access: Access to healthcare must be universal, guaranteed for all on an equitable basis. Healthcare must be affordable and comprehensive for everyone and its accessibility must be need-based.

Availability: Adequate healthcare infrastructure such as, hospitals, community health facilities, efficient healthcare professionals and goods such as, drugs, equipments and services such as, primary care, mental health must be available in all areas of a country so that each and every person living even in the interior places can avail of the services.

Accessibility and Dignity: Healthcare institutions and providers must respect human dignity, provide culturally appropriate care, be responsive to needs based on gender, age, culture, language and different ways of life and abilities. Respect for medical ethics by the service providers is also very important.

Quality: All healthcare services must be quality services and provided in timely, safe and patient oriented manner.

Non-discrimination: Healthcare services must be accessible to all irrespective of race, ethnicity, age, sex, disability, language, religion, nationality, income, social status etc.

Transparency: Healthcare service must maintain transparency.

Participation: Participation or cooperation of all individuals and communities in the decision-making and decision-implementing that affect the health of the individuals is necessary.

Accountability: Provision must be made to ensure accountability of the service providers through rules and regulations and other suitable devices.

Healthcare as a Human Rights Campaign now exists in several states of United States, inspired by the example of Vermont, which in 2011 became the first state to pass a law for a universal, publicly financed healthcare system.

(https:/www.nesri.org/programs/what-is-the-human-right-to-health-and-health-care)

In 2000, the United Nations' Committee on Economic, Social and Cultural Rights issued general comment, which addresses "substantive issue arising in the implementation of the International Covenant on

Economic, Social and Cultural Rights" with respect article 12 and "the right to the highest attainable standard of health." It is more explicit, operational language on the freedoms and entitlements included in a right to health.

The general comment clarifies that "the right to health is not to be understood as a right to be healthy. Instead, the right to health is articulated as asset of freedoms and entitlements which accommodate the individual's biological and social conditions as well as the state's available resources, both of which may include a right to be healthy for reasons beyond the influence or control of the state. Article 12 tasks the state with recognizing that each individual holds an inherent right to the best feasible standard of health, and itemizes the 'freedoms from' and 'entitlements to' that accompany such a rights; however, it does not charge the state with ensuring that all individuals, in fact, are fully healthy, nor that all individuals have made full recognition of the rights and opportunities enumerated in the right to health.

The right to health is closely related to and dependent upon the realization of other human rights to food, work, housing, life, non-discrimination, human dignity. Similarly, the comment acknowledges that "the right to health embraces a wide range of socio-economic factors that promote conditions in which people can lead a healthy life, and extends to the underlying determinants of health."

The general comment also makes additional reference to the question of health equity, a concept not addressed in the initial International Covenant. The documents note, "the Covenant proscribes any discrimination in access to healthcare and underlying determinants to health, as well as to means and entitlements for their procurement." Moreover, responsibility for ameliorating discrimination and its effects with regard to health is delegated to state: "states have a special obligation to provide those who do not have sufficient means with the necessary health insurance and healthcare facilities and to prevent any discrimination on internationally prohibited grounds in the provision of healthcare and health services." Additional emphasis is placed on non-discrimination on the basis of gender, age, disability or membership in indigenous communities.

The obligations of nations are placed into three categories: obligations to respect, obligations to protect and obligations to fulfill the right to health. These include preventing discrimination in access or delivery of care; refraining from limitations to contraceptive access or family planning; restricting denial of access to health information; reducing environmental pollution; restricting coercive and/or harmful culturally based medical practices; accreditation of medical facilities, personnel, and equipment. International obligations include allowing for the enjoyment of health in other countries; preventing violations of health in countries; cooperating in the provision of humanitarian aid for disasters and emergencies; and refraining from use of embargoes on medical goods or personnel as an act of political and economic influence.

Article 12 of the 1979 United Nations Convention on the Elimination of All Forms of Discrimination against women outlines women's protection from gender discrimination when receiving health services and women's entitlement to specific gender-related healthcare provisions. The full text of Article 12 states: 1. States Parties shall take all appropriate measures to eliminate discrimination against women, access to healthcare services, including those related to family planning; 2. Notwithstanding the provisions of paragraph I of this article, States Parties shall ensure to women appropriate services in connection with pregnancy, confinement and the post-natal period, granting free services, as well as, in which it includes health services, rehabilitation, preventive care. Article 14 outlines child health in detail, and stresses, "Parties recognize the right of the child to the enjoyment of the highest attainable standard and to facilities for the treatment of illness and rehabilitation of health. States shall strive to ensure that no child is deprived of his or her right to access."

Health is mentioned on several instances in the Convention on the Rights of the Child (1989). Article 3 calls upon parties to ensure that institutions and facilities for the care of children adhere to health standards. Article 17 recognizes the child's right to access information that is pertinent to his/her physical and mental health and well-being. Article 23 makes specific reference to the rights of disabled children, in which it includes health services, rehabilitation, preventive care. Article 24 outlines child health in detail, and states "Parties recognize the right of the child to the enjoyment of the highest standard of health and to facilities for the treatment of illness and rehabilitation of health. States shall strive to ensure that no child is deprived of his or her right to access to such healthcare services." Towards implementation of this provision, the Convention enumerates the following measures:

- To diminish infant and child mortality;
- To ensure the provision of necessary medical assistance and healthcare to all children with emphasis on the development of primary healthcare;

- To combat disease and malnutrition, including within the framework of primary healthcare, through, *inter alia*, the application of readily available technology and through the provision of adequate nutritious foods and clean drinking water, taking into consideration the dangers and risks of environmental pollution;
- To ensure appropriate pre-natal and post-natal healthcare for mothers;
- To ensure that all segments of society, in particular parents and children, are informed, have access to education and are supported in the use of basic knowledge of child health and nutrition, the advantages of breastfeeding, hygiene and environmental sanitation and the prevention of accidents;
- To develop preventive healthcare, guidance for parents and family planning education and services.

(*http://en.wikipedia.org/wiki/Right_to_health_equity 8.12.2014)*

The right to health encompasses all categories of people covering the life of an individual from birth to death. Different kinds of health issues/problems relating to diverse social groups with multiplicity of culture and religion have been addressed by this right making its scope very wide. For example, treatment of disease of the ailing people who are within the hospital system or those who are admitted in the hospital, preventive measures for non-spread of infectious diseases, physically and mentally disabled persons, senior people with age related health problems, maintenance of general health of the people who are not patients, production and administration of medicine, equipment, medical education and training, protection of environment congenial for health of the people, resource distribution etc.

The Free Encyclopaedia stated that public health is "the science and art of preventing disease, prolonging life and promoting health through the organized efforts and informed choices of society, organizations, public or private, communities and individuals. The dimensions of health encompass "a state of complete physical, mental and social well-being and not merely the absence of disease or infirmity" as defined by UNO's World Health Organization. "Public health also incorporates interdisciplinary approaches of epidemiology, biostatistics and health services, environmental health, community health, health economics, public policy, insurance medicine, occupational safety and health are other important sub-fields."

Modern public health practice requires multidisciplinary teams of public health workers and professionals including physicians specializing in health/community medicine/infectious disease, psychologists, epidemiologists, biostatisticians, medical assistant, public health nurses, medical microbiologists, environmental health officers/public health inspectors, pharmacists, dental hygienists, dietitians and nutritionists, veterinarians, public health engineers, public health lawyers, sociologists, community development workers, communication experts, bioethicists, and others.

The public health intervention is nothing but prevention and management of diseases, injuries and other health conditions through surveillance of cases and promotion of healthy behaviour, communities and environments. It may be mentioned that many diseases are preventable through simple and non-medical methods. For example, cleanliness, regularity in taking food, pure drinking water, good living conditions, self-discipline etc.

Public health plays an important role in disease prevention efforts in both developed and developing nations. The governmental as well as non-governmental agencies are engaged in these activities at the national and local levels. The World Health Organization stands as an apex body at the global level to coordinate these diverse efforts. However, it is found that the developing countries are still struggling to remove the constraints of trained and honest manpower, adequate resources and other facilities, ignorance of the worst consequences of modernization.

(http:/en.wikipedia.org/wiki/Public_health)

The process of globalization naturally brings to its fold medical services of India. The physicians of India cannot ignore competitive character or private administration, the globalizing process, modern information technology, invention of sophisticated equipment which are appearing in-between the physicians and the patients, invention of new medicine for administration on patients etc. The provision for modern facilities in the private/corporate hospitals, frequent appeals from the industrialists for use of modern technologies and medicine provoke even the honest service providers dragging them to a difficult situation to say 'No' to it. While adopting these facilities there is the scope of slipping away from the path of reaching humanity and which may convert the physician from a 'Man of Need' to a 'Man of Greed'. The new and unexpected offers always knock at him making the physician indecisive and in this stage of immaturity they may be the victim of emotion or the process of imitation. There are instances of leaving the Government job for job in the Private hospital by the physicians even after rendering service for several years. Sometimes, the Private hospitals motivate them to serve those hospitals in addition to their additional duty and responsibility in the original hospital. Indian healthcare system cannot be an exception to it. It is natural that exposure to this modern world with development of science and technology will influence the medical service providers like other service providers. The most dangerous trend is the influence of money power which is very serious threat to human rights of both the providers of service and the receivers of service. Both are the important components of the nation.

Right to Leisure: Leisure is a free time. During this time a person is not engaged in any work. Every human being has the right to leisure. The right to leisure is directly related to health issue to each one of us. But it plays a significant role in the case of both patient and physician. The World Leisure Board of Directors approved a Charter for Leisure in July 2000. The original version of it was adopted by the International Recreation Association in 1970 and subsequently revised by its successor, the World Leisure and Recreation association in 1979.

The Charter for Leisure, in its introduction stated that consistent with the Universal Declaration of Human Rights (Article 27), all cultures and societies recognize to some extent the right to rest and leisure. Personal freedom and choice are central elements of leisure, individuals can freely choose their activities, many of them leading to substantial benefits for person and community. The articles of the Charter are:

(1) All people have a basic human right to leisure activities that are in harmony with norms and social values of their compatriots. All Governments are obliged to recognize and protect this right of all its citizens.
(2) Provisions for leisure for the quality of life are as important as those of health and education. Governments should ensure their citizens a variety of accessible leisure and recreational opportunities of the highest quality.
(3) The individual is his/her best leisure and recreational resource. Thus, Governments should ensure the means for acquiring those skills and understandings necessary to optimize leisure experiences.
(4) Individuals can use leisure opportunities to self-fulfillment, developing personal relationships, improving social integration, developing communities and cultural identity as well as

promoting international understandings and co-operation and enhancing quality of life.

(5) Governments should ensure the future availability of fulfilling leisure experiences by maintaining the quality of their country's physical, social and cultural environment.

(6) Governments should ensure the training of professionals to help individuals acquire skills, discover and develop their talents and to broaden their range of leisure and recreational opportunities.

(7) Citizens must have access to all forms of leisure information about the nature of leisure and its opportunities, using it to enhance their knowledge and inform decisions on local and national policy.

(8) Educational institutions must make every effort to teach the nature and importance of leisure and how to integrate this knowledge into personal lifestyle.

Leisure may be viewed as "just a spare time", time not consumed by the necessities of living. It may also be viewed leisure as a force that allows individuals to consider and reflect on the values and realities that are missed in the activities of daily life. Thus, it is an essential element of personal development and civilization. This direction of thought has been extended to the view that leisure is the purpose of work, and a reward in itself, and leisure life reflects the values and character of a nation.

Closely connected to leisure is play, recreation and work. Recreation is difficult to separate from the general concept of play. The term play is generally associated with the children in common parlance. The children learn things while playing. It is said that the play or recreational activities are the outlets or expression of excess energy, channeling it into socially acceptable activities that fulfill individual as well as social needs without being constrained by compulsion and providing satisfaction and pleasure to the participants. A traditional view holds that work is supported by recreation. Recreation improves work performance. Work may be said as an activity generally performed out of economic necessity or family compulsions and useful for society. However, it cannot be denied that sometimes the concept of recreational activity may vary from person to person. Many activities may be work for one person and recreation to another.

Recreation has many health benefits, and, accordingly, recreational therapy has been developed to take advantage of this effect. Such therapy is applied in rehabilitation, and in the care of the elderly, the disabled, or people with chronic disease.

http://en.wikipedia.org/wiki/Recreation

Modernity and progress should improve the quality of life of the masses and a wider sense of well-being or happiness. And according to various well-being surveys in recent years (Happy Planet Index, World Values Survey and the Human Development Index), the key to achieving such things may well lie in good health, decent education, greater level of social equality, self-sustaining communities and the people living with the limits set by the nature.

Referring to public health it is found that one of the most revealing pieces about the impact of chemical-based agriculture in the face of globalization appeared in Bangalore Deccan Herald Newspaper. Gautam Dheer writes that contamination of drinking water by pesticides is a major cause of cancer in India's Punjab state. At this point, although various other factors may also be to blame, it is worth noting that cancer is on the rise in many of India's urban centers. The links between pesticides and cancers and illness in Western countries are well documented (for instance, Dr. Mery Hammond Campaign for Alternatives to pesticides told a Canadian Parliament Committee in 2009 that a draft of studies published Prestigious peer-reviewed journals pointed out the strong associations between chemical pesticides and a vast range of serious life-threatening health consequences).

India is one of the world's largest users of pesticides. Ladyfinger, cabbage, tomato and cauliflower in particular may often contain dangerously high levels and fruits and vegetables are sprayed and tampered with to ripen and make them colourful. Research by the School of Natural Sciences and Engineering at the National Institute of Advanced Studies in Bangalore reported in 2008 that many crops for export had been rejected internationally due to high pesticides residues.

In his speech Gautam Dheer argues that Punjab stare at an inevitable crisis. Agriculture has become increasingly unsustainable and the model practiced by desperate debt-ridden farmers has only meant more indiscriminate use of pesticides, something in Punjab which is now being linked to the alarmingly high incidents of cancer.

(www.global research.ca/globalization-and-social-destruction-stealing-wealth-and-health-in-india/5322132)

Now public service in India is exposed to a new environment in the face of 'globalization', 'privatization' and 'good governance'. There is the need of revival of ethical principles and human values, especially in health and education sectors in India as these two services occupy the position next to the security of the nation from foreign aggression. The author makes an attempt to analyze in this book the ethical principles and human values in medical services in the face of it by considering the Indian philosophy and religion.

Globalization may be defined differently depending on the context and on the person. Further, the precise definition of globalization is still not available. However, here mention may be made of a few definitions given by some eminent persons. Stephen Gill defines globalization as the reduction of transaction cost of transborder movements of capital and goods.

(economics.about.com/globalizationtrade/aaglobalization.htm)

Guy Brainbant says that the process of globalization not only includes opening up of world trade, development of advanced means of communication, internationalization of financial markets, growing importance of Multi-National Companies, population migration and more specifically increased mobility of workers, students, patients along with goods, capital, data and ideas is found. With this infections, diseases and pollution also move from place to place.

The term globalization refers to the integration of economies of the world through uninhibited trade and financial flows, as also through mutual exchange of technology and knowledge. Ideally, it contains intercountry movement of labour. In the context of India, this implies opening up of the economy to foreign direct investment by providing facilities to foreign companies to invest in different fields of economic activity in India, removing constraints and obstacles to the entry of Multi-National Companies in India, allowing Indian companies to enter into foreign collaboration and also encouraging them to set up joint ventures abroad; carrying out massive import liberalization programmes by switching over from quantitative restrictions to tariffs and import duties, therefore globalization has been identified with the policy reformed of 1991 in India.

(www.fibre2fashion.com/industry-article/8738/impact-of-globalization1.asp)

Globalization also implies the development of local and nationalistic perspectives to a broader outlook of an interconnected and interdependent world with free transfer of capital, goods and services across national frontiers. However, it does not include unhindered movement of labour and as suggested by economists, may hurt smaller or fragile economies if applied indiscriminately.

(www.businessdictionary.com/definition/globalization.html)

UN defines globalization as "increased and intensified flows of goods, services, capital, ideas, information and people between countries, which produce national cross-broader integration of a number of economic, social and cultural activities." (UN, 2001: World Public Sector Report: Globalization and the State, 2001, New Work).

Thus, India opened up the economy in the early nineties following a major crisis that led by a foreign exchange crunch that dragged the economy close to defaulting loans. The response was a slew of domestic and external sector policy measures partly prompted by the immediate needs and partly by the demand of the multilateral organizations. The policy regime radically pushed forward in favour of more open and market oriented economy.

Major measures initiated as a part of the liberalization and globalization strategy in the early nineties included scrapping of the industrial licensing regime, reduction in the number of areas reserved for the public sector, amendment of the Monopolies and Restrictive Trade Practices Act, start of the privatization programme, reduction in tariff rates and change over to market determined by exchange rates.

(economics.about.com/globalizationtrade/aaglobalization.htm)

Thus, Globalization, briefly refers to the growing interdependence among nations compelling the sorting out of economic, social, environmental and human rights issues at the international level. It is based on the acceptance of the market forces, which intensifies international competition. It compels reconciliation of global imperatives with local needs and requirements. Around the late 1960s, the bureaucracy received a lot of criticism from economists like Gordon Tullock, Anthony Downs, William Niskanen etc. These scholars strongly advocated the market as an efficient alternative to bureaucracy and paved the way for the emergence of what has come to be known as New Public Management in public administration. In his work '*The Politics of Bureaucracy*', published in 1965, Gordon Tullock propounds the principal thesis that bureaucrats are motivated primarily by selfishness. Anthony Downs, another scholar, in his work, '*Inside Bureaucracy*', published in 1967, demonstrates that bureaucrats are motivated by survival instincts. Osborne and Gaebler's '*Re-inventing Government*' entered in the United States Government *via* Al Gore's Report on the National Performance Review (NPR) 1993. The NPR is the outcome of an in-depth six month study of the US Federal bureaucracy carried out by 250 public employees under the leadership of the then American Vice-President Al Gore. Some of the suggestions of the committee for developing entrepreneurship in government are:

- Government must promote competition between service-providers.
- It must empower citizens by pushing control out of the bureaucracy into the community.
- It must measure the performance of their agencies focusing on outcomes, not on inputs.
- It redefines clients as customers and offers them choices.
- It must prevent problems before they emerge, rather than simply offer them services afterwards.
- It must prefer market mechanisms to bureaucratic mechanisms.

The report of Al Gore's National Performance Review (1993) prefers the term 'democratic governance' to 'good governance' and its distinguishing attributes lie in certain 'values', such as justice, democracy etc. (author: S.R. Maheswari; book: *Administrative Theory*; 2nd edition; published by MacMillan India Ltd., Delhi, 2002.

Another aspect of developing nations is the mobility of rural youths to urban areas in the plea of job and business. It is also alleged that these youths are motivated to take up some illegal activities like transportation of drugs, and similar items from place to place in lieu of some amount of money, engagement in the process of mobilizing people to invest money in fake financial organizations, use of youths as human traffickers for commercial purposes in both medical and non-medical purposes by giving wrong information to fulfill the requirement for the purpose, sex service providers etc. Under these circumstances, the rural youths' mobility to urban areas is found. These activities bring to the youths the problems of drug addiction, alcoholism, victimization of various kinds of diseases due to tension, irregularities of food, lack of rest, fear complex, unhygienic living conditions etc. Further e-media has also brought different kinds of health related problems which come within the arena of public health. In India due to these problems public health is affected to a great extent.

Article 25 of the Convention on the Rights of Persons with Disabilities (2006) specifies that "persons with disabilities have the right to the enjoyment of highest attainable standard of health without discrimination on the basis of disability." The sub-clauses of Article 25 state that States shall give the disabled the same "range, quality, and standard" of healthcare as it provides to other persons, as well as those services specifically required for prevention, identification, and management of disability. Further provisions specify that healthcare for the disabled should be made available to local communities and that care should be geographically equitable, with additional statements against the denial or unequal provision of health services (including "food and fluids" and "life insurance" on the basis of disability.

Hendricks criticizes the failure of the Convention to define specifically "disability"; he contends further that "the absence of a clear description may prejudice the uniform interpretation, or at least place in jeopardy the consistent protection the Convention seeks to guarantee." He does, however, acknowledge that the lack of a clear definition for "disability" may benefit the disabled by limiting the ability to limit extension of the Convention's provisions to specific populations or those with certain conditions.

While most human rights are theoretically framed as negative rights, meaning that they are areas upon which society cannot interfere or restrict by political action, Mervyn Susser contends that the right to health is a particularly unique and challenging right because it is often expressed as a positive right, where society bears an obligation to provide certain resources and opportunities to the general population.

Susser further sets out four provisions that he sees as covered under a right to health: equitable access to health and medical services; a "good faith" social effort to promote equal health among different social groups; means to measure and assess health equity; and equal socio-political system to give all parties a unique voice in health advocacy and promotion. He is careful to note here that, while this likely entails some minimum standard of access to health resources, it does not guarantee or necessitate an equitable state of health for each person due to inherent biological differences in health status. This distinction is an important one, as some common critiques of a "right to health" are that it establishes a right to an unreachable standard and it aspires to a state of health that is too subjectively variable from person to person and from one society to the next.

While Susser's discussion centers on healthcare as a positive right, Paul Hunt refutes this view and makes the argument that right to health also encompasses certain negative rights such as a protection from discrimination and the right not to receive medical treatment without the recipient's voluntary consent. However, Hunt does concede that some positive rights, such as the responsibility of society to pay special attention to the health needs of the unreserved and vulnerable, are included in the right to health.

Paul Farmer addresses the issue of unequal access to healthcare in his article, "*The Major Infectious Diseases in the World—To Treat or Not to Treat*". He discusses the growing "outcome gap" between the populations receiving health interventions and the ones that are not. Poor people are not receiving the same treatment, if any at all, as the more financially fortunate. The high costs of medicine and treatment make it chief human-rights dilemma of healthcare in the twentieth century.

An alternative way to conceptualize one facet of the right to health is a "human right to healthcare." Notably this encompasses both patient and the provider rights in the delivery of healthcare services, the latter being similarly open to frequent abuse by the states. Patient rights to healthcare delivery include: right to privacy, information, life, and quality care, as well as freedom from discrimination, torture, and cruel, inhumane, or degrading treatment. Marginalized groups, such as migrants and persons who have been displaced, racial and ethnic minorities, women, sexual minorities may be segregated into poorer quality wards, disabled persons may be forced into virginal examinations and may be denied life-saving abortions, suspected homo-sexual men may be forced into anal examinations and women of marginalized groups and transgender persons may be forcibly sterilized.

Provider rights include the right to quality standards of working conditions, the right to associate freely, and the right to refuse to perform a procedure based on their morals. Healthcare providers often experience violations of their rights. For instance, particularly in countries with weak rule of law, healthcare providers are often forced to perform procedures which negate their morals, deny marginalized groups the best possible standards of care, breach patient confidentiality, and conceal crimes against humanity and torture. Furthermore, providers who do not oblige these pressures are often persecuted. Currently, especially in the United States, much debate surrounds the issue of "provider consciousness", which retains the right to providers to abstain from performing procedures that do not align with their moral code, such as abortions.

Some scholars have questioned or criticized the concept of a right to health. Philip Barlow writes that healthcare should not be considered a human right because of the difficulty of defining what it entails and where the 'minimum standard' of entitlements under the right ought to be established. Additionally, Barlow holds the social responsibility for the right to health. John Berkeley, in agreement with Barlow, critiques further that the right to health does not consider adequately the responsibility that an individual has to uphold his or her own health.

It is difficult to conceptualize the minimum standard of health as it is difficult to determine the minimum needs of a modern man. With the process of modernization and industrialization the needs of man are also increasing. It is also because of the complex problems caused by the negative impact of the progress of science and technology. The more are the facilities/comforts provided by the state more are the expectations of the people. With this values in the society are also changing influencing the needs of man.

Richard D. Lamm vehemently argues against making healthcare a right. He defines a right as one that is to be defended at all costs, and a concept that is defined and interpreted by the judicial system. Making healthcare a right would require Governments to spend a large portion of its resources to provide its citizens with it. He asserts that the healthcare system is based on the erroneous assumption of unlimited resources. Limited resources inhibit governments from providing everyone with adequate healthcare, especially in the long term. Attempting to provide "beneficial" healthcare to all people utilizing limited resources would lead to economical collapse

(http://en.wikipedia.org/wiki/Right_to_health_equity 8.12.2014).

In the face of above discussion if we look to India it is found that in India the discussion on the right to healthcare may be traced from the time of *Vedas*. *Vedas* said that it was the duty of the king to see that the people of his kingdom were free from all kinds of diseases. He should provide required facilities for maintenance of health of the citizens. Mala Pyasi in her article, *"Duties Before Rights"* cited a hymn of *Veda* as, "O Protector and Caretaker of the houses, Vayan ! You are the destroyer of diseases. You are our friend and you give us happiness (*Rigveda* 7-55-11)". It reveals the healthcare provisions provided by the King for the people. (Pyasi: 2002) With the increase of population and progress of education and development of science and technology the state will be able to care of public health only with the cooperation of the public. Depending heavily on the state machinery without doing our duties enjoyment of rights is not at all possible. In India this experience is found in average people.

Democracy and Human Rights: The word 'democracy' has become a common word used by the citizens of a modern state. They have enough faith in the democratic principles. But experience in India shows that in reality average people do not practice them in their lives though they have faith in them and express the need of these principles in public speeches and writings. Adherence of democratic principles or to follow a democratic way of life is not an easy task, it requires perseverance, mental strength and commitment to the cause of humanity. It is also a difficult task as the whole concept of democracy centers round human being and success of democracy depends on activism of human power along with other qualities.

The freedom struggle under the leadership of Mahatma Gandhi may be called as the struggle for democratic way of life in all fields of man's life—political, social, economic, legal, religious—both within and outside the family—public or private. After gaining independence, the framers of the Constitution of India took utmost care to see that it would provide a wide path on which all Indians, irrespective of caste, creed, place of birth, sex etc. can travel without difficulty to reach the destination of establishing a democratic society in India. But the human power of commitment to the efforts of the framers of the Constitution and the freedom fighters could not be sustained by both the rulers and the ruled in independent India. Nani A. Palkhiwala, an eminent personality in the field of law pointed out four costly failures of the Government and the people which are the direct causes of it as below:

1. Failure to maintain law and order. We have too much Government and too little administration: too many public servants and too little public service; too many controls and too little welfare; too many laws and too many justice;
2. Failure to bring the unbounded economic potential of the country to fruition;
3. Failure to make human investment—investment in education, family planning, nutrition and public health, in contradiction to physical investment in factories and plants. Gross national happiness;
4. Failure to provide moral leadership. (Palkhiwala: 1984)

The responsibility for this state of affairs must be shared by both the rulers and the ruled. While discussing this issue we have to underline the state as the largest component of the Indian governance, which belongs, along with others, to the socially, economically and educationally backward classes also and to those who are exploited by political leaders, moneylenders, social workers, administrators, private businessmen, etc. The emergence of large number of false educational institutions at higher levels and false financial organizations are appearing as a serious threat to humanity, the key to democracy. The leading personalities in the fields of politics, administration, education, social work, religions constitute very significant component of the Indian governance. They are the role models for the rest of the society. Unfortunately, experience shows that most of them maintain multi-standards of life which is not easily understandable by the common men. They hide their inner motive very skillfully while approaching the general masses for participation in their programmes. They have become slaves of money and move as directed by money power. Naturally, they lose the capacity to judge what is good and what is bad even for their own lives. Criminalization of politics is a serious ailment in Indian democracy affecting the human rights of the people at every walk of life. The administration is not responsive, responsible and accountable to the public even for genuine causes. The common people are exploited and cheated by falsehood and dishonesty in various forms. As mentioned above, it is not because of lack of laws or rules and regulations and institutions to safeguard human rights of different sections of the people. What is lacking is the obedience to human values and human dignity. To-day priority is given to accumulation of money by any means and any amount without limitation and building of huge property—movable or immovable at the cost of human rights of our own people. Now, the question before us is how to save the human beings from this new form of slavery caused by the money and muscle power in modern India. Disraeli said, "Money is not the measure of a man, but it is often the means of finding out how small he is." It is difficult no doubt but not impossible to redirect the society towards humanity so that each individual can be relieved from uncomfortable stay in the domain of monetary slavery.

Nani A. Palkhiwala rightly said, "In a vast democracy like India, many citizens are bound to be undimensional. But no lawyer has any excuse for being undimensional. By his training and equipment and by his professional competence he is better qualified than the rest of the citizenry to take an active part in the making of laws and the formulation of public policies. He would be failing to serve his country if he did not do this duty." This is applicable to every public service provider. To-day ethical vacuum in every walk of life is causing deviation from the real path of human progress.

Acharya J.B. Kripalani spoke in the Constituent Assembly on 17th October, 1949, "I want this House to remember that what we have enunciated are not merely legal, constitutional and formal principles, but moral principles; and moral principles have to be lived in life. They have to be lived, whether it is in private life, or it is in public life, whether it is in commercial life, political life of an administrator. They have to be lived throughout." But very soon these principles are withering away.

The concept of democracy cannot be understood fully without reference to human rights. The journey of a man from the status of cave-man who was exposed to all kinds of natural calamities and attacks of wild animals to that of democratic man, who is safeguarded on every aspect of his life was piloted by faith in human rights and dignity. During this period man had to struggle against the violent forces of nature and wild animals in every walk of life. This journey will always remind us that human rights are not created in thin air. These are the results of untiring and long struggle of man for survival. In course of journey man has realized the dignity of human being. And explicit expression of it is found in the emergence of the concept of democracy. (Palkhiwala: 1997)

Charles E. Merriam said, "Democracy is not a set of formulas or blueprint of organization, but a cast of thought and a mode of action directed toward the common weal as interpreted and directed by the common will." (Merriam: 1939) Merriam's weal embraces a wide range of material objectives and spiritual ideals; raising the standard of living, cultivating and enriching human personality and diffusing the "mass gains" of common wealth resulting from increased economic and social productivity throughout the community.

The UN Charter, though does not mention the term Democracy, it emphasizes on the key elements of democracy in wider perspective. The objective of UN is to establish world peace and security through international cooperation for promoting and encouraging respect for human rights and fundamental freedom to all, irrespective of race, religion, sex and language.

International Labour Organization also makes continuous efforts to create democratic environment in the workplace by affirming basic human rights of the employees.

Human Rights Education: A global and serious thought was given, after the worldwide efforts during Second World War to safeguard human rights of the peoples, on the eve of the thirtieth anniversary of the Universal Declaration of Human Rights, UNESCO, with the close co-operation of the Government of the Federal Republic of Austria, convened the first International Congress on the Teaching of Human Rights. The Congress served dual purposes—first, it marked this anniversary with a stock-taking of the situation in the world concerning education for human rights, thirty years after the General Assembly proclaimed the Universal Declaration of Human Rights, "as a common standard of achievement for all peoples and all nations, to the end that every individual and every organ of society, keeping this Declaration constantly in mind, shall strive by teaching and education to promote respect for these rights and freedoms...." Secondly, it provided an opportunity for specialists in human rights teaching research, together with those responsible for education policies of UNESCO member states, to exchange their views and experience freely to adopt a series of conclusions and recommendations.

The sequence of events leading to the convening of the Congress began with the proposal for such a meeting made by Willibald Pahr, Federal Minister of Foreign Affairs of the Republic of Austria, to the Nineteenth General Conference of UNESCO, held in Nairobi, Kenya in November 1976. Ultimately, United Nations Commission on Human Rights, in Resolution No. 3 at its 33rd session (February-March 1977), recommended that education for human rights be chosen as an appropriate theme to mark the thirtieth anniversary year of the Universal Declaration of Human Rights.

The International Congress on the Teaching of Human Rights was set for 12th-16th September, 1978 in the Kongresszentrum of the Hofburg Palace, Vienna. Experts from all regions of the world were invited by the Director-General to participate in their individual capacities. Representatives from organizations of the United Nations system and observers from non-governmental organizations in consultative status with UNESCO were invited to attend the Congress. The Congress was opened on 12th September by Amadou-Mahtar M' Bow, Director General of UNESCO.

The Congress along with other recommendations relating to teaching and research in human rights, suggested the following: "The concept of human rights should not be formulated in traditional or classical terms, but should include the historical contributions of all peoples, particularly in relation to the major contemporary problems such as self-determination and all forms of discrimination and exploitation.

Human Rights education and teaching must aim at:

(i) Fostering the attitudes of tolerance, respect and solidarity inherent in human rights;
(ii) Providing knowledge about human rights, in both their national and international dimensions, and the institutions established for their implementation; and

(iii) Developing the individual's awareness of the ways and means by which human rights can be translated into social and political reality at both the national and international levels.

Further, it was also suggested that human rights must be seen as an aspect of professional, ethical and social responsibility in all fields of research, study, teaching and work.

Referring to the teaching of human rights and professional ethics in the faculties or schools of medicine, it is found that a world survey on the subject was carried out, at UNESCO's request, by the International Institute of Human Rights in 1977-78. The surveyors made it clear that without slackening the attention paid to law and political science, efforts were made to discover the importance attached to this question in the framework of the teaching of medicine and medical sciences in order that it may be possible to evaluate what needs to be done and what resources are required to develop medical ethics in the faculties of schools concerned. Further UN Commission on Human Rights has been regularly considering the topic of Human Rights and Scientific and Technological Developments. The relationship between human rights and medical ethics occupies a prominent place in the discussion at the international level and India cannot remain isolated from it as the progress of science and technology in the field of medicine and medical sciences is entering into the process of healthcare process of the country (UNESCO: 1978).

Human Rights Education begins with the origin and development of the concept of human rights. However, as an academic discipline it emerged with its incorporation in the agenda of the International Conference on Human Rights held in Teheran in 1968. On 12th May of that year, the Conference adopted a resolution entitled, "Education of Youth in Respect for Human Rights and Fundamental Freedoms." In the resolution, the Conference called upon all states to ensure that all means of education should be employed for this purpose so that youths grow up and develop in a spirit of respect for human dignity and equal rights without discrimination as to race, colour, language, sex or faith. UNESCO was invited to develop a programme aimed at.

Provision 13 of the Declaration on the Rights of Disabled Persons provides that disabled persons, families and communities shall be fully informed by all appropriate means of the rights contained in the Declaration. One year after the proclamation of the Disabled Persons Declaration, the United Nations Commission on Human Rights vide its Resolution B (XXXII) of 11th February, 1976 appealed UN organs, specialized agencies, and NGOs as well as Governments to promote within their respective spheres of competence, measures for the development of youth in human rights, including development of a special curriculum on human rights for use in various educational institutions.

In 1988, the UN convened an International Congress on the teachings of Human Rights at Vienna (Mahanty: 2000).

The 1993 United Nations World Conference on Human Rights held at Vienna underlined the need of Human Rights education. On 25th June, 1993 representatives of 171 states adopted a resolution by consensus towards this end. The World Conference on Human Rights in the Vienna Declaration and Programme of Action stated that human rights education, training and public information were essential for the promotion and achievement of stable and harmonious relations among communities and for fostering method of understanding, tolerance and peace. The Conference recommended that states should strive to eradicate illiteracy and should direct education towards the full development of human personality and strengthening of respect for human rights and fundamental freedoms. It called on all states and institutions to include human rights, humanitarian laws, democracy and rule of law as subjects in the curricula of all learning institutions in formal and non-formal settings. The Declaration of Human Rights Education Decade was made on 23rd December, 1994.

The significance of UN Decade for Human Rights Education has been highlighted very well by John Pace, Director, United Nations Center for Human Rights in his keynote address in the symposium on Human Rights Education organized by HURIGHTS OSAKA on July 29th, 1995. The edited version of the address may be stated as below.

The aim of the United Nations is to translate the international human rights norms into national day-to-day reality. The process of achieving this goal has been very slow. In order to expedite the whole process, the United Nations has taken the responsibility of executing the ideals of human rights instead of being mere recommending agency. In 1987, the United Nations set-up a Voluntary Fund for technical cooperation in the field of Human Rights. This has been considered as a new effort to offer voluntary contribution in the technical field. In 1988, the World Public Information Campaign for Human Rights was launched by the UN spreading over five types of programmes—

1. Production, dissemination of printed information and reference materials;

2. Workshops, seminars and training courses;
3. Fellowships and internships;
4. Special human rights observances; and
5. Media and promotional activities.

The main purpose of this Campaign was to make the international human rights norms as a part of the administrative process of a state. In 1989, UN decided to hold the World Conference on Human Rights. Thus, it created an environment congenial enough to declare UN Decade for Human Rights Education in December 1994.

The United Nations' programme for implementing international human rights norms has three dimensions—protection, promotion and prevention. Promotional and preventive actions were added to the protection mechanism that had been worked out in the earlier years in the conventional and extra-conventional fields. The addition of the two latter parts is due to a realization that awareness and education is a prior condition for any meaningful implementation of human rights standards.

The United Nations is seeking to build a universal culture of human rights based on the charter and the international bill of human rights. As phrased by the United Nations Secretary General, human rights should become the "Common Language of Humanity". Human rights education is the means to attain this.

In the United Nations World Conference on Human Rights, human rights education received the greatest concurrence by governments. The Vienna Declaration and Programme of Action contains a significant number of statements on human rights education.

The Decade of Human Rights Education has a Plan of Action that sets out a complete strategy for education activities. It has the following objectives:

1. To assess the needs and formulate effective strategies for the furtherance of human rights education at the international, regional, national and local levels;
2. To build and strengthen programmes and capacities for human rights education at these levels;
3. To coordinate the development of human rights education materials;
4. To strengthen the role and capacity of mass media in the furtherance of human rights education;

5. To disseminate globally the Universal Declaration of Human Rights in the maximum levels of literacy and for disabled.

(http://www.hrights.or.jp/archives/focus/section2/the-significance-of-the-un-decade-for-human-rights-education-its-background-and-future.html 4.1.2015

A significant effort towards the development of human rights education is the creation of the office of the High Commissioner by the United Nations. It is found that during the time of drafting of the Universal Declaration of Human Rights in 1948 Rene Cassin, the French representative first conceived the idea of an Attorney General. This was a revolutionary view expressed by him before the Assembly and was not welcomed by the people and could not occupy any place in the discussions or debates at the international level.

At the 5th session of Commission on Human Rights in 1950 Australia appealed with a proposal for the establishment of an international court of human rights that would ensure protection of human rights. However, it failed to have its way. In the same year Uruguay submitted a proposal to the General Assembly requesting creation of a permanent body of the United Nations either in the form of an office of High Commissioner or Attorney General which would function within the framework of the International Covenant of Human Rights. Though the proposal appeared in the seventh session of the Commission, finally it was rejected in its tenth session.

After about fifteen years, i.e. in 1965, the issue was raised by a Latin American country, Costa Rica at the 28th session of the General Assembly with a draft resolution entitled, “Election of the United Nations High Commissioner for Human Rights.” The proposal was approved by the Commission after several rounds of debates and discussion. But it was in dark for about twenty years without any official declaration. The World Conference on Human Rights held at Vienna in 1993 was successful in bringing into existence the office of the High Commissioner. On 31st January, 1994, the Secretary General appointed Jose Aya La Lasso of Equador as the first United Nations High Commissioner (Srivastava: 2002).

Office of the United Nations High Commissioner for Human Rights: The office of High Commissioner works for the promotion and protection of human rights guaranteed by international law and incorporated in the Universal Declaration of Human Rights adopted on 10th December, 1948. The office is headed by the High Commissioner for Human Rights. He is also the coordinator of the human rights activities within the UN systems. At present, the High Commissioner is Prince Zeid bin Ra'ad who assumed his duties as seventh High Commissioner on 1st September, 2014.

The mandate of the office of the High Commissioner for Human Rights is derived from Article 1, 13 and 55 of the Charter of the United Nations, the Vienna Declaration and programme of Action and General Assembly Resolution 48/141 of twentieth December, 1993 by which Assembly established the office. On fifteenth September, 1997, the Centre for Human Rights was merged with the office of the UN High Commissioner for Human Rights.

What are the aims of the Office of the High Commissioner? The aims of the office are to:

1. Promote universal enjoyment of all human rights by giving practical effect to the will and resolve of the world community as expressed by the United Nations;
2. Play the leading role on human rights issues and emphasize the importance of human rights at the international and national levels;
3. Promote international cooperation for human rights;
4. Stimulate and coordinate action for human rights throughout the United Nations system;
5. Promote universal ratification and implementation of international standards;
6. Assist in the development of new norms;
7. Support human rights organs and treaty monitoring bodies;
8. Respond to serious violations of human rights;
9. Undertake preventive human rights action;
10. Promote the establishment of normal human rights infrastructures;
11. Undertake human rights field activities and operations; and
12. Provide education, information, advisory services and technical assistance in the field of human rights.

The High Commissioner is accountable to the Secretary General. He is responsible for all the activities of the office of the United Nations High Commissioner for Human Rights, as well as its administration and carries out the functions.

The High Commissioner for Human Rights, with the support of the United Nations Centre for Human Rights, will promote and coordinate the implementation of the Plan of Action. Governments, national human rights institutions, national NGOs, various United Nations agencies and other international organizations working on human rights will be involved.

The Plan of Action aims to bring the objectives of the Decade to as wide an audience as possible through both formal and non-formal education and encourages an approach which is designed to build permanent capacity, including the training of trainers. Activities will provide special attention to women, children, the aged, minorities, refugees, indigenous peoples, persons in extreme poverty and other vulnerable sectors as well as to police, prison officials, lawyers, judges, teachers and curriculum developers, the armed forces, international civil servants, development officers and peacekeepers, NGOs, the media, Government officials, parliamentarians and other groups which are in a position to effect the realization of human rights.

Educational institutions and programmes, and appropriate institutions in society will be encouraged to incorporate human rights education into the formal and non-formal education systems respectively.

The Plan of Action envisages the designation of national focal points for human rights education in each state which will be charged with identifying national human rights education needs, developing a national plan of action, raising funds, coordinating with regional and international bodies and reporting to the High Commissioner.

Each state is encouraged to establish a national human rights resource and training center capable of engaging in research, training of trainers etc. Where such centers exist the Plan encourages states to work toward their strengthening.

The concept of human rights education appears in a number of international human rights instruments including the Universal Declaration of Human Rights (Article 26), the International Covenant on Economic, Social and Cultural Rights (Article 13), the Convention on the Rights of the Child (Article 29), and most recently, the Vienna Declaration and Programme of Action.

Human rights education may thus be defined as training, dissemination and information efforts aimed at the building of a universal culture of human rights through the imparting of knowledge and skills and the molding of attitudes which are directed to:

- The strengthening of respect for human rights and fundamental freedoms;
- The full development of human personality and the sense of its dignity;
- The promotion of understanding, tolerance, gender equality and friendship among all nations, indigenous peoples, racial, ethnic and religious groups;
- The enabling of all persons to participate effectively in a free society; and
- The furtherance of the activities of the United Nations for the maintenance of peace.

The task of the United Nations is to bring these lessons for life to the world.

Thus, John Pace highlighted the significance of human rights education.

(http://www.hrights.or.jp/archives/focus/section2/the-significance-of-the-un-decade-for-human-rights-education-its-background-and-future.html 4.1.2015

In ancient India men of learning were honoured by Kings and Emperors. Men of knowledge and intellectuals received highest honour in the society. Curiosity to acquire knowledge even by the Kings and emperors was very strong. Example of this has been given by Nani A. Pakhliwala while delivering his convocation address in the University of Bangalore on fifteenth January in 1972. He pointed out that King Janaka, himself was a philosopher and journeyed on foot into the jungle to discourse with Yajnavalkya on high matters of state. In the eighth century, Sankaracharya travelled on foot from Kerala to Kashmir and from Dwarka in the west to Puri in the east. He could not have changed the minds of men and established centres of learning in remote areas of India, but for the great esteem and reverence which intellectuals enjoyed. "Unfortunately", today the very word, "intellectual" have been devalued. Today it means "a man who is intelligent enough to know on which side his bread is buttered." Less emphasis is given on the major two functions of education in modern India—to enlighten the understanding and to enrich the character. The processes of earning money, education, employment in public services have simplified to such an extent in most cases that one get confused to make a distinction between the earner of money and collector of money, between degree or marks awarding system and education system, between merit based job market and price bargain based vegetable market.

Rule of Law: The Rule of Law is one of the basic principles of democracy. The Rule of Law (also known as Nomocracy) is the legal principle that law should govern a nation, as opposed to arbitrary decisions by individual Government officials. It may primarily refer to the influence and authority of law within a society, particularly as a constraint upon behaviour, including the behaviour of Government officials. The phrase can be traced back to sixteenth century England and it was popularized in the nineteenth century by British jurist A.V. Dicey. The concept was familiar to ancient philosophers such as Aristotle, to whom law should govern.

Rule of Law implies that every citizen is subject to law, including law makers themselves. In this sense, it stands in contrast to an autocracy, collective leadership, dictatorship or oligarchy where the rulers are above the law. Lack of the rule of law generally figures in dictatorships. It also occurs due to ignorance of the law and ignorance is worst consequence of non-adherence of law, corruption, or lack of corrective mechanisms for administrative abuse.

A Secretary General of United Nations defined Rule of Law as a principle of governance in which all persons, institutions and entities, private and public, including the state itself, are accountable to laws that are publicly promulgated, equally enforced and independently adjudicated, and which are consistent with international human rights norms and standards. It requires as well measures to ensure adherence to the principles of supremacy of laws, equality before law, accountability to the law, fairness in the applicability of law, separation of powers, participation in decision making, legal certainty, avoidance of arbitrariness and procedural and legal transparency.

(http://en.wikipedia.org/wiki/Rule_of_law 6.12.2014)

Now, let us have a look to what Dicey, the British jurist talked of Rule of Law. Dicey discussed the concept of Rule of Law in the context of the concept of Administrative Law. Dicey identified Administrative Law with French Droit Administratif. It is a special mechanism under which the official wrong doers are tried, who committed wrong in official capacity. It consists of experienced administrative officials. It is an advisory body with judicial powers. It can set aside any administrative decision which affects individual's interest and pay compensation to aggrieved person. It advises the Government on important matters and entertains complaints from the citizens. The Council has the authority to see not only "that the administration observes the highest standards of behaviour, but also that they arrive at a correct decision or a reasonable decision....and that they observe a fair and formal procedure."

In contrast to French system, to Dicey England had Rule of Law. In support of what was said by him, Dicey brought out three distinguishing features of both Rule of Law and Administrative Law as below:

(1) Droit Administratif provides a special set of laws to determine the rights of state and it is not applicable to common citizens;
(2) Ordinary courts have no jurisdiction in cases in which state or officials are a party in official capacity; and
(3) A special protection is given to officials in France for wrongful acts done while on duty.

In contrast to above Dicey pointed out three significant features of Rule of law as below:

(1) Under Rule of Law absolute supremacy of ordinary law prevails. Under this special protection for wrongful acts by the officials in official capacity;
(2) Equal subjection of all classes of people—official or non-official to the ordinary law of the land; and
(3) The primacy of the rights of the individuals, which as defined and enforced by the courts are the source of administrative law instead of the latter being the source of the former.

What is Administrative Law? Administrative Law may be defined as a body of laws which concerns the functions of administration and its relationship with the individuals and other state agencies. In broader sense, any law relating to administration may be called as administrative law which exists in all countries from the inception of administration and it embraces the statutes, charters, resolutions, rules and regulations including the constitution of a country which have relations with administration.

The administrative laws occupy a prominent place in the administration of a state with the expansion of the functions of the Government and also awareness of human rights by the citizens of modern State. In eighteenth and nineteenth centuries there existed the police state which performed mainly the negative role concern for the administrative laws was insignificant. The maintenance of law and order, collection of taxes and protection of life and property of the citizens were the main concerns of the police state. However, with the development of the concept of welfare state and impact of industrialization and modernization or urbanization of human civilization the state's role has become positive as a service provider resulting increase of its functions and responsibilities and bringing administration to the doors of the citizens covering the whole span of a man's life.

In the police state, the individuals or social groups were self-dependent for livelihood, there was less interference from the state authorities on their rights. The traditional societies were administered by local or community's own customs and traditions. As the traditional society was basically agricultural in nature the economic power was also rested with each family or social group. The industrial revolution brought drastic change to it under which a handful of persons or industrialists became the possessors of economic power. In the factories, the owners required large number of workers for production in large scale. With the emergence of the factories, the process of urbanization started. The factory owners' sole objective was to make profit. To achieve this goal they become very cruel to the workers and compelled them to accept and tolerate all kinds of inhuman treatment. The workers were helpless under this situation. Simultaneously, greedy landlords started exploiting the tenants. During 1950s, most colonies of the world gained independence making the citizens of those countries assertive of their rights. The impact of the progress of science and technology has made the man's life comfortable but very complicated making it dependent on state service. Today emergence of the concept of globalization has brought the culture of private administration close to Government agencies creating a very complex administrative processes. The concepts like "public interest", "good governance", "welfare", "development" etc. are evolving concepts inviting more interference by the State. These also demand expert guidance from the administrators with innovative ideas and commitment to the cause of the nation. Thus, the State's interference is increasing day by day. All these concepts demand some kind of flexibility in the administrative process for translating the ideals behind them into reality. This need can be met by administrative laws not by legal rules passed by the legislature. Here lies the need of moral leadership.

One has to admit that gradually the administration of a nation has become a very complex affair. For example, the concepts like welfare, good governance and development invites dynamism, innovation and changeability in public policies. These require the administrative agencies to formulate new or additional rules or laws considering the demand of the situation and needs of different groups of people.

Status of Rule of Law in India: India was under the British rule for a long time and its administration was shaped by the British. The independence of India did not relieve its administration from the British ideals. The British legacy is visible in several vital areas of Indian administration even to-day. Further independent India has to undertake developmental programmes in large scale.

The Constitution of India deals with administration in the context of laws through the articles 13, 136, 226, 227 and 300. It also incorporates a chapter on civil service spreading from article 309 to article 315.

The Law Commission of 1955 touched different areas of Administrative Law. It insisted on judicial control over administrative agencies and enforcement of Rule of Law to avoid monopoly and misuse of power by the administrators so that the rights of the citizens are not jeopardized. The Commission realized that the absence of the system of judicial review in France was compensated by French Droit Administratif, but in India situation is different. In India the Apex Court of the country is competent to provide relief to a citizen who is a victim of administrative action not merely on the ground of violation of the constitution, but also on the grounds such as—ultra virus, malafides, unfair, abuse of power or discretion etc. This power is not enjoyed by Counsel d'Etat in France.

The delegated legislation, administrative adjudication and judicial review are the three major components of administrative law. It indicates that the administration, besides performing the administrative functions is empowered to undertake quasi-legislative and quasi-judicial functions.

The existence of written Constitution in India provides the scope for judiciary to ascertain that administrative activism is based on rule of law and within the framework of the constitution. The administrative tribunals are special arrangements with some judicial functions. The Directive Principles of State Policy incorporated in the Constitution entrust very wide and diverse responsibilities to the administrative agencies which require some kind of special arrangement to settle the problems of judicial in nature arising in course of their functions. In 1985, the Parliament made provision for establishment of Administrative Tribunal to expedite the process of settlement of disputes by passing the Administrative Tribunals Act. At the instance of the 42nd Amendment of the Constitution provides for creation of tribunals by appropriate legislatures on subjects like taxation, foreign exchange, labour disputes, land reforms, election, essential goods, offences and other relevant issues. These tribunals are free to follow any procedure according to their conveniences provided they follow the rules of natural justice and fair play. However, these tribunals are under the appellate jurisdiction of the Supreme Court under article 136. The jurisdiction of the High Courts may also be extended to administrative tribunals under articles 226 and 227 whenever necessity arises. (Sadana: 2004)

Social Justice: The Free encyclopaedia refers social justice as "justice in terms of the distribution of wealth, opportunities, and privileges within a society." Classically, "justice" referred to ensuring that individuals both fulfilled their societal roles, and received what was due from society. "Social Justice" is generally used to refer to a set of institutions which will enable people to lead a fulfilling life and be active contributors to their community. The goal of social justice is generally same as human development. The relevant institutions can include education, healthcare, social security, labour rights, as well as a broader system of public services, progressive taxation and regulation of markets, to ensure fair distribution of wealth, equality of opportunity, and no gross inequality of outcome.

As a student of Political Science I have the temptation to bring to light in this context what Plato (429-347 B.C.) talked of Justice. To him "Justice is the having and doing what is one's own." Plato, unlike his predecessors tried to establish that justice is something internal. It exists in individual and in the state. The justice in the state is social justice which can be best explained by referring to the four virtues—wisdom, courage, temperance and justice. In every state there should be a class of persons to undertake deliberative functions. These functions can be performed only by the men of knowledge. The knowledge will enable the possessors to sacrifice his interests for the sake of others. This knowledge is possessed only by a few. These persons should be the rulers of the State. Second virtue is courage. That is, there should be another class of persons with a sense of danger. They will be able to meet any situation to safeguard the security of the State. The third virtue is temperance or self-control or discipline. This section of people would be able to control their bad elements by their good elements.

Justice exists in a state when all citizens occupy their respective positions and perform their duties without interfering the affairs of others. Thus, social justice is nothing, but a principle of society, consisting of producing class, military class and ruling class. The collective efforts of them can bring common good.

On the same line, every man has three elements in him—reason, appetite and spirit. The appetite and spirit must be controlled by reason. In this way Plato justified, justice is a principle of life. It is nothing but inner quality of man. (Rao: 1980) Although every man has these three elements in him, all men do not have them on equal degree—some are controlled by appetite, some by courage or spirit and some by reason. On the basis of degree of the strength of these elements the citizens may be classified as men of reason, men of spirit and men of appetite. (Gupta: 1972)

While the concept of social justice can be traced through ancient and renaissance philosophy, from early twentieth century it was embedded in international law and institutions, starting with the Treaty of Versailles 1919. The preamble to establish the International Labour Organization recalled that "universal and lasting peace can be established only if it is based upon social justice". In the later twentieth century, social justice was made central to the philosophy of the social contract, primarily by John Rawls in *A Theory of Justice* (1971), the Vienna Declaration and Programme of Action treats social justice as a purpose of the human rights education.

The term "social justice" first appeared in United Nations texts during the second half of the 1960s. At the initiative of the Soviet Union and with the support of the developing countries, the term was used in the Declaration on Social Progress and Development, adopted in 1969.

The same document reports, "From the comprehensive global perspective shaped by the United Nations Charter and the Universal Declaration of Human Rights, neglect of the pursuit of social justice in all its dimensions translate into *de facto* acceptance of a future marred by violence, repression and chaos." The report concludes, "Social justice is not possible without strong and coherent redistributive policies conceived and implemented by public agencies."

The same UN document offers a concise history; the notion of social justice is relatively new. None of history's great philosophers—not Plato or Aristotle, or Confucius or Averroes, or even Rousseau or Kant—saw the need to consider justice or the redress of injustices from a social perspective. The concept first surfaced in Western thought and political language in the wake of the industrial revolution and the parallel development of the socialist doctrine. It emerged as an expression of protest against what was perceived as the exploitation of labour and as a focal point for the development of measures to improve the human condition. It was born as a revolutionary slogan embodying the ideals of progress and fraternity. Following the revolutions that shook Europe in the mid-1800s, social justice became a rallying cry for progressive thinkers and political activists.... By the mid-twentieth century, the concept of social justice had become central to the ideologies and programmes of virtually all the leftist and centrist political parties around the world.

Social justice is also a concept that is used to describe the movement towards a socially just world, for example, Global Justice Movement. In this context, social justice is based on the concepts of human rights and equality, and can be defined as, "the way in which rights are manifested in the everyday lives of people at every level of society."

The term "social justice warrior" has been used to describe people who work for social justice issues: Mahatma Gandhi may be considered as a social justice warrior.

Social justice has more recently made its way into the field of bioethics. Discussion involves topics such as affordable access to healthcare, especially for low income households and families. The discussion also raises questions such as whether society should bear healthcare costs for low income families, and whether the global marketplace is a good thing to deal with healthcare. Ruth Faden and Madison Powers of the John Hopkins Berman Institute of Bioethics focus their analysis of social justice on which inequalities matter the most. They develop a social justice theory that answers some of these questions in concrete settings.

Social injustices occur when there is a preventable difference in a health state among the people. These social injustices take on the form of health inequities when negative health states such as, malnourishment, and infectious diseases are more prevalent among impoverished nation. These negative health states can often be prevented by providing social and economic structures such as primary healthcare which ensure the general population has equal access to healthcare services regardless of income level, gender, education or any other stratifying factor.

(http://en.wikipedia.org/wiki/Social_Justice 8.12.2014)

The efforts of the framers of the Constitution of India to establish social justice cannot be ignored. Independent India makes all possible arrangements for welfare of individual as well as different social groups. It attempts to reduce the gap due to caste, place of birth, race, creed, sex and status. Through the reservation of seats in services and educational institutions for weaker sections an attempt has been made to establish social justice in the country. Provision for free education up to the age of 14 years is a very significant or bold step in Indian democracy towards this end.

It must be remembered that India occupies a unique position in asserting, since the time of *Vedas*, that duty precedes right and to believe that duty is synonymous to *Dharma*. *Dharma* does not mean a particular religion, caste or community, it means a code of conduct to make a man to be dutiful. The *Vedas* which talked of three paths for self-realization—*Karma Yoga, Bhakti Yoga* and *Jnana Yoga*. Duty, devotion and knowledge are the keys to enjoy human rights. Creation, distribution and use of economic means are controlled by *dharma*. *Manusmriti* and *Yajnavalkya Smriti* described rules of trade. Wealth earned through righteous, genuine and incorrupt means is classified as *Purushartha*. Wealth acquired otherwise is declared illegal and attracts punishment. *Mahabharata* advised to observe *dharma* for acquiring wealth. The wealth acquired otherwise will cause tension and loss of peace of mind. (Chaturvedi: 2002)

Human Rights and Good Governance

The concept of governance is an old one. It is as old as human civilization. It has occupied and is occupying a prominent place in the discussion of scholars and administrative reformers since 1990s. The book titled, *"Re-Inventing Government"* authored by David Osborne and Ted Gaebler in 1992 focused very clearly the criteria for Good Governance. Some of the features of it are applicable to medical service also as sub-governance. These are: (a) Driven by Mission; (b) Be Result-oriented; and (c) Invest in preventing problems rather than curing crises. *www.Scottlondon/Osborne.html*

In 1997 Osborne, Gaebler and Peter Plastrik identified five strategies in connection with re-inventing Government—effectiveness, entrepreneurship, responsiveness, creativeness, and accountability. If we look into the Social Capital Theories of which Robert Putnam is associated as one of the leading advocates we find that it underlines the citizens' participation.

www.mildredwarner-org/govt-restructuring/re-inventing-govt.
www.unpan.org/DPADM/Events/GlobalForumReinventinggovernment/tabid/441/language/en-US/default.aspx.

The normative concept of governance is a value laden concept. It may be termed as Good Governance. The norms of a society are ultimately an expression of its values—socially shared ideas about what is good, right, and desirable. The difference between values and norms is that values are abstract and general concepts, whereas norms are behavioural rules or guidelines for people in particular kinds of situations. In India to-day health of a person is valued most. Therefore, it is noticed that self healthcare, practice of *Yoga*, diet control and morning walk, periodic health check-up, taking care of food nutrition of the children, revival of the system of midday meal in school, taking advice periodically from the family doctors etc. are the indicators giving value in priority to the health. However, most rural areas have yet to be sensitized in this regard. The World Bank realized from experiences of several developing countries that good governance is key not only to creating and sustaining an environment which fosters strong and equitable development, but it is also an essential complement to sound economic policies. Three distinct aspects can well be identified in the conceptualization of 'governance': (a) nature of political regime; (b) the process by which authority is exercised in the management of a country's economic and social resources; (c) ability of the Government to formulate and implement policies. (M. Bhattacharya: 1999)

Participation: Participation in the administration of a country by both men and women is the key cornerstone of good governance. Participation may be direct or indirect. Setting aside the members of the Government and the administrators, personnel of other professions contribute indirectly to the process governing the State. The physicians, teachers, social workers, religious leaders, different associations or organizations play significant role in policy formulation and implementation process. The physicians constitute an important group of participants in the governance. The high quality of performance of the physicians or other professionals can contribute to build-up Good Governance.

Rule of Law: Good governance requires fair legal frameworks that are enforced impartially. It also requires protection of human rights. Just as impartial enforcement of laws requires independent and impartial police force and bureaucracy, for satisfactory medical services there is the need of skilled physicians with human qualities. On the other hand, state must provide atmosphere and ways to motivate them to be committed to this noble service to humanity (discussed above).

Transparency: It means that information is freely available and directly accessible to those who will be affected by such decisions and their enforcement. It also means that enough information is provided and that it is provided in easily understandable forms and media. This is the fundamental requirement in the medical services for mainly three reasons—1. Skilled of the physician is his own monopoly, which the patients and attendants cannot acquire; 2. Patient has immense faith on the doctor; 3. The attendants suffer from acute anxiety and always want early recovery of the patient. Generally, conflict between police and public arises as the police meet people mostly in the controversial situations.

Similarly, doctors always meet people who are vulnerable due to illness accompanied the tension ridden attendants. Therefore, the transparency and easily understandable communication of the status of the patient and the nature of the treatment may reduce anxiety of the attendants which may help disappearance of conflicting situation.

Responsiveness: Good governance requires that institutions and processes try to serve all stakeholders within a reasonable timeframe.

Consensus oriented: There are several actors in the process of governing a state. Good governance requires to reach a broad consensus in a society on what is in the best interest of community and how this can be achieved. It also requires a broad and long-term perspective on what is needed for sustainable human development and to achieve the goals of such development. This is possible from an understanding of the historical, cultural and social contexts of a given society.

Equity and Inclusiveness: A society's well-being depends on ensuring that all its members feel that they have a stake in it and do not feel excluded from the mainstream of the society. It requires all groups, but particularly the most vulnerable, have opportunities to improve and maintain well-being.

Effectiveness and Efficiency: Good governance means the processes and institutions produce results that meet the needs of society while making the best use of resources at their disposal. The concept of good governance also covers the sustainable use of natural resources and the protection of the environment.

Accountability: Accountability is a key requirement of good governance. Not only the Government institutions, but the private and civil society organizations must be accountable to the public and to their institutional stakeholders. Accountability cannot be enforced without transparency and rule of law.

www.unescap.org/pdd/prs/ProjectActivities/Ongoing/gg/governance/.asp

The World Bank identified seven parameters of good governance which are relevant to both developed and developing countries as:

Legitimacy of the political system which can best be achieved through regular elections and political accountability.

Freedom of association and participation by various socio-economic, religious, cultural and professional groups in the process of governance.

An established legal framework based on the rule of law and independence of judiciary to protect human rights, secure social justice and guard against exploitation and abuse of power.

Bureaucratic accountability including transparency.

Freedom of expression required for formulation of policies, monitoring and evaluation of government performance.

A sound administrative system leading to efficiency and effectiveness.

Co-operation between the government and civil society organization.

www.unescap.org/pdd/prs/ProjectActivities/Ongoing/gg/governance/.asp

According to UN Economic and Social Commission for Asia and Pacific (UNESPACP) Good Governance has eight characteristics: (1) Participation, (2) Rule of Law, (3) Transparency, (4) Responsiveness, (5) Consensus oriented, (6) Equity and Inclusiveness, (7) Effectiveness and Efficiency, and (8) Accountability.

A Global Forum to address Government for re-invention was first organized by the Government of United States in 1999. Since then it has emerged as one of the most significant global events to address the issue. Subsequent Forums have been organized by the Governments of Brazil, Italy, Morocco, Mexico met regularly. The seventh meeting of the Global Forum was held in UN at the instance of the Under Secretary General of it. It also highlighted several features of good governance, such as effectiveness, efficiency, accountability etc.

www.mildredwarner-org/govt-restructuring/re-inventing-govt.

Priority of duties is referred to in *smritis*. The eleventh chapter of *Gautama Smriti*, a King is considered not fit to levy taxes on the citizens if he does not perform his duties faithfully, diligently and consciously. G.S. Misra, in his article, *Limits of Statutory Rights* said, "Moral conduct and obligation to discharge one's duties was considered essential for both king and the people. The spirit of devotion to duty was therefore instilled in all the citizens in various ways. It was done not only through education but also by making it an integral aspect of the traditional value system which were absorbed even while one was growing up. A society which was built upon such foundations inherently guaranteed the human rights. These were the very notions which made India a land of true action or *Karma Bhumi*."

During freedom struggle Gandhi also stated in support of the above tradition of the country that true source of right is duty. The framers of the Constitution has provided enough scope for its realization. The human rights cannot be enjoyed by an individual without human duties. In other words, these are not absolute in nature. The limitation originates from the fact that each human being has similar rights. (Baxi:1994)

But in independent India neither the rulers nor the ruled honoured this Indian tradition. They have started giving weightage to rights only. Negligence of duty has become the law of the average people. The political leaders have become more concern of the security of their political positions, nation's interest has been neglected to a great extent.

Shirin Abadi said, "People are different, and so are their cultures; People live in different ways, and civilizations also differ; People speak in a variety of languages; People are guided by different religions; People are born different colours, and many traditions influence their lives with varying colours and shades; People dress differently and adapt to their environment in different ways; People express themselves differently. Music, literature and art reflect different styles as well. But despite these differences, all people have one single common attribute: they are all human beings—nothing more, nothing less. And however different they may be all cultures embrace certain common principles. No culture tolerates the exploitation of human beings. No religion allows the killing of the innocent. No civilization accepts violence or terror. Torture is abhorrent to the human conscience. Brutality and cruelty are appalling in every tradition.

In short, these common principles, which are shared by all civilizations, reflect our fundamental human rights. These rights are treasured by everyone, everywhere.

So, cultural relativity should never be used as a pretext to violate human rights, since these rights embody most fundamental values of human civilizations. The Universal Declaration of Human Rights is needed universally, applicable with to both East and West. It is compatible with every faith and religion. Failing to respect our human rights only undermines our humanity.

Let us not destroy this fundamental truth; if we do, the weak will have nowhere to turn." (Shirin Abadi, 2003 Nobel Peace Prize Winner, Human Development Report, 2002, UNDP)

Dr. Sapru pointed out in an international conference held in 1986 at Delhi that, it is no denying a fact that the evolution of societal forms of living throughout the animal world has been an innate response to the compulsions of self-preservation. However, unlike rest of the animal world, the human attribute of reason has permitted our species to break the biological barriers and subjugate, to some extent, nature to human will. This has opened up several dimensions for societal development within the human species far beyond those found in the rest of the animal world. Even to-day self-preservation is the basis of social living. Dr. R.P.

Sapru has indicated two major components of self-preservation—security and sound health.

The concept of healthcare has evolved to mean a comprehensive scheme which promotes good health, prevents ill health, cures the sick and rehabilitates the disadvantaged. It is a scheme which involves interaction between economic uplift, social uplift, public health, health education, targeted prevention and cure as well as physical, social, and economic rehabilitation. It is obvious that the limited resources of poor nations cannot provide for wide ranging needs. As a result some prioritization is inevitable. Social justice on the other hand, requires universalization of healthcare, even across the geographical boundaries.

The journey from agricultural society to industrial society or from traditional society to modern society creates confusion and indecisiveness as regards the adherence of old traditions in the days of specialization and expertness. The modern scholars have discarded the amateur philosophy of learning. Average educated or enlightened parents do not feel comfort to accept the value of ethical principles and humanity. There is a feeling that competition and morality do not go together. The Governments in India are investing a large amount of money on education. The number of educational institutions and educated people is increasing. In spite of Governmental efforts the experience of last more than a decade reveals that government run schools in most cases fail to attract the students from the families with affordable financial capacity. These families send their children to private schools. Similar picture may appear in the case of Government hospital systems. There is not one reason for this state of affairs. However, it may be said most of the Government policies are failing at the implementing stage in which implementing agencies and the people are directly associated. Politicization and selling of jobs are the two major factors for distortion of essentials of administration and to make the path of entry into the service wide and smooth for the yes men/ yes women and moneyed people. This act of leadership not only destroys the ideals of human society, it appears as a threat to the leadership itself.

While appreciating the increasing emphasis and need of quality of skill or professional expertise of the physicians as asserted by Dr. Sapru the need of taking care of human values and ethical principles cannot be ignored in the case of both the service providers and the beneficiaries, i.e., the patients. Medical service has its own uniqueness by its very nature of work and working situation and receivers of the service.

The encounter of a doctor with fellow human being occurs at a time when the later is most vulnerable; the patient-doctor relationship is indeed a symmetric. As a consequence, the responsibility of the doctor is twofold—first to offer services and alleviate suffering, and secondly, not to exploit the vulnerable position of the patient, however, tempting the circumstances may be. As a trustee of the patient's health, the doctor is enjoined to provide the best skills irrespective of the economic status or social position of the patient. Exhortations to this effect form part of the Hippocratic Oath and more recently the Geneva Convention Code of the World Medical Association (1949).

In India, the emerging problem is that the safeguard of human rights is considered as the responsibility of the Government agencies and people have no responsibility for it. Democracy as a way life must be practiced for safeguard of human rights. Education is the sole means of safeguarding human rights. The ancient Indian tradition always reminds us that the main source of our rights is our duty.

Education is the strongest device to develop inherent powers of men. It provides wide scope and courage to take steps for development of one's own capacities. Education cultivates the mind of a man. As mentioned above one may think of enjoying human rights through the device insisted in India since ancient time, i.e. rights are conferred automatically through commitment to one's own duty which demands love, dedication and peace efforts to serve the human society.

References

Abadi, Shirin 2003: Nobel Peace Prize Winner, Human Development Report. 2002. UNDP.

Annan, Kofi: United Nations Secretary General: Human Development Report 2002 UNDP Human Development and Human Dignity.

Agarwal, R.C.: *Constitutional Development of India and National Movement*; S. Chand & Co, New Delhi, 1986.

Anand, Dr. V.K. 2001: Allahabad Law Agency, 16/2, Mathura Road, Plot No. 33, Faridabad.

Bakshi, P.M. 2004: *The Constitution of India With Selective Comments*; 5th edition, Universal Law Publishing House Co. Ltd.

Basu, Acharya, Dr. Durga Das 2007: *Commentary on the Constitution of India:* Eighth edition 2007: Wadha & Company Publisher: Agra, Nagpur and New Delhi.

Baxi, Upendra: *Inhuman Wrongs and Human Rights*, Har Anand Publications, New Delhi, 1994.

Bhardwaj, Rekha 2000: Significance of Scriptures in Highlighting Human Rights, *Human Rights: Global Perspective* edited by Hemlata Talesa, Nalini

Pansholy and Mangi Lal Nagda; Rajasthan Council of Educational Administration and Management, Udaipur.

Canley, Simon and Peter Jones (ed.) 1945: *Human Rights and Global Diversity*, Frank Cass, London, 1945.

Chatterjee, Aneek 2010: International Relations Today: Longman (Pearson) Kolkatta.

Chaturvedi, Urmila: Priority to Duties in Indian Tradition; *Governance and Human Rights*, edited by Jhunjhunwala, Kalpaz Publications, Delhi, 2002.

Dias, R.W.M. 1994: *Jurisprudence*, Aditya Book Pvt. Ltd., New Delhi.

Ebenstein, W., *Introduction to Political Philosophy.*

Gupta, M.G.: *History of Political Thought*, Chaitanya Publishing House, Allahabad, 1972.

IWCOHR Occasional paper No. 4 on Human Rights in India: An Overview; January 1997.

Jha, Vidyananda (2002): Priority given to Human Rights in Ancient Indian Tradition: *Governance and Human Rights*, edited by Bharat Jhunjhunwala, Kalpaz Publications; Delhi, 2002.

Kapur, A.C. 1989: *Indian Political System*, S. Chand & Company Pvt. Ltd., Delhi.

Krishna Iyer, Justice V.R. 1995: *Human Rights—A Judge's Miscellany*, B.R. Publishing Corporation, A Division of D.K. Publishers & Distributors, Delhi.

Laski, Harold J. 1960: *A Grammar of Politics*, London, 4th edition, 1960 reprint.

Mahanty, Jaganath; *Human Rights Education*, Deep & Deep Publications, 2000.

Maheswari, S.R., *Administrative Theory*, 2nd edition; MacMillan India Ltd., Delhi, 2002.

Merriam, Charles A. 1939: *The New Democracy and the New Despotism*, McGraw-Hill Book Company, New York.

Misra, Sridhar (2002), The Element of Social Good in Indian Tradition, *Good Governance and Human Rights*, edited by Bharat Jhunjhunwala, published by Kalpaz Publications, Delhi-110052.

Naseema, C. 2002: *Human Rights Education: Conceptual and Pedagological Aspects*; Kanishka Publisher Distributors, New Delhi.

Nehru, Jawaharlal 1946: *The Discovery of India*, New Delhi, 1946, 12th impression 1992, Delhi referred in IWCOHR Occasional paper No. 4 on Human Rights in India: An Overview; January 1997.

Nirmal, C.J. 1999: *Human Rights in India*, Oxford University Press.

Palkhiwala, Nani A., *We The People*, UBS Publisher' Distributors Ltd., New Delhi, 11th print 1997.

Pyasi, Mala: Duties Before Rights; *Governance and Human Rights*, edited by Bharat Jhunjhunwala; Kalpaz Publications, Delhi, 2002.

Rao, B. Shiva: *The Framing of India's Constitution*; Vol. II, 1967, The Indian Institute of Public Administration, New Delhi.

Rao, V.V., *A History of Political Thought*, S. Chand & Company, Delhi, 1980.

Roy, A.C., *International Relations Since 1919*, World Press, Calcutta, 9th edition.

Sabine, G.H., 1949; *A History of Political Theory*; 3rd edition, 1949.

Sadana, B.L. and M.P. Sharma, *Public Administration in Theory and Practice*, Kitab Mahal, Allahabad, 2004.

Sapru, S.P. The Conflict of Ethics and Social Justice in Developing Countries, (Dr. R.P. Sapru, Associate Professor, Dept. of Cardiology, Postgraduate Institute of Medical Education and Research, Chandigarh) Published under the auspices of Indian Council of Medical Research the Conference papers. The International Conference was held in New Delhi in 1986. The topic was Health Policy: Ethics and Human Values. It was held in collaboration with the Council of International Organization of Medical Sciences (Geneva). Compiled by Dr. P.C. Bhatta, Secretariat, IMA House, May, New Delhi).

Sharma, Gakuleh 2000: *Human Rights and legal Remedies*, Deep & Deep Publication Pvt. Limited, New Delhi.

Singh, Dr. Deepa 2002: *Human Rights and Police Predicament*, The Bright Law House, Delhi-110 006.

Singh, Nagendra (1981): *Human Rights and The Future of Mankind*: Varsity Books, 1981.

Singh, S. 1966, *A History of Political Thought*, Rastogi & Company, Meerut, 1966, pp. 280-320.

Sunanda Raj 1999; Awakening of Human Rights; *Human Rights in India*, ed. by C.J. Nirmal, Institute of Indian and International Studies, Oxford University Press.

Srivastava, V.P. and R.S. Narayan: *United Nations on Human Rights*, Vol. 1, 1st Publication 2002.

Vij, D.R. 2000: United Nations Decade (1995-2004) For Human Rights Education: A Challenge and Opportunity for the Educators; *Human Rights: Global Perspective*, edited by Hemlata Talesa, Nalini Pansholy and Mangi Lal Nagda; Rajasthan Council of Educational Administration and Management, Udaipur.

FIVE
Social Relationship

Social relationship exists both within and outside an organization, irrespective of its nature of work and goals. Every organization may be called social organization, because in the ultimate analysis of it there remain human beings. Outside the organization also every individual has to maintain social relationship for fulfilling his or her fundamental requirements. This relationship is inevitable in an organization as well as outside it. It begins at home immediately after the birth of a child and continues till the end of his or her life along with the relations with other social groups. This relationship influences a person's behaviour, thought process and style of living. In a man's life human relationship plays a significant role, especially at the very young age, from the time of birth when the child is at the helpless stage to adulthood when he comes out of the stage of helplessness becomes self-dependent for his daily activities.

A baby depends fully on others for its very survival. Then again at his old age he/she requires help from others for day-to-day affairs or survival. At this stage he/she also needs family members around him/her not only for carrying out the daily activities, but also for mental strength and peace. Their close association increases self-confidence of an individual at the old age. Further whenever a man falls ill, he becomes helpless at stage of his life and needs an attendant. While approaching a doctor for treatment generally a patient is accompanied by one or two family members. Only in the case of absence of the family members he is accompanied by others. In addition to medical treatment a patient needs some mental strength and confidence for quick recovery which patient acquires from the very presence of the attendants or family members. Thus, at every stage of man's life social or human relationship plays a very significant role for the survival of the human beings.

In an organization social relationship is of two kinds—formal and informal. Maximilian Carl Emil Weber, popularly known as Max Weber is well known for his advocacy for formalism or impersonal relationship in an organization. To him formal rules, regulations, selection of personnel on the basis of merit etc. are enough to achieve the goals of an organization. To him informal or personal relationship or human element does not appear as a factor to be taken care for maintaining efficiency in any organization.

This human aspect of organization was highlighted by the Hawthorne Study made by a group of researchers under the leadership of George Elton Mayo (1880-1949). Elton Mayo was born at Adelaide, Australia. He was educated at Queen's School and the Collegiate School of St. Peter. He joined the University of Adelaide to study medicine. But soon he left the university and went to UK to study at medical school of Edinburgh and London. There also he could not continue his study and left for West Africa and ultimately he returned to Adelaide and he studied psychology and philosophy and became famous for his contribution towards development of organizational theory in administration.

Hawthorne experiment has showed that an organization is a social system with group relationship and group attitudes. It reflects the informal aspect of an organization. An organization is a complex system as it depends for its success on interdependence of individuals, their motives, attitudes, behaviour etc. Besides formal rules and regulations informal relationship is an inalienable part of an organization. It generally originates in continuous interactions, contacts and relationships which are not at all a part of formal system. These contacts may be incidental or accidental to organized activities or may arise from personal desire or gregarious instincts. Thus, the employees who come from different places and with different family backgrounds form social groups according to their liking and disliking while working together.

These informal relations are necessary to the operation of formal organizations as a means of communication, cohesion and protecting the personality and integrity of the individual. This informal relationship serves certain objectives—(a) helps attainment of personal objectives; (b) provides social satisfaction; (c) makes communication easy; and (d) ensure social control of behaviour etc.

It is true that formal organization cannot be replaced by informal organization. But it fills the gaps in an organization and helps effective functioning of it. S.R. Maheswari, in his book titled, '*Administrative Theory*' emphasized the need of informal organization to meet the deficiencies of rules or policies. These rules generally lack dynamism unless interpreted by the personnel working in the organization to ensure effective implementation with the human spirit of the laws or policies. (Maheswari: 2002).

In the medical care services informal or social relationship occupies a prominent place spreading over to several areas, such as, the relationship between the service providers and the patients, functional group consisting of physicians, nurses, other medical and non-medical personnel attending patients in one ward, personnel belonging to same faculty or specialization etc.

This informal relationship helps development of 'science of work' as advocated by Frederick Winslow Taylor while explaining the Scientific Management Theory of organization. Taylor talked of following principles of Scientific Management:

- Development of true science
- Scientific selection of the workers
- Scientific education and development of workers
- Intimate and friendly cooperation amongst the employees (Bhaskara Rao: 2010)

True science means 'organized knowledge'. In the context of the personnel system in an organization it may be understood that each person occupies a position which is the smallest unit of a service or an organization setting aside infrastructure, equipment and finance. Each position has mainly three components—duties and responsibilities, technique required to carry out the duties and responsibilities attached to the position and certain conditions of service. A 'duty' consists of certain tasks to be performed by the incumbent.

The employees must be selected scientifically which requires standardization of qualifications of the incumbent with the duties and responsibilities attached to the position. During the service life of an employee provision must also be made for development of his or her career by giving enough scope to undergo training and to avail the educational facilities based on aptitude and performance survey through effective supervision. Further provision must also be made to motivate an employee to work hard with dedication through rewards and recognition either in kind or coin. This kind of scientific approach is very essential in the medical care services to create a healthy social environment so that mutual trust, free and frank interaction or exchange of ideas become possible.

Doctor-Patient Relationship: Every organization may be termed as social or human organization as stated above for the simple reason that it is by the human beings and its ultimate goal is also service to humanity. Any organization which fails to fulfill this goal has no justification of its existence. Because it will become a burden of the society and gradually it will destroy the human fabric of social relationship. Social relations are always human oriented. And again it is the human being who is to generate human culture in the organization to achieve its ultimate goal to serve people. He is not only the creator of human culture in the organization he is also the sustainer of this culture in the organization when it faces turbulent social, political and economic changes and problems. The changes have to be regulated with normative approach and the problems must be solved with human approach. He has to direct the society to climb up in the escalator of human welfare and progress with the help of scientific innovation. Dilution of human power in the process of direction or leadership or organizational activism may allow the science to start the process of dehumanizing the human organization. This is applicable to all organizations, whether public or private. Because both have to serve the interest of the people. For example in the school, the relationships between teachers and students, in hospital between physicians and patients, in administration between administrator and administered, at home between parents and children are rooted in human values.

Another significant aspect of social relationship has been indicated by Mahatma Gandhi in his own way that the control of self-interest of the individual is an essential prerequisite to the transformation of social relationship in terms of the ultimate values. The values must be inculcated in the individual before they can find true social expression. He emphasized the need for a private moral on the part of the individual before he can qualify himself for social action. In order to engage in the task of transforming social relationships, the individual must observe, he said, the five vows enjoined by the ancient Indian scriptures, namely, *Satya* (truth), *ahimsa* (non-violence), *asteya* (non-stealing), *aparigraha* (non-possession) and *brahmacharya* (control of animal passion). (Tripathi: 1980)

One person or individual is not a society. To be a society there must be at least two individuals. Gandhi prescribed that the simple social virtues of truth and non-violence should be practiced and tried. If two persons wish to live together, benefit from each other, prosper together and seek the highest good from each other, only two social disciplines necessary are truth and non-violence. Each should be sure that the other speaks the truth and means no harm—they may belong to any race or clan or religion. They may be of different sexes. This applies to all multiples of two, be they groups or nations.

This formula he tried and perfected for himself and has placed it before humanity to try and see the result. This does not require any religion to sanction it nor any philosophy to uphold it. It has come to us not as a revelation nor as a word from scriptures, but from one who tried in scientific spirit to experiment with truth.

Regarding *ahimsa* or non-violence, there is a beauty about it; though negative in form it has a positive effect—security and safety in the presence of it. To-day the whole of humanity, the poorest and the richest, the weakest and the strongest are full of fear of violence.

In Gandhi's case *ahimsa* or non-violence could not remain a negative virtue. It evolved itself into the positive power of love, 'the cohesive force' which holds the constituents of an atom together and the atoms themselves together to form any recognizable thing or substance.

Every rational human being's *Dharma*, i.e. duty is to promote the positive forces of light, life and love. While violence destroys social-living and multiplies violence, non-violence builds through mutual security social living and ensures the progress of positive forces. (Diwakar: 1986)

Human relationship flourishes first in the family with human warmth primarily of mother followed by other members of the family in which a baby is born. Then in the school teachers help improvement of human traits in a child. They occupy a position next to the parents of the children. Thus, the process of socialization begins at home and then this responsibility is handed over to school. But society changes. India being a developing country social transformation takes place prominently and very quickly. On several occasions changes take place through imitation. The movement of the traditional society towards modernization and industrialization affects not only the process of socialization, but also social values inviting contradictions and confusions in the minds of the youths.

Background of Physician-Patient Relationship in India

Family is the primary social institution. This institution is based on the natural love and the members are emotionally united. The children are protected and taken care of by the parents and other members by providing food, cloth, shelter and satisfying other emotional needs of the children.

The most notable aspect of the child's life is the process of socialization which begins at home. The seeds of social virtues like sympathy, fellow-feeling, love and cooperation are sown in their minds by the members of the family. Family is like a cultivating field of personal and social virtues of a child. This field must be fertile for the healthy growth of the personality of a child. The children develop love and reverence for their parents, learn obeying the instructions of their parents and pick-up the nature of the ways of living from those of the parents. The spirit of self-sacrifice and community life or mutual sharing and adjustment with brothers and sisters begins at home itself. Therefore, utmost care has to be taken by the parents not to influence their minds by narrow mental outlook or other elements like hatred to others, selfishness, ego and other cruel behaviour to others in the midst of which the children spend their time. The human touch of the parents cannot be provided by any other persons and the institutions as is the case with the parents and the family.

A baby is not born with the sense of morality. It is inculcated in him through the process of socialization which begins at home. Lipi Mukhopadhyay, in her article, '*Social Conditioning and Deviant Behaviour*' rightly pointed out that a baby has no conscience and is ignorant of values. He is neither moral nor immoral. He starts learning moral codes at home from the parents followed by teachers and peer groups. Though it is a lifelong process to learn, to confirm and reconfirm the faith on these moral codes, the foundation for it is laid down in the mind of a child very well at home itself.

The baby judges what is good or bad in the context of pleasure and pain, attitude and behaviour of others towards him rather than what is right and what is wrong. Gradually his moral codes develops in the environment of the family to which he belongs, where he spends more time and with whom he is more attached.

It is said in the article by Mukhopadhyay, "whether a child will be creative or conformist in his outlook and behaviour is influenced by his home training; democratic child-training methods encourage leadership ability, creativity and authoritarian methods tend to foster conformity. Family relationships play a more important role in developing personality. What one thinks of himself as a person is a direct reflection of what he believes the different family members think of him as judged by the way they treat him" (Mukhopadhyay: 2002).

Similarly, the parents should not be deprived of the love, affection and the human care from the children which are extremely essential for their mental peace and security at the old age or even otherwise. Family is only social institution which can satisfy these human need. Because the family is the primary social unit and this was not a problem in the traditional society where there existed joint family system.

Significantly, in India realizing the need of the human care for the elderly people the Maintenance and Welfare of Parents and Senior Citizens Act, 2007 was passed in Parliament. The Act in its introduction, objects and reasons makes it clear that the ageing has become a major social challenge because of decline in the joint family system. A large number of elderly persons, particularly widowed women are not being looked after by their families. They are forced to spend their twilight years all alone and are exposed to emotional neglect and are not being provided financial support. To combat this social challenge, there is a need to give more attention to the care and protection for the older persons. Though there is a provision in the Code of Criminal Procedure, 1973 under which parents can claim maintenance from their children, but the procedure is time consuming and expensive. It is desired that simple, inexpensive and speedy provisions may be made to claim maintenance by the suffering parents. To cast an obligation on the persons who inherit the property of their aged relatives to maintain them and to make provisions for setting up old age homes for providing maintenance to the senior indigent older persons and to provide better medical facilities to the senior citizens and to make provisions for protection of their life and property, the Bill was introduced in the Parliament.

A specific mention may be made of the Chapter IV (Article) 20 which deals with the medical care of the senior citizens. It states: the State Government shall ensure that—

(i) The Government hospitals or hospitals funded fully or partially by the Government shall provide beds for all citizens as far as possible;
(ii) Separate queues be arranged for senior citizens;
(iii) Facility for treatment of chronic, terminal and degenerative diseases is expanded for senior citizens;
(iv) Research activities for chronic elderly diseases and ageing is expanded; and
(v) There are earmarked facilities for geriatric patients in every district hospital duly headed by a medical officer with experience in geriatric care.

It is difficult to deny that the environment of a family may not always congenial for the development of the personal qualities of a child in the right direction to make him the possessor of human qualities and to dedicate his/her self for acquiring expert knowledge in the field of his choice as student and as service provider to the society. In the contemporary Indian society experience shows that average families are struggling to socialize their children develop the human qualities.

In traditional Indian society religion, social custom and tradition played a significant role in the functioning of the family as the socializing agency. The significant features of the family environment were—*first*, it was not influenced by outside world as the mobility of the people was very low; *second*, blind faith on social customs and tradition; *third*, every act of family was performed in the name of God or was related to religion; and *fourth*, parental as well as social control over the behaviour of the children was very strong. Gradually with the spread of education, improvement of communication facilities at a rapid rate, high mobility of the modern man, emergence of the concept of democracy and awareness of the rights of man and woman the role of the family as well its structure change. To-day both the father and the mother of a child are the earner of money outside the four walls of their habitation in different capacities, old joint family system in most cases replaced by the nuclear family system. Side by side awareness of human rights and multiplication of these rights, for rapid development of information and communication technology a child of today need not wait for the parents to choose things relating to their way of life, the domestic caretaker of the children takes the help of television to control or console them, as it is her contract with the parents of the children, the service holder-parents try to compensate the human touch of theirs to the children by providing them things they demand or like most. The institutional devices or play school are found in the contemporary India with expert teachers to educate the children. While accepting all these devices a serious thought has to be given to strengthen the moral life of the children by providing some more comprehensive and effective devices to inculcate human qualities in them. However, India has already undertaken formulation of policies like Domestic Violence Act (Sinha: 2006).

In India traditional society experienced joint family system in which a child was socialized by the parents with active cooperation of other members like grand-parents, uncle-aunts etc. of a child as they live in the same family. Here begins the social control over the child. The family as the primary social institution played a very significant role in inculcating social values in the child or in the process of being to becoming of a baby. This is the case in all the societies. Two reasons for it are forwarded by Ian Robertson in his book, *Sociology*. These are—*first*, family is a place where children establish their first close emotional ties, learn language and begin to internalize cultural norms and values. The impact of certain unintentional elements like behaviour of family members, the ways of the daily life, inter-personal relationship, conversation amongst the family members, values adhered by them also leave deep impact on a child. *Second*, the location of the family is another important factor to be counted. Because an inclusive of sub-culture of race, community, religion, ethnicity etc. the children from the time of their birth receive ascribed values prevalent in race, community, religion, ethnicity etc.

The joint family system is gradually disappearing in the process of development of the nation. Its place is occupied by nuclear family system. The old agricultural society has changed making joint family system almost irrelevant, unmanageable and more conflict oriented than peace oriented social institutions. In independent India in the face of political development, spread of education, political participation, employment, fundamental rights, directive principles of state policy, progress of science and technology etc. Indians prefer nuclear family system. Government favoured small nuclear family in the economic interest and also in the interest of population strength. It affected the process of socialization of the children in the perception of human values and human dignity. Further, the socializing process has been constrained by employment of both father and mother in the job. Generally, educated mother is always in search of job. She prefers salaried job instead of remaining as house maker within the four walls of her habitation. Thus, there begins the change of values in the family life. Enhancement of monetary power of the family to equip the house with modern paraphernalia for social status and comfortable day to day life has become the primary goal of the parents in Indian families. The children are also socialized with this perception. Gradually, most people have failed to make a distinction between 'need' and 'greed'. Under this situation, the children get confused regarding social values.

In ancient India *Gurus* played a very significant role in shaping the character of the disciples who were to stay in the *Guru Griha* (house of the teachers). There the disciples learned lessons from *Vedas* and their character and social relations were shaped by the *Gurus*. Gradually, with the spread of education by the British changes emerged in the pattern of education and later with independence of the country the implementation of the constriction has brought further changes in the process of socialization by the school. Now with the innovation of television and internet the impact of traditional classroom has changed. The students have started acquiring information from these sources and these constitute another device of socializing the students. But these have more negative impact on most students instead of shaping their character on positive direction. So, the paternalistic authority of both the parents and the teachers is diminishing gradually. With it human relationship in the family and the school is becoming very fragile. The members of the young or new generation are in the new world of space segregating themselves from social reality.

The rapid progress of information technology has helped them to get all information about the happenings in any part of the world in a moment. In addition to it serials and advertisements of different articles in electronic media influence the younger generation to a great extent. What is taught in the class room, what is advised at home and what is insisted by traditional social ideals are found irrelevant to the youths. There emerges contradictions in the minds of the students. They have also found—what is taught in the class is not practiced at home or in public life either by the teachers or by others. They notice the disintegration in the advice and the acts of the teachers, administrators, politicians and the parents, contradictions between customs and traditions of old society and those of the modern one. Under this changing situation, role of the family as a socializing agency in the perception of well-established ethical and human values faces serious challenges. Similar is the case with regard to the school and other social organizations. Both the school and the family have considered training of the children on skill to get highly paid job with social status attached to job. Human aspect of the process of humanization of an individual at the early stage itself has been thrown out in modern India.

Socialization is the process of social interaction through which people form personality and learn the way of their social life. It helps an individual to learn the norms, values, language, skills, beliefs and other patterns of thought and action required for social living. Personality of an individual is the offshoot of the process of socialization. Personality refers to the fairly stable patterns of thought, feeling, and action that are typical of an individual. Personality has three components, as analyzed by Ian Robertson—*Cognitive*, *Emotional* and *Behavioural*. The *Cognitive* component consists of thought, belief, perception, memory and other intellectual, capacities; the *Emotional* component consists of love, hate, envy, sympathy, anger, pride and feelings; the *Behavioural* component accommodates skills, aptitudes, competence and other abilities. Nobody is born a great scientist and skilled carpenter, they may have potential to become any of these, but generally what they become is basically the unique socialization process.

Coming to the role of the teachers in the school as agents of socialization of the children it cannot be denied that main concern of the school is teaching skill and knowledge. Both invite the capacity of the teachers to carry out this responsibility. Along with these there are several other implicit things the impact of which go long way to the life of an individual and which are reflected in the behaviour and social relationships of the persons in their service life. For example, maintenance of cleanliness, regularity in attending classes, respect for elders who are their teachers, to be good listener, participation in discussion with permission of the teacher, waiting silently for his or her turn, expression of their ignorance freely etc. Further in school students come under similar rules, individual student is not considered as somebody special, which may generally happen in the family. It helps injecting feeling of oneness in the children coming from different families. Coming from different family backgrounds they start learning lessons in the same class room under the same environment and from the same teacher. Their academic achievements and failures constitute permanent record to be applicable in their future lives. They are exposed to a formal and wide world.

In an organization interactions, contacts and face-to-face relationships amongst the personnel are natural and continuous. Interestingly, these relationships do not constitute a part of or governed by formal organization nor it is possible to regulate these relationships by formal rules and regulations. These relationships may grow due to some personal interests and gregarious instinct of the human beings. These contacts in course of time emerge as informal organization within the formal organization and becomes an activating wheel of the formal organization.

The informal organization, i.e. social relationship is an inalienable part of formal organization and it produces two kinds of influence on formal organization. It establishes certain norms, attitudes, understandings, habit etc. and *secondly*, it creates an environment in which the formal organization has to function. Social norms and customs are very powerful with wide coverage of personnel system for smooth functioning of a formal organization. The environment created by social relationship is a precondition for accepting or rejecting common strategies, determination of means of communication, secure cooperation etc. (Robertson:1980)

In USA during 1960s scholars under the leadership of Dwight Waldo talked of value-based public administration by rejecting value-neutrality concept in it. Herbert A. Simon, H. Donald Smithburg and Frank J.

Thompson pointed out that inadequacy of formal organization creates vacuum making informal or social organization inevitable and irresistible. Katz and Kahn elaborated it by saying, "No organization chart and no book of policies and procedures can specify every act and prescribe for every contingency encountered in a complex organization." Professor Douglas McGregor's work, *The Human Side of the Enterprise* published in 1960 marked the watershed in the history of management movement dominated by the writings of his predecessors. He said, "It would not in any sense be an exaggeration to assert that any large organization would come to a grinding halt within a month if all its members began behaving strictly in accordance with the structure of responsibility and authority defined by the formal organization chart, the position classification and formal comforts." (Maheswari: 2003)

In 1920s, the Hawthorne experiment made by George Elton Mayo and his team on working of industries suggested a new mix of managerial skills. In addition to technical skills, the management should handle human situations, motivate, lead and communicate with workers. In his study he concentrated in fatigue, accidents, production levels, rest periods, working conditions, sentiment etc. of the industrial workers. (Mayo: 2007)

In India traditional social culture was rooted in human values and dignity and human relations. The administrative organizations were influenced by it. Public while appreciating an organization for its services used to give weightage to informal relationship also, such as offering a seat and a cup of tea while talking whenever a visitor comes, except those who have daily working relations. Sometimes more weightage was attached to it leading to annihilation of efficiency in the organization, which is to be avoided. Even now its flavour exists, though in a very mild and limited way, in spite of the deep impact of science and technology on the society. Most notable point to be remembered is the contribution made by Mahatma Gandhi who led the freedom movement in India to the human culture. He championed freedom of the individuals and induced Indians to fight with the weapons of *Satyagraha* and Non-violence against British Rule. The contributions of Radhakrishnan, Raja Ram Mohun Roy, Dr. B.R. Ambedkar and several other political leaders and social reformers helped strengthening human aspect in Indian culture. All these have notable impact or reflection in the Constitution of independent India.

It may be said that the social and political history of India provides wide scope to learn about the human culture by the modern Indians. Unfortunately, the society is moving other way round causing rampant corruption in all services without any exception, most members of the society engage themselves to acquire money power at any cost, accountability and responsibility have been driven out, slave mentality has emerged in spite of high mobility of persons across the country and also outside the country. In the face of it, rules and regulations of the services become fragile. Service holders as well as common peoples' apathy to cooperation in efficient implementation of public policies is a clear indication of ethical vacuum in the social relationship. There are enough instances of deviation from the constitutional provisions of the country.

The social relationship in medical services is of great importance due to its unique nature. Further most patients in India are inhabitants of rural area without much exposure to the outside world and without sufficient education and experience of conversation with expert professionals or high officials. Therefore, social relationship is to be emphasized as an important part of the process of achieving the goal of an organization.

The relationship between physician and patient is known as *Fiduciary* relationship. The word *Fiduciary* derives from the Latin word "confidence" or "trust". The patients trust the physician, i.e. on his professional capacity to cure his or her disease and to maintain secrecy of the information disclosed to him by the patient.

The professional capacity of the physician is the first priority of the patients. Then they think of personal qualities, i.e. character of the physician, especially his behaviour towards patient, particularly in the case of female patient and maintenance of secrecy of the information communicated to him or her about the disease. Generally, it is noticed that the patients and family members in India do not want to disclose anything about the deadly diseases or the diseases which are difficult to cure or infectious diseases. Reasons may be psychological, i.e. they do not want others to know about their distress or problems. As regards the infectious diseases, there is the fear of segregation of social relationship or these may stand a hindrance to accessibility to public places or public institutions accessibility not only of the patients but also the patient's family members. Since ancient time in India most people emphasized on confidentially from this point of view, they were not aware of the right to privacy. Only in the recent times the educated and urban people, the rural people who have the exposure to e-media as well as print media have become aware of the right to privacy in the perspective of medical treatment.

Trust in Physician is a motivating factor to encourage the patients to be free to disclose information about their ailments in detail which help the physician to take decision for treatment. The trust in professional capacity of the physicians was not questioned until the development of medical sciences in India with specialities in different areas of it and the increase in the number of physicians and hospitals, nursing homes etc. in the same area. For example, a patient with eye ailment, today will try to be sure which eye specialist/eye hospital he/she should approach for cure of eye ailment. The choice depends on the efficiency of the physician on this task which determined by most new patients from the exit patients. However, the known or close physicians also help them on this act of theirs.

Relationship in the Process of Treatment: In order to make accurate diagnoses and provide optimal treatment recommendations, the patient must communicate all relevant information about his ailments or suffering. The trust in physician is a strong motivating factor to secure required information. The physicians are obliged to refrain from divulging confidential information. Generally this relationship is based on medical ethics. The history of the disease and the family of the patient is necessary to understand the cause and the nature of the problem of the patient.

In order to secure accurate and open communication, the physician may take certain common approaches like:

- Attend to patient comfort
- Establish eye contact
- Listen without interrupting
- Show attention with nonverbal cues, such as nodding
- Allow silences while patients search for words
- Acknowledge and legitimize feelings
- Explain and reassure during examinations
- Ask explicitly if there are other areas of concern.

(https://depts.washington.edu/bioethx/tpoics/physpt.html)

Physician-patient relationship begins when the patient meets the physician in the Out Patient Department (OPD) of the hospital or in the private chamber of a physician or when physician visits the patient at his or her residence. Every patient is habituated some kind of social relationship in which he or she is born and brought up, therefore, it is natural that the patient expects the known behaviour and attitude from the physician also. Generally, the patient wants sympathetic attitude, attention to be paid to him or her; the physician listens with patience to the patient and answers to their queries. With the increase in the number of patient population and lack of required number of physicians in most cases the physicians in the urban/city hospitals cannot afford to spend more time on one patient as large number of patients stay in the Que. In addition to the increased number of population the language problem is another barrier between physicians and patients in India. Further, the progress of technologies for investigation has simplified the conversation between the physician and patient. Now long conversation is not required to understand the nature of ailment from the confusing narration of ailments from the patients and to a great extent the language problem is minimized as the machine speaks about the nature of ailment not the patients nor the physicians. The physicians can read the result produced by the machine and communicate to the patients for treatment.

The relationship between the patient and the physicians is also highly influenced by the role played by the attendants not only in the case of minors, but also in the case of adult provided they are very seriously ill and not in a position to talk and take decision.

After entry into hospital every patient has to agree when the physicians claim that the setting and judging of working conditions for taking care of patients is their sole monopoly. To be very precise one has to admit the paternalistic authority of the physicians over the treatment system. Patients and other laymen cannot have any say on it. The patient is a layman, unless he/she is a doctor-patient he or she cannot judge competently his or her requirements. However, the physicians as service providers have to take care of patients' comfort and need as the cure of the patient is the ultimate goal of the physicians. This makes the physicians to adjust according to the requirement of the patients. Medicine, food, cleanliness and other allied services needed daily by a patient including the progress report are the common requirements of the patients. It is for the physicians how efficiently these have to be provided to the satisfaction of the patients so that a healthy relationship can be maintained between physicians and the patients to achieve the ultimate goal of the medical services. Here lies the mutual cooperation between patient and physician.

In this context, it is found that patients in India are not legally obliged to approach physician for cure. A patient has the right to self-determination in this context. A person may or may not approach a physician to be relieved of his/her suffering. He may also undergo self-treatment. Law in India has nothing to do with it. Even the physician cannot compel a patient to avail of his services. Though there is no legal compulsion to avail of the physician's care, there is social pressure which the patient cannot ignore, especially, family members, neighbours and close friends always motivate the patient to approach physicians. In the recent years with the availability of medical service facilities (though in a limited way) even in the interior places of India people become aware of these services and their benefit. Therefore, though the physician and law of the country have no control over the decision of a patient to consult physician, social environment and awareness of healthcare induce a patient to approach physician for cure. The physicians have the monopoly only to decide the need and nature of medical services to be provided to a patient when a patient is under his or her custody. Physicians working in an organization enjoy monopoly only within the framework of the statutes and administrative requirements of the organization.

Mutual Influence in Physician-Patient Relationship: In the Physician-patient relationship there is every scope for mutual influence on each other. Particularly in the face-to-face interaction it is noticed. On the part of the physician through convincing communication of instructions and the way they use to make investigation and know the progression and digression of patient's condition they can influence the patient. Similarly, the patient through his or her behaviour, obligation to directions or cooperation with the medical service providers can influence the physicians. During the pre-entry into the process of treatment patient may ask the physicians several questions, such as, *Is there any alternative treatment? How long the treatment will continue? etc.* These questions are asked when the treatment recommended by the physician is not acceptable to the patient due to financial crunch, non-availability of attendant, geographical distance or communication problem, risk factor, fear psychosis etc.

However, observations of consultations reveals that in general the overt patient behaviour tends to be passive compared to that of the Physicians, and most frequent types of exchanges being physician initiated information- seeking exchanges, rather than patient-initiated information-giving exchanges. The patients generally wait for the physician to initiate the conversation. They are constrained by fear, tension or sometimes may be physically and mentally very weak to take decision how to start, what to tell, what the physician will think etc.

Another area where the patient may control is the utilization of treatment. When the patient is an indoor patient he/she has no other way but to carry out the instructions of the physicians as these are administered through nurses and other junior assistants. The presence of nurses cannot be ignored by the patient. But in the case of exit patients who are released from the hospital with certain specific conditions as regards the medicine to be used and instructions to be followed after being released from the hospital problem of control by the physicians over the patients arises. Patients may not oblige the physicians at this stage. Patients may take decisions not to take a drug or follow instructions when patients are not satisfied with the instructions or the patient feel difficult to follow them. At this stage doctor fails to persuade the patients to accept his advices unless the patients come to the physicians at their own initiative. Therefore, there is enough scope for the exit patient to neglect the treatment as advised by the physicians at the time of release.

The number of patients who do not obey the physician's order, whether these treatments are drugs or referral to hospital is quite big. Physicians are unable to know this aspect of patient-doctors relationship unless the patient volunteers to inform the physicians. The physicians rarely know that the patients have not used the treatment as directed after going out of the hospitals.

However, it must be said that the concern to maintain autonomy involves both the parties to control each other. From a client perspective the ability of patients to exert control over the doctor and over the medical care they receive—by not consulting, by choosing which doctor to consult, by influencing the interaction in the consultation, and by the utilization of treatment in a limited way. Controls that patients do exert are small-scale, individualistic, covert, and met by counter strategies by the physicians and the staff.

Today in between the physician and the patient there emerges physio-therapist. During pre-operation, and mainly during post-operation stages the physiotherapist enter into the process of treatment. He may become a mediator and thus may influence the patient to take decision and also help the physician to decide depending upon the experience of the therapist. (Gallagher: 1976)

History of Physician-Patient Relationship: The history of physician-patient relationship reveals that in ancient India the relationship began with the full faith on the professional capacity of the doctor. The question of suspicion of the patient on the professional authority of the doctor did not arise. There were several reasons for it. Most rural people were ignorant and less mobile and agriculturalists by profession. The number of medical service providers was also limited. The patients had no choice in selecting the doctors to approach, they generally used to go to a doctor who was easily accessible to them. They consider the position of a doctor next to God. Under that circumstance, it was quite natural to have paternalistic authority over the patients by the doctors.

In course of time wide development of medical services and education took place in the country. Healthcare has become the minimum need of the Indians. The people also become aware of this development and as a result they started to choose the hospital/doctor for their treatment. Closely related to it is the awareness of the human rights by the citizens due to the effort of UNO and the constitutional provisions for fundamental rights of the citizens. Gradually, issues like 'patient's autonomy', 'patient's safeguard', 'patient's informed consent' etc. emerged. In other words, the whole process of treatment has become democratic to certain extent.

Recently, the dominating role of the science and technology in the world of medical services is influencing the relationship between a doctor and a patient. Along with it the social values have changed. Public services in India are allowing the principles commercialization and competition in delivery of service to the people.

(https://depts.washington.edu/bioethx/tpoics/physpt.html accessed on 28.7.2014)

Change of social values causes corruption in the administration influencing medical services also. Naturally, earlier paternalistic authority of the doctor has changed. The patient himself or herself has become a part of decision making process. The patients today are conscious about the financial or otherwise benefit to be gained from a particular doctor or hospital, risks of alternative treatment etc.

http://www.ama-assn.org/ama/pub/physician-resources/medical-ethics/opinion10001.page accessed on 28.7.2014

Human Rights as the basis of Physician-patient relationship: Physician and patient relationship cannot be divorced from the basic human rights. This aspect is considered in almost all nations of the modern world under the umbrella of United Nations of Organizations. Here mention may be made of what is stated by American Medical Association in a report adopted in June 1990. The American Medical Association emphasizes on the right of the patients as:

> "From ancient times, physicians have recognized that the health and well-being of patients depends upon a collaborative effort between physician and patient. Patients share with physicians the responsibility for their own healthcare. The patient-physician relationship is of greatest benefit to patient when they bring medical problems to attention of their physicians in a timely fashion, provide information about their medical condition to

the best of their ability, and work with their physicians in a mutually peaceful alliance. Physicians can best contribute to this alliance by serving at their patients' advocate and by fostering those rights:

1. The patient has the right to receive information from physicians and to discuss the benefits, risks and costs of appropriate treatment alternatives. Patients should receive guidance from their physicians as to the optimal course of action. Patients are also entitled to copies or summaries of medical records, to have their questions answered, to be advised of potential conflicts of interest that their physicians might have and to receive independent professional options.
2. The patient has the right to make decisions regarding the healthcare that is recommended by his or her physician. Accordingly, patients may accept or refuse any recommended medical treatment.
3. The patient has the right to courtesy, respect, dignity, responsiveness and timely attention to his or her needs.
4. The consent of the patient, unless provided for by law or by the need to protect the welfare of the individual or the public interest. Patient has the right to confidentiality. The physician should not reveal confidential communications or information without the consent of the patient.
5. The patient has the right to continuity of healthcare. The physician has an obligation to cooperate in the coordination of medically indicated care with other healthcare providers treating the patient. The physician may not discontinue treatment of a patient as long as further treatment is medically indicated, without giving the patient reasonable assistance and sufficient opportunity to make alternative arrangement for care.
6. The patient has a basic right to have available adequate healthcare. Physicians along with the rest of the society, should continue to work toward this goal. Fulfillment of this right is dependent on society providing resources so that no patient is deprived of necessary care because of an inability to pay for the care. Physician should continue their traditional assumption of a part of responsibility for the medical care of those who cannot afford essential health.

Physicians should advocate for patients in dealing with third parties when appropriate."

http://www.ama-assn.org/ama/pub/physician-resources/medical-ethics/opinion10001.page accessed on 28.7.2014

The above discussion shows that the physician-patient relationship in ultimate analysis is human relationship and based on human rights. The quality of the patient-physician relationship is important to both parties. This quality of relationship depends on mutual respect, knowledge, trust, shared values and perspectives about disease and life and time available. The amount and quality of information about the patient's disease communicated in both directions. Further, the capacity of the physician to make accurate or correct diagnosis of the disease and to convince the patients of the honesty and sincerity of the doctor is also an important factor to command respect and trust of the patients.

http://en.wikipedia.org/wiki/Doctor%E2%80%93patient_relationship accessed on 28.7.2014

The World Medical Association while discussing Physicians and Patients relationship underlines six issues that arise in their daily practice:

1. Respect and Equal Treatment
2. Communication and Consent
3. Decision-making for incompetent patients
4. Confidentiality
5. Beginning of Life Issues
6. End of Life Issues.

Respect and Equal Treatment: The belief that all men are equal by birth and to be treated equally, that is, as human beings is applicable to the doctor and patient relationship also. The emergence of this belief is relatively a recent one. In most societies disrespectful and unequal treatment of individuals and group was accepted as normal and natural. Slavery was one such practice that was not eradicated in the European colonies and the USA until the nineteenth century and still exists in some parts of the world. The end of institutional discrimination against non-whites in countries such as South Africa is much more recent. Women still experience lack of respect and unequal treatment in most countries. Discrimination on the basis of age, disability or sexual orientation is widespread. Clearly there remains considerable resistance to the claim that all people should be treated as equals. In India, caste systems, untouchabilty, *Sati Pratha*, Child marriage etc. were serious ailments of the societies which violated the human rights of the people.

The gradual and still ongoing conversion of humanity to a belief in human equality began in the seventeenth and eighteenth centuries and Europe and North America. It was led by two opposed ideologies: a new interpretation of Christian faith and an anti-Christian rationalism. The former inspired the American Revolution and Bill of Rights. The latter, the French Revolution and related political developments. Under these two influences, democracy very gradually, took hold and began to spread throughout the world. It was based on the belief in a political equality of all men and the consequent right to have a say who should govern them.

The World Medical Association. B.P.63,o1212Femey-Voltaire Codex, France, website www.wma.net

Even before that in the thirteenth, fourteenth and fifteenth centuries and later on, there was the rise of the *Bhakti* cult, and the various saints, teachers and social reformers in India preached the gospel of human equality in the spiritual field. They made protest against priestly claims of superiority and caste arrogance. Mystics like the Alwars and Nandas in the south, Kabir and Soordas in the north, Meera and Narsimha in Gujarat and Eknath and Tukaram in Maharashtra sang songs preaching the oneness of God and human beings as His children.

The nineteenth century under the influence of British produced a galaxy of reformers, *Bahma Samajists* in Bengal and *Arya Samajists* in Punjab. Ram Mohun Roy, Dayananda, Vivekananda and several others worked for the emancipation of the suppressed classes.

These were followed by Mahatma Gandhi's effort to stage war against social inequality and humiliating conditions to which the so-called untouchables were exposed in Indian society. (Mrs. Bhattacharya: 1981)

Gandhi championed the cause of human equality. He was born on 2nd October, 1869 at Porbunder in Kathiawar district of Gujarat. He went to England in 1887 where he qualified for the Bar. He returned to India and started his practice. In 1893, he went as legal representative of an Indian firm to South Africa where he stayed for twenty years. There he fought relentlessly for racial equality. He himself had bitter experiences of colour-prejudice. He started *Satyagraha* against apartheid or colour discrimination. (Agarwal: 1986)

Gandhiji believed in the spiritual oneness of all persons. This belief led him to oppose 'Untouchability'. He felt that the virus of untouchability was only a prominent phase of the devil of social arrogance and chauvinism.

Gandhi's influence succeeded in abolishing untouchablity by laws. The representation of untouchables has been guaranteed in the legislatures. Provision has been made to take special care of them at the entry point to public services through reservation. This provision for reservation has also been made for women in India.

The constitution has incorporated fundamental rights of the citizens and subsequently several Acts have been passed in Parliament safeguarding the rights of children, women, weaker sections, elderly persons etc. Further Human Rights Commissions, Women Commissions etc. are also constituted for implementing human rights related laws in the country. But the unfortunate aspect is that more we are giving importance on human rights more we are experiencing violation of human rights through domestic violence, human trafficking, exploitation of vulnerable people, illegal transaction of human organs, drugs, etc.

In twentieth century there was considerable elaboration of the concept of human equality in terms of human rights. One of the first acts of the newly established United Nations was to develop the Universal Declaration of Human Rights on 10th December, 1948. Article 1 of the Declaration says, "All beings are born free and equal in dignity and rights."

The medical profession while accepting the above statement has entered into controversies or some dilemmas on patient's equality and rights over the years. On one hand, the physicians have been told not to permit considerations of age, disease or disability, creed, ethnic origin, gender, nationality, political affiliation, race, sexual orientation, or social standing to intervene between his/her duty and his/her patient by Declaration of Geneva. At the same time, the physicians have claimed the right to refuse to accept a patient, except in an emergency. However, this may be allowed on certain legitimate grounds, such as, lack of educational qualifications or specialization, ill health or some genuine personal problems which are unavoidable. Here there is a scope of discrimination provided there is no provision of ensuring accountability or answer from physicians for such refusal. In such cases one has to depend upon the honesty of the physicians and they must be accountable to their own conscience for such an act.

Even if physicians do not offend against respect and human equality in their choice of patients, they can still do so in their attitude towards the patients, which is reflected or felt by the patient, such as way they look at the patients, enquiring about their health, facial expression etc. the patient is after all a human being he or she can easily read the facial expression and body language of the physicians. Therefore, enough care has to be taken to adopt compassionate attitude towards the patients. Here one has to realize that what is reflected in attitude, behaviour and thinking process of the physicians in maintaining relationship with the patients is nothing but the values and culture injected in them during childhood through socializing process or family or social environment. Every physician has to think that compassion is one of the core values of medicine and is an essential element of a good therapeutic relationship. It is based on respect for the patient's dignity and values but goes vulnerability in the face of illness and/or disability. If patients sense the physician's compassion, they will be more likely to trust the physician to act in their best interests, and this trust can contribute to the healing process. A physically and mentally weak patient always eagerly looks for compassionate behaviour from the service providers whether physicians or attendants.

The trust that is essential to the physician-patient relationship has generally been interpreted to mean that physicians should not desert patients whose care they have undertaken. The WMA's International Code of Medical Ethics implies that the only reason for ending a physician-patient relationship is if the patient requires another physician with different skills. "A physician shall owe his patients complete loyalty and all the resources of his science. Whenever an examination or treatment is beyond the physician's capacity he should summon another physician who has the necessary ability." However, there are many other reasons for a physician wanting to terminate a relationship with patient, for example, physician's moving or stopping practice, the patient's refusal or inability to pay for the physician's services, dislike of patient and physician to each other, the patient's refusal to comply with the physician's recommendations etc. The reasons may be entirely legitimate, or they may be unethical. When considering such an action, physicians should consult their Code of Ethics and other relevant guidance, documents and carefully examine their motives. They should be prepared to justify their decision, to themselves, to the patient and to a third party if appropriate. If the motive is legitimate, the physician should help the patient find another suitable physician or, if this not possible, should give the patient adequate notice of withdrawal of services so that the patient can find alternative medical care. If the motive is not legitimate, for example racial prejudice, the physician should take steps to deal with this defect.

Many physicians, especially those in the public sector, often have no choice of the patients they treat. Some patients are violent and pose a threat to the physician's safety. Others can only be described as obnoxious because of their antisocial attitudes and behaviour. Have such patients forsaken their right to respect and equal treatment, or are physicians expected to make extra, perhaps heroic efforts to establish and maintain therapeutic relationships with them? With such patients, physicians must balance their responsibility for their own safety and wellbeing and that of their staff with their duty to promote the well-being of the patients. They should attempt to find ways to honour both these obligations. If this is not possible they should make alternative arrangements for the care of the patients.

The trust that is essential to the physician-patient relationship has generally been interpreted to mean that physicians should not desert patients whose care they have undertaken. Trust is the basis of democratic way of life. It democratizes the physician and patient relationship. With the transformation paternalistic authoritarianism to democratization of relationship between physician and patient responsibility of the patient/ attendant has been increased. This is no longer noticed under the paternalistic authority of the physician. He is gradually becoming a part of the decision making process on treatment. It also enhances the responsibility of the patient. It is an ethical approach to this relationship". *The World Medical Association. B.P.63,o1212Femey-Voltaire Codex, France, website www.wma.net*

Radhakrishnan talked of the ethical approach to democracy. To him democracy is a faith. Democracy asks us to adopt persuasion, restraint and consent in the settlement of the problems. Naturally these elements have become a part of the physician and patient relations. (Radhakrishnan: 1992).

Another challenge to the principle of respect and equal treatment for all patients arises in the care of infectious patients. The focus here is often on HIV/AIDS, not only because it is life-threatening disease but also because it is often associated with social prejudices. However, there are many other serious infections including some that are more easily transmissible to healthcare workers than HIV/AIDS. Some physicians hesitate to perform invasive procedures on patients with such conditions because of the possibility that they, the physicians, might become infected. However, medical codes of ethics make no exception for infectious patients with regard to the physician's duty to treat all patients equally. The WMA's statement on the Professional Responsibility of Physicians in Treating AIDS Patients put it this way: "AIDS patients are entitled to competent medical care with compassion and human dignity.

A physician may not ethically refuse to treat a patient whose condition is within the physician's current realm of competence, solely because the patient is seropositive.

Medical ethics do not permit categorical discrimination against a patient based solely on his or her seropositivity. A person who is afflicted with AIDS needs competent, compassionable treatment. A physician who is not able to provide the care and services required by persons with AIDS should make an appropriate referral to those physicians or facilities that are equipped to provide such services. Until the referral can be accomplished, the physician must care for the patient to the best of his or her ability.

The intimate nature of the physician-patient relationship can give rise to sexual attraction. A fundamental rule of traditional medical ethics is that such attraction must be resisted. The Oath of Hippocrates includes the following promise: "Whatever houses I may visit it will come for the benefit of the sick, remaining free of all intentional injustice, of all mischief and in particular of sexual relations with both female and male persons...." In recent years many medical associations have restated this prohibition of sexual relations between physicians and patients. The reasons for this are as valid today as they were in Hippocrates' time, 2500 years ago. Patients are vulnerable and put their trust in physicians to treat them well. They may feel unable to resist sexual advances of physicians for fear that their treatment will be jeopardized. Moreover, the clinical judgment of a physician can be adversely affected by emotional involvement with a patient.

The later reason applies as well to physicians treating their family members, which is strongly discouraged in many medical codes of ethics. However, as with some other statements in codes of ethics, its application can vary according to circumstances. For example, solo practitioners working in remote areas may have to provide medical care for their family members, especially, in emergency situations."

The World Medical Association. B.P.63,o1212Femey-Voltaire Codex, France, website www.wma.net

While looking to the equal treatment with regard to healthcare in India, it is found that some are more equal than others for the government. Under the Central Government Health Scheme (CGHS) which covers Central Government employees, including serving and retired officials, current and ex-members of Parliament and the Judiciary, the annual per capita expenditure is more than Rs. 5,000. In contrast, the National Rural Health Mission (NRHM), which caters to the rural masses, spends just Rs. 180 per head.

The CGHS is financed mainly through the Centre's tax revenues. Though beneficiaries do contribute a share of their wages towards premium, ranging from Rs. 600 to Rs. 6,000 a year depending on their pay scale, this accounts for just about 5 per cent of the total expenditure. The government sells out the remaining 95 per cent.

A Planning Commission report of January 2011 titled, "A Critical Assessment of the Existing Insurance Models in India" noted that Employees State Insurance Scheme (ESIS) was probably managing to keep costs down because it relied on its own facilities in most cases. CGHS, on the other hand, provided 100 per cent inpatient care through a private network of hospitals and was driven by high-end tertiary care provided largely by big corporate hospitals.

The CGHS also had the highest hospitalization rate among the state-funded insurance schemes (22 per 1000 beneficiaries). Though this was lower than that of private insurance (64 per 1000 beneficiaries), the average hospitalization expenditure per beneficiary was the highest under CGHS, higher than even the commercial insurers. And though the central government-funded hospitals, including premier ones like AIIMS are available to beneficiaries, a majority of them chose corporate hospitals.

"In CGHS a few million people are being given huge benefits. One of the big drivers of cost under CGHS is prescription drugs", pointed out by a public health expert. "While the central government promotes generic drugs for all government facilities and schemes, a look at the list of drugs procured by CGHS reveals that for its own employees it buys mostly branded generics and patented drugs, which are very expensive and drive up average health expenditure."

There is also total lack of transparency on how the CGHS operates. "The CGHS collect information on coverage, infrastructure and utilization of its dispensaries but it does not publish the same. It neither reports financial nor other type of performance publicly," pointed out the Planning Commission report.

http:/times of india.indiatimes.com/india/Healthcare-pie-Rs 5000-for-a-bureaucrat-or-politician-Rs- 1180-for -villagers/articleshow/38703674.cms accessed on 27.7.2014

This kind of behaviour in the medical services is a clear deviation from the Constitution, the highest law of the country as well as Gandhi's teachings and the socio-political history of the country itself. In short, it is an indication of failure of a significant group of Indian governance to realize the basics of Indian democracy as a way of life in each and every profession.

The framers of the Constitution incorporated several provisions in it to translate the ideals of Welfare State into reality. The Preamble to the

Constitution reflects the basic aim of the Welfare State and the Part IV of the Constitution Directive Principles of State Policy. Democracy not only requires equality but also justice. Equality of status and opportunity are not available unless all sections of people are equally in a position and circumstances to benefit from the social order that prevails. The Constitution of India prohibits discrimination on grounds of birth, sex, religion, caste and creed but also adequately provides for the promotion of the interests of the Backward Classes and areas. It seeks to remove all inequalities in possession of wealth and opportunity, race, caste and religion, by providing just and human conditions of work, maternity relief, leisure and cultural opportunity to every individual, prevention of exploitation in labour and industry.

The significance of Directive Principles was appreciably realized by almost all the members of the Constituent Assembly. They firmly believed that certain social values, especially those related to economic rights, embodied in Part III of the Constitution, were meaningless to large sections of people of poverty. (Kapur: 1989)

Closely connected with the ideals of Welfare State is the Gandhi's concept of *Sarvodaya*, i.e. well-being of all. Here Gandhi gave importance on internal aspect of life to organize institutions. He did not believe that revolution or evolution when imposed from outside would bring about any fundamental change in human nature or in society. The entire responsibility of reconstruction in social, economic and political aspects must start with the individual himself; without the individual's consistent and constant effort for reorientation no amount of effort will bring the socialistic order. The Gandhian idea of *Sarvodaya* is the apex of Gandhian socialism. *Sarvodaya* does not mean that majority alone is enough; the growth and uplift of everyone is necessary. (Gupta: 2006)

The word *Sarvodaya* was coined by Mahatma Gandhi. It is a compound of two Sanskrit words: *sarva* means all and *udaya* means uplift or welfare or prosperity. Thus *Sarvodaya* means the uplift of all. Gandhi first used this word *Sarvodaya* in a booklet he published in his own language (Gujarati) after he was inspired by an essay by the Englishman, John Ruskin. This essay was titled as, "Unto This Last."

Gandhi used the word *sarvodaya* to highlight some principles to be observed by us while making efforts to build ourselves, our communities and nations. He felt very strongly that the soundest foundation on which the societies should be built were qualities of truth, love and compassion in both personal and public lives. The theory of trusteeship, elimination of exploitation in every shape; a classless society which offers no privileges by birth or wealth or talent; mutual cooperation and not individual competition being the driving force of motivation and behaviour; and above all, securing the welfare of all without any distinction whatsoever by race, religion, political affiliation, or else. (Kempadoo)

Each service provider's first responsibility is to build up our mental set up to realize the need of learning from the history first, from his or her own country itself and to proceed to the outside world.

This is urgently needed in India as the human aspect of Indian society is fast withering away in the face of modernization and commercialization of social relationships. To Radhakrishnan escape from decline and catastrophe depends not on scientific ideas and material forces but on the perceptions and ideas of men and women, on the moral judgment of the community. If we choose rightly, the achievements of science may lead to such a degree of material wealth and abundance of leisure as has never before been possible in human history. All this will be possible only if we achieve a revolution in the inner compulsions that control us. (R.C. Gupta)

Communication and Consent

Herbert A. Simon looks at communication as a process whereby decisional premises are transmitted from one member of an organization to another. To him "without communication there can be no organization, for there is no possibility of the group influencing the behaviour of the individual." What is Communication? Communication is a process of sending and receiving information between two parties. The word communication is derived from the Latin word *Communis* which means 'common'. In a communication process, the sender of information seeks to establish a commonness with the receiver of information. On the basis of it, Mohit Bhattacharya tried to define communication as the use of words, letters symbols or some other means to have common information about any object of attention. Three major aspects of communication may be identified—*first*, when interacting with others, words, letters etc. are used; *second*, two or more persons are involved in communication; and *third*, the interaction process is motivated by sharing of information toward a common goal.

In the whole communication system another significant feature is that the sender of information turns as receiver and *vice versa*. The sender receives the feedback from the other end which receives the information. This feedback may change the premises of decision. Further free flow of feedback of reaction, ideas etc. can influence the behaviour and assumption of both the parties. It helps handling of a problem with more confidence and effective way. This system of communication between the physician and the patient is an important component of a hospital system. Because the immediate target group of the medical service is the ailing population of the nation approaching the hospital for service. This successful communication between them will be followed by other required arrangements based on communication to the relevant groups in course of time or change of receiving group. Here what is important is the determination or identification of channel by the sender of information. While sending a message there may be need of decoding or interpretation of message to make it understandable without difficulty by the receiver. One has to take care so that information sent are not distorted and are received in the exact nature. (Bhattacharya: 1987)

Informed consent is one of the central concepts of present day medical ethics. The right of patients to make decisions about their healthcare has been enshrined in legal and ethical statements throughout the world. The WMA Declaration on the Rights of the Patient state: "Patient has the right to self-determination to make free decisions regarding himself or herself. The physician will inform the patient of the consequences of his/her decisions. A mentally competent adult patient has the right to give or withhold consent to any diagnostic procedure or therapy. The patient has the right to the information necessary to make his/her decisions. The patient should understand clearly what is the purpose of any test and treatment, what the results should imply and what would be the implications of withholding consent."

The World Medical Association. B.P.63,o1212Femey-Voltaire Codex, France, website www.wma.nett

Another point to be noted is that showing respect to patient also requires the physician to be truthful in informing the patient of their health and to be direct in asking for the patient's consent before giving treatment. Historically in many cultures there has been a shift from paternalism or "doctor knows best" to the idea that patients must have a choice in the provision of their care and be given the right to make informed consent to medical procedures. The issues like how to handle informed consent in a doctor-patient relationship, for example who do not want to know about their condition.

http:/en.wikipedia.org/wiki/Doctor%E2%80%93patient_ relationship accessed on 28.7.2014

Consent is a key word in democracy. In functioning of democracy, a responsible citizen is one who has opinions and expressed them. Boorstin said, "In the United States we tend to talk not about the wise, the knowledgeable, or the prudent citizen, but rather about the 'well informed' citizen." In medical services 'Informed Consent' is talked of. (Boorstin: 2000)

A necessary condition for informed consent is effective communication between physician and patient. There was a time when physicians had paternalistic authority over the patient. It was almost one way traffic in the sense that the physicians directed administered medicine and the patient was the silent receiver of his or her services. Medical paternalism was normal because in the traditional society there prevailed prescriptive values. The customs and traditions were transmitted from one generation to other without facing the question "Why" from the receiving or accepting end. Naturally communication was very simple; it consisted of the physician's orders to the patient to comply with such and such a treatment. But with the change of society from traditional to modernity, the new generation is influenced by achievement oriented values. It makes the transmitting of social values from one generation to other. The medical services are also influenced by these achievement oriented values due to which the task of the physician in conversation with the patient has become not only time consuming but also challenging. Today patients expect more information and also as required by them communication. They must provide patient with all the information they need to make decisions. This involves explaining complex medical diagnoses, prognoses and treatment regimes in simple language, ensuring that the patients understand the treatment options including the advantages and disadvantages of each, answering any question they may have and understanding whatever decision the patient has reached and if possible, the reasons for it. Effective communication is a skill and do not come naturally to most people, they must be developed and maintained with conscious effort and periodic review.

Two major obstacles to good communication between physician and patient are differences of language and culture. If the physician and the patient do not speak the same language, an interpreter is required to make the conversation understandable to both the parties. This is essential with regard to the patients from rural areas, who speak only the regional language instead of either English or Hindi. Unfortunately, in India the practice of appointing formal and qualified interpreters has yet to develop. However, it is found that with the use of English as medium of instruction in educational institutions, especially at the school most young patients do not face the language problem and they may fill the gap of the need of formal interpreters to their elders who are patients. The language is only a part of culture. It raises additional issues to be raised in the conversation between the patients and the physicians. Diversity of culture creates some complexity in the process of diagnosis to explore causes and effect on the health. Further, this aspect is foreign to modern equipment to be used for investigation of the diseases. In such circumstances physicians should make every reasonable effort to probe their patient's understanding of health and healing and communicate their recommendations to the patients as best they can.

If the physician has successfully communicated to the patient all the information the patient needs and wants to know about his or her diagnosis, prognosis and treatment options, the patient will then be in a position to make an informed decision about how to proceed. Although the term 'consent' implies acceptance of treatment, the concept of informed consent applies equally to refusal of treatment or to choice among alternative treatments. Competent patients have the right to refuse treatment, even when the refusal will result in disability or death.

Evidence of consent can be explicit or implicit (implied). Explicit consent is given verbally or in writing. Consent is implied when the patient indicates a willingness to undergo a certain procedure treatment by his or her behaviour. For example, consent for venipuncture is implied by the action of presenting one's arm. For treatments that entail risk or involve more than mild discomfort, it is preferable to obtain explicit rather than implied consent.

There are two exceptions to the requirement for informed consent by competent patients:

1. Situations where patients voluntarily give over their decisions making authority to the physician or to the third party. Because of the complexity of the matter or because the patient has complete confidence in the physician's judgment, the patient may tell the physician, "Do what you think is best". Physicians should not be eager to act on such requests but should provide patients with basic information about the treatment options and encourage them to make their own decisions. However, if after such encouragement the patient still wants the physician to decide, the physician should do so according to the best interests of the patient.
2. Instances where the disclosure of information would cause harm to the patient: the traditional concept of "therapeutic privilege"

is invoked in such cases; it allows physicians to withhold medical information if disclosure would likely to result in serious physical, psychological or emotional harm to the patient.

In some cultures, it is widely held that the physician's obligation to provide information to the patient does not apply when the diagnosis is a terminal illness. It is felt that such information would cause the patient to despair and would make the remaining days of life much more miserable than if there were hope of recovery. Throughout the world, it is not uncommon for family members of patients to plead with physicians not to tell the patients that they are dying. Physicians do have to be sensitive to cultural as well as personal factors when communicating bad news, especially of impending death. Nevertheless, the patient's right to informed consent is becoming more and more widely accepted and the physician has a primary duty to help patients exercise this right.

In keeping with the growing trend towards considering healthcare as a consumer product and patients as consumers, patients and families not infrequently demand access to medical services that, in the considered opinion of physicians, are not appropriate. Some patients claim a 'right' to any medical service that they feel can benefit them, and often physicians are only too willing to oblige, even when they are convinced that the service can offer no medical benefit for the patient's condition. This problem is especially serious in situations where resources are limited and providing 'futile' or 'no beneficial' treatments to some patients means that other patients are left untreated.

Futile and non-beneficial treatment can be understood as follows: In some situations a physician can determine that a treatment is 'medically' futile or non-beneficial because it offers no reasonable hope of recovery or improvement or because the patient is permanently unable to experience any benefit. In other cases, the utility and benefit of a treatment can only be determined with reference to the patient's subjective judgment about his or her overall well-being. As a general rule a patient should be involved in determining futility in his or her case. In exceptional circumstances such discussions may not be in the patient's best interest. The physician has no obligation to offer a patient futile or non-beneficial treatment.

The principle of informed consent incorporates the patient's right to choose from among the options presented by the physician. To what extent patients and their families have a right to services not recommended by physicians is becoming a major topic of controversy in ethics, law and public policy. Until the matter is decided by governments, medical insurance providers and/or professional organizations, individual physicians have to decide for themselves whether they should accede to requests for inappropriate treatments. They should refuse such requests if they are convinced that the treatment would produce more harm than benefit. They should also feel free to refuse if the treatment is unlikely to be beneficial, even if it is not harmful, although the possibility of a placebo effect should not be discounted, if limited resources are an issue, they should bring this to the attention of whoever is responsible for allocating resources.

The World Medical Association. B.P.63,o1212Femey-Voltaire Codex, France, website www.wma.net

The concepts of communication and consent are two basic ingredients of democracy. These are applicable to political democracy as well as social democracy. Daniel J. Boorstin in his book, *Democracy and Discontents* gives an interesting explanation of the word, 'communicate'. He said that 'communicate' is a very old word. Its history reflects many meanings of it. He referred to Starkey's *History of England* in 1538 in which the word 'communicate' is defined as a quality of Supreme Being or God. Starkey said, "God is He who 'communicate' His goodness to all others." In origin, 'communicate' is related to the word, 'common' or 'community', it means to make common or to share.

Boorstin went to the extent of saying that rise of civilization is nothing but rise of communication—"improvement of ways of sharing and improvement of that which is already shared." While the progress of civilization is an improvement in what we share and in the process of sharing, there is another commonly forgotten essential is 'willingness of people not to say and not to do many things they might want to say or do,' as pointed out by Sigmund Freud. This is also one way of maintaining good manners towards building a decent society. Good manners consist not only in our willingness to say what we are expected to say, but just as much in our self-control in keeping ourselves away from saying what we really feel and really want to tell, but which might hurt others. (Boorstin: 1974)

Decision-making for Patients: Herbert Alexander Simon, an eminent administrative thinker considers decision-making as a process of drawing conclusions from premises. He equated administration with decision-making and laid emphasis on how decisions are made and how they be made more effectively.

Basically an organization consists of decision-makers. To Simon at all levels of an organization decisions are made with variation in the jurisdiction of application and importance. Decisions are not made in vacuum. These are made on some premises. To Simon some of these premises have decision-maker's preferences, some are guided by social conditions, some have communications from the organization itself.

While talking about facts and value, Simon provides no place for value in the scientific approach to the facts. He asserts on concentration on facts, precision and clarity of definition of terms, strictness in analysis. The science of administration must concern with the factual statements. It does not invite any ethical or value statements.

On the basis of the factual statements decisions are taken. The decision-making process involves choice between alternative plans. Here begins the relationship between the facts and values. A fact is a statement of reality. Factual premise can be ascertained by observation and several other modern devices. But this is an expression of preferences.

To take a right decision physical and mental health of a person is required. An individual who suffers from serious ailments generally cannot have the capacity to take right decision. Further he may not understand the consequences of each different treatment procedures communicated to him by his physician. Decision-making for ailing person is a difficult task except for a few. So, they are not competent enough to take decision even for their own good. (Umapathy: 2010)

In addition to above there are many who are not competent to make decisions for themselves. Examples as indicated by WMA Medical Ethics Manual, include young children, individuals affected by certain psychiatric or neurological conditions and those who are temporarily unconscious or camotose. These patients require substitute decision-makers, either physician or another person. Ethical issues arise in the determination of the appropriate substitute decision-maker and in the choice of criteria for decisions on behalf of incompetent patients.

In traditional society there prevailed medical paternalism under which the physician was the decision-maker for the incompetent persons. However, they might consult the family members about the options. Physicians might consult with Physicians have been gradually losing this authority in many countries as patients are given the opportunity to name their own substitute decision-makers to act for them when they become incompetent. In addition, some states specify the appropriate substitute decision makers in descending order (e.g. husband or wife, adult children, brothers and sisters). In such cases, physicians make decisions for patients only when the designated substitute cannot be found, as often happens in emergency situations. The WMA Declaration on the Rights of the Patient states the physician's duty in this matter as follows:

> "If the patient is unconscious or otherwise unable to express his/her will, informed consent must be obtained, whenever possible from a legally entitled representative, where legally relevant. If a legally entitled representative is not available, but the medical intervention is urgently needed, consent of a patient may be presumed unless it is obvious and beyond any doubt on the basis of the patient's previous firm expression or conviction that he/she would refuse consent to the intervention in that situation."

Problems arise when those claiming to be the appropriate substitute decision-makers, for example different family members, do not agree among themselves or when they do agree, their decision is, in the physician's opinion, not in the best interests of the patients. In the first instance, the physician can serve a mediating function, but if the disagreement persists, it can be resolved in other ways, for example, by letting the senior member of the family decide or by voting. In cases of serious disagreement between the substitute decision-maker and the physician, the Declaration on the Rights of the Patient offers the following advice: "If the patient's legally entitled representative, or person authorized by the patient, forbids treatment which is, in the opinion of the physician, in the patient's best interest, the physician should challenge this decision in the relevant legal or other institution."

The principal criteria to be used for treatment decisions for an incompetent patient are his or her preferences, if these are known. The preferences may be found in an advance directive or may have been communicated to the designated substitute decision-maker, the physician and other members of healthcare team. When incompetent patient's preferences are not known, treatment decisions should be based on the patient's best interests, taking into account:

(a) The patient's diagnosis and prognosis;
(b) The patient's known values;
(c) Information received from those who are significant in the patient's life and who could help in determining his or her best interests; and
(d) Aspects of the patient's culture and religion that would influence a treatment decision.

This approach is less certain than if the patient has left specific instructions about treatment, but it does enable the substitute decision-maker to infer, in light of other choices the patient has made and his or her approach to life in general, what he or she would decide in the present situation.

Competence to make decisions is difficult to assess, especially in young people and those whose capacity for reasoning has been impaired by acute or chronic illness. A person may be competent to make decisions regarding some aspects of life but not others. A person may be lucid and oriented at certain times of the day and not at others. Although such patients may not be legally competent, their preferences should be taken into account when decisions are being made for them. The Declaration on the Rights of the Patient states the matter thus: "if a patient is a minor or otherwise legally incompetent, the consent of a legally entitled representative, where legally relevant, is required". Nevertheless, the patient must be involved in the decision-making to the fullest extent depending on his or her capacity.

Not infrequently, patients are unable to make a reasoned, well thought-out-decision regarding different treatment options due to the discomfort and distraction caused by their disease. However, they may still be able to indicate their rejection of a specific intervention, an intravenous feeding tube, for example. In such cases, these expressions of dissent should be taken very seriously, although they need to be considered in light of the overall goals of their treatment plan.

Patients suffering from psychiatric or neurological disorders raise particularly difficult ethical issues. It is important to honour their human rights, especially the right to freedom, to the greatest extent possible. Nevertheless, they may have to be confined and/or treated against their will in order to prevent harm to themselves or others. A distinction can be made between involuntary confinement and involuntary treatment. Some patient advocates defend right of these individuals to refuse treatment even if they have to be confined as a result. A legitimate reason for refusing treatment could be painful experience with treatments in the past, for example, the severe side effects of psychotropic medications. When serving as substitute decision-makers for such patients, physician should ensure that the patients really do pose a danger, and not just an annoyance, to others or themselves. They should try to ascertain the patient's preferences regarding treatment and the reasons for these preferences, even if in the end the preferences cannot be fulfilled.

Confidentiality: The medical ethics requires a physician to keep all information regarding patient confidentially. This has been considered as a duty of the physician since the time of Hippocrates. The Hippocratic Oath states, "What I may see here in the course of the treatment or even outside of the treatment in regard to the life of men, which on no account one must spread abroad, I will keep to myself holding such things shameful to be spoken about." The Oath, and some more recent versions, allow no exception to this duty of confidentiality. For example, the WMA's International Code of Medical Ethics requires that, "A physician shall preserve absolute confidentiality on all he knows about the patient even after the patient has died." However, other codes reject this absolutist approach to confidentiality. The possibility that breaches of confidentiality are sometimes justified calls for clarification of the very idea of confidentiality.

The high value that is placed on confidentiality has three sources: autonomy, respect for others and the trust. Autonomy relates to confidentiality in that personal information about an individual belongs to him or her and should not be made known to others without his or her consent. When an individual reveals personal information to another, a physician or nurse for example, or when information comes to light through a medical test, those are bound to keep it confidential unless authorized to divulge it by the individual concerned.

Confidentiality is also closely related to the human dignity which must be honoured besides being related to autonomy. One important way of showing them respect is by preserving their privacy. Here it has to be mentioned that in medical care services maintenance of privacy has different meaning. The concept of privacy in medical care service is just to prevent unnecessary intrusions into a person's private life. Since, individuals differ regarding their desire for privacy, we cannot assume that everyone wants to be treated as we would want to be. Care must be taken to determine which personal information a patient wants to keep secret and which he or she is willing to have revealed to others.

Trust is an essential part of the physician-patient relationship. In order to receive medical care, patients have to reveal his personal information to physicians and others who may be total strangers to them—information that they would not want anyone to know. They must have good reason to trust their caregivers not to divulge their information. The basis of this trust is the ethical and legal standards of confidentiality that healthcare professionals are expected to uphold. Without an understanding that their disclosures will be kept secret, patients may withhold personal information. This can hinder physicians in their efforts to provide effective interventions or to attain certain public health goals.

The WMA Declaration on the Rights of the Patient summaries the patient's right to confidentiality as follows:

- All identifiable information about a patient's health status, medical condition, diagnosis, prognosis and treatment and all other information of a personal kind, must be kept confidential even after death. Exceptionally, the patient's relatives may have a right of access to information that would inform them of their health risks.
- Confidential information can only be disclosed to other healthcare providers only on a strictly "need to know" basis unless the patient has given explicit consent.
- All identifiable patient data must be protected. The protection of data must be appropriate to the manner of its storage. Human substances from which identifiable data can be derived must be likewise protected.

As this WMA Declaration states, there are exceptions to the requirement to maintain confidentiality. Some of these are non-problematic, others raise very difficult ethical issues for physicians.

Routine breaches of confidentiality occur frequently in most healthcare institutions. Many individuals—physicians, nurses, laboratory technicians, students etc.—require access to a patient's health records in order to provide adequate care to that person and, for students, to learn how to practise medicine. Where patients speak a different language than their caregivers, then there is a need of interpreters to facilitate communication. In case of patients who are not competent to make their own medical decisions, other individuals have to be given information about them in order to make decisions on their behalf or to take care for them. Physicians routinely inform the family members of a deceased person about the cause of death. These breaches of confidentiality are usually justified but they should be kept to a minimum and those who gain access to confidential information should be aware of the need not to spread it any further than is necessary for the patient's benefit. Where possible, patients should be informed that such breaches occur.

Another generally accepted reason for breaching confidentiality is to comply with legal requirements. For example, many jurisdictions have laws for mandatory reporting of patients who suffer from designated diseases, those deemed not fit to drive, and those suspected of child abuse.

Physicians should be aware of the legal requirements for the disclosure of patient information where they work. However, legal requirements can conflict with the respect for human rights that underlies medical ethics. Therefore, physicians should view with a critical eye any legal requirement to breach confidentiality and assure themselves that it is justified before adhering to it.

If physicians are persuaded to comply with legal requirements to disclose their patient's medical information, it is desirable that they discuss with the patients the necessity of any disclosure before it occurs and enlist their cooperation. For example, it is preferable that a patient suspected of child abuse call the child protection authorities in the physician's presence to self-report or that the physician obtains his or her consent before the authorities are notified. This approach will prepare the way for subsequent interventions. If such cooperation is not forthcoming and the physician has reason to believe any delay in notification may put a child at risk of serious harm, then the physician ought to immediately notify child protection authorities and subsequently inform the patient that this has been done.

In addition to those breaches of confidentiality that are required by law, physicians may have an ethical duty to impart confidential information to others who could be at risk of harm from the patient. Two situations in which this can occur are when a patient tells a psychiatrist that he intends to harm another person and when a physician is convinced that an HIV-positive patient is going to continue to have unprotected intercourse with his spouse or other partners.

Conditions for breaching confidentiality when not required by law are that the expected harm is believed to be imminent, serious (and irreversible), unavoidable except by unauthorized disclosure, and greater than the harm likely to result from the harms, the physician needs to assess and compare the seriousness of the harms and the likelihood of their occurrence. In cases of doubt, it would be wise for the physician to seek expert advice.

When the physician has determined that the duty to warn justifies an unauthorized disclosure, two further decisions must be made. Whom should the physician tell? How much should be told? Generally speaking, the disclosure should contain only that information necessary to prevent the anticipated harm and should be directed only to those who need the information in order to prevent the harm. Reasonable steps should be taken to minimize the harm and offence to the patient that may arise from the disclosure. It is recommended that the physician should inform the patient that confidentiality might be breached for his or her own protection and that of any potential victim. Patient's cooperation should be enlisted if possible.

In the case of HIV-positive patient, disclosure to a spouse or current sexual partner may not be unethical and, indeed, may be justified when the patient is unwilling to inform the person at risk. Such disclosure requires that all of the following conditions are met: the patient is at the risk of infection with HIV and has no other reasonable means of knowing the risk; the patient has refused to inform his or her sexual partner; the patient has refused an offer of assistance by the physician to do so on the patient's behalf; and the physician has informed the patient of his or her intention to disclose the information to the partner.

The World Medical Association. B.P.63,o1212Femey-Voltaire Codex, France, website www.wma.net.

The UN report stated in 2014 that India has the third-highest number of people living with HIV in the world with 2.1 million Indians accounting for about four out of 10 people infected with the deadly virus in the Asia-Pacific region.

The report by UNAIDS, the United Nations programme on HIV/AIDS, said that 19 million of the 35 million people living with the virus globally do not know their HIV/AIDS-positive status and so ending the AIDS epidemic by 2030 will require smart scale-up to close the gap.

Six countries—China, India, Indonesia, Myanmar, Thailand and Vietnam—account for more than 90 per cent of the people living with HIV in the region. "India has the third-largest number of people living with HIV in the world—2.1 million at the end of 2013—an account for about 4 out of 10 people living with HIV in the region," said the report. It said HIV treatment coverage is only 36 per cent in India, where 51 per cent of AIDS-related deaths occur. (*The Assam Tribune*: 18th July, 2014)

The medical care of suspected and convicted criminals poses particular difficulties with regard to confidentiality. Although physicians providing care to those in custody have limited independence, they should try their best to treat these patients as they would any others. In particular they should safeguard confidentiality by not revealing details of medical condition to prison authorities without first obtaining the patient's consent.

The World Medical Association. B.P.63,o1212Femey-Voltaire Codex, France, website www.wma.net

Here reference may be made of two of issues partner notification and HIV infection discussed in the writings of, four medical scientists, A. Abraham, J. Prasad, A. Joseph and K.S. Jacob in the context of India.

HIV infection has close relationship with poverty and illiteracy in India and other developing countries. In India partner notification is very sensitive issue due to low awareness and limited capacity to act. Most people, especially rural areas are poor, uneducated and unemployed. At the same time partner notification is important to these categories of people. They require special care.

The limitation of resources in developing countries is a severe hindrance to partner notification. The contact tracing is expensive and it is also difficult to choose the strategy for contact tracing. No one strategy can be adopted due to regional variations. It is said that the tracing of contact will benefit the partners who are not infected. But the partners who are infected and asymptomatic will not be able to use the various treatment options due to the high cost of therapy.

The National AIDS Control Organization's guidelines for HIV counselling stated that there may be situations where partner notification is permissible. However, it does not indicate the issues and specific criteria for disclosure.

The Supreme Court of India has ruled on the issue of the right to confidentiality of subjects with HIV infection and breach of confidentiality in order to protect the health of third parties. The opinion of the court was that the right to privacy and confidentiality is not absolute. The right may be lawfully restricted in situations where third parties are at risk. The judgment went on to state that the persons with HIV infection, who knowingly expose others to health risk, are guilty of an offence and punishable under law. The court ruling maintained that HIV-infected subjects did not have the right to marry. However, NGOs and human rights activists have pointed out that the law should look at the larger issues arising out of it.

Efforts to maintain confidentiality in order to prevent discrimination have formed the cornerstone of public health. Confidentiality is a means to prevent discrimination in the treatment of fellow members in a society. However, it has to be admitted that if such principle has adverse result then it loses its validity. The right to privacy needs to honoured in the interest of the welfare or safeguard of mankind or not at the cost of it. No right of an individual is absolute. What is important is that without disregarding the sentiment of the patient with infectious disease may be prepared mentally by explaining the situation under which disclosure is to be made. Efforts have to be made to convince the patient that breach of confidentiality is needed in the interest of both the patient and other people. Efforts may be made through the attendants who are close to the patient. The physicians who enjoy the privilege of having access to such information are not in a position to afford time and energy to do that and therefore this responsibility may be carried out by the family members and thereby extending their cooperation to the noble medical service indirectly and ultimately to the humanity. In the case of the HIV infected or any such patients who come forward voluntarily may realize the situation to give consent to this effort of the medical service providers. The protection of public health also demand not to adopt right to privacy in its absolute form. (Abraham and Others: 2000)

Trust is the basis of patient and physician relationship. However, the poverty has tempted the people in India to breach of trust between the two. Instances are found of exploitation of poor people by tempting them to sell kidneys to the patients who require transplantation of kidneys. The poor people come forward to do so either out of ignorance of the organ transplantation laws or otherwise. They used to tell lie before the medical authority about their relationship or with regard to other related matters as directed by the buyers of the kidneys. In a recent case, the CID has unearthed a racket in which poor people from four Bengal districts in India "donated" their kidneys to patients in Uttar Pradesh and Rajasthan.

It is alleged that while unearthing another such racket where poor people from Punjab and Chhattisgarh were brought to the city for "donating" their kidneys in lieu of cash it was found that Lalbazar detective had found how the "poorest of the poor" from Punjab and Chhattisgarh were promised Rs. 10,000-70,000 for a kidney and brought to Kolkata as donors using the loopholes in organ transplantation laws. But in the latest case, the CID sleuths at Bhawani Bhawan say they have traced several poor land tillers and daily wage earners in four Bengal districts who have' donated' their kidneys for a price to patients from Uttar Pradesh and Rajasthan. All these operations took place in private hospitals close to EM Bypass.

A fax sent to the Bengal home department by UP Chief Secretary, in April 2014 alerted the state to the racket, prompting the health department to launch a probe. The CID officers were shocked by the questionable documents in each kidney transplant case that "certified" that the donor was a blood relation of the recipient. While the Lalbazar officers suspected the veracity of the "clearance" from the ethics committees of states such as Punjab, Chhattisgarh and Jharkhand CID officials claim the papers from the districts of Bengal—carrying signatures of senior health functionaries—are forged or have been misused.

It was found that around 40 per cent of all kidney transplants done in the city involve financial transactions. Over last few years there is beeline to Kolkata transplants. A TOI report says that in Chhattisgarh largest number of 'unrelated donors' were from Bengal. Thus, it is noticed that even the patients exploit the situation for their benefit by giving false information to the physicians and thus involve them in the unethical and illegal acts of them. The principle of mutual trust is not honoured by the people, especially those who are poverty ridden. The allegations relating to this kind of medical care stand as serious challenge to ethics and human values in medical sciences, especially in the area of physician-patient relationship.

http:/timesofindia.indiatimes.com/india/How-Bengals-poor-sell-kidneysin-other-states/articleshow/39772460.cms

Beginning-of-Life Issues: Many significant issues in medical ethics relate to the beginning of human life. Following are some of the significant issues highlighted in the WMA Medical Ethics Manual:

- *Contraception*: Although there is increasing international recognition of a woman's right to control her fertility, including the prevention of unwanted pregnancies, physicians still have to deal with difficult issues such as requests to contraception from minors and explaining the different methods of contraception.
- *Assisted Reproduction*: For couples (and individuals) who cannot conceive naturally there are various techniques of assisted reproduction, such as artificial insemination and in-viro fertilization and embryo transfer, widely available in major medical centres. *Surogate or substitute gestation* is another alternative.
- *Prenatal Genetic Screening*: Genetic tests are now available for determining whether an embriyo or foetus is affected by certain genetic abnormalities and whether it is male or female. Depending on the findings, a decision can be taken whether or not to proceed with pregnancy. Physicians need to determine when to offer such tests and how to explain the results to patients.
- *Abortion*: This has long been one of the most divisive issues in medical ethics, both for physicians and public authorities. The WMA Statement on Therapeutic Abortion acknowledges the diversity of opinion and belief and concludes that 'This is matter of individual conviction and conscience which must be respected.'

- *Severely Compromised Neonates:* Because of extreme prematurity or congenital abnormalities, some neonates have a very poor prognosis for survival. Difficult decisions often have to be made whether to attempt to probing their lives or allow them to die.
- *Research Issues*: These include the production of new embryos or the use of 'spare' embryos to obtain stem cells for potential therapeutic applications, testing of new techniques for assisted reproduction, and experimentation on foetuses.

End-of-Life-Issues: End-of-Life Issues range attempts prolong the lives of dying patients through highly experimental technologies, such as the implantation of animal organs, to efforts to terminate life prematurely through euthanasia and medically assisted suicide. In between these extremes lie numerous issues regarding the initiation or withdrawing of potentially life-extending treatments, the care of terminally ill patients and the advisability and use of advance directives.

Two issues deserve particular attention. Euthanasia and assistance in suicide:

A. Euthanasia: Euthanasia means knowingly and intentionally performing an act that is clearly intended to end another person's life and that includes the following elements: the subject is a competent informed person with an incurable illness who has voluntarily asked his or her life ended; the agent knows about the person's condition and desire to die, and commits the act with the primary intention of ending the life of that person, and the act is undertaken with compassion and without personal gain.

B. Assistance to Suicide: It means knowingly and intentionally providing a person with the knowledge or means or both required to commit suicide, including counselling about lethal doses of drugs, prescribing such lethal doses or supplying the drugs.

Euthanasia and assisted suicide are often regarded as morally equivalent, although there is a clear practical distinction, and in some jurisdictions a legal distinction, between them.

Euthanasia and assisted suicide, according to these definitions are to be distinguished from the withholding or withdrawal of inappropriate, futile or unwanted medical treatment or the provision of compassionate palliative care, even when these practices shorten life.

Requests for euthanasia or assistance in suicide arise as a result of pain or suffering that is considered by the patient to be intolerable. They would rather die than continue to live in such circumstances. Furthermore, many patients consider that they have a right to die if they so choose, and even a right to assistance in dying. Physicians are considered as most appropriate instruments of death since they have the medical knowledge and access to the appropriate drugs for ensuring a quick and painless death.

Physicians are understandably reluctant to implement requests for euthanasia or assistance to suicide because these are illegal in most countries and are prohibited in most medical codes of ethics. This prohibition was part of the Hippocratic Oath and has been emphatically related by the WMA in its Declaration on Euthanasia: "Euthanasia that is the act of deliberately ending the life of a patient even at the patient's own request or at the request of close relatives, is unethical. This does not prevent the physician from respecting the desire of a patient to allow the natural process of death to follow its course in the terminal phase of sickness."

The rejection of euthanasia and assisted suicide does not mean that physicians can do nothing for the patient with a life-threatening illness that is an advanced stage and for which curative measures are not appropriate. In recent years there have been great advances in palliative care treatments for relieving pain and suffering and improving quality of life. Palliative care can be appropriate for patients of all ages, from a child with cancer to a senior nearing the end of life. One aspect of palliative care that needs greater attention for all patients is pain control. All physicians who care for the dying patients should ensure that they have adequate skills in this domain, as well as, where available, access to skilled consultative help from palliative care specialists. Above all, physicians should not abandon dying patients but should continue to provide compassionate care even when cure is no longer possible.

The approach of death presents many other ethical challenges for patients, substitute decision-makers and physicians. The possibility of prolonging life through recourse to drugs, resuscitative interventions, radiological procedures and intensive care requires decisions about when to initiate these treatments and when to withdraw them if they are not working.

As discussed above in relation to communication and consent, competent patients have the right to refuse any medical treatment, even if the refusal results in their death. Individuals differ greatly with regard to their attitude towards dying; some will do anything to prolong their lives; no matter how much pain and suffering it involves, while others so look forward to dying them alive, that they refuse even simple measures that are likely to keep them alive, such as antibiotics for bacterial pneumonia. Once physicians have made every effort to provide their likelihood of success, they must respect the patients' decisions about the initiation or continuation of any treatment.

End-of-Life decision-making for incompetent patients presents greater difficulties. If patients have clearly expressed their wishes in advance, for example in an advance directive, the decision will be easier, although such directives are often very vague and need to be interpreted with respect to the patient's actual condition. If patients have not adequately expressed their wishes, the appropriate substitute decision-maker must use another criterion for treatment decisions, namely, the best interests of the patient.

In between physician-patient relationship there arise the nurses who use to provide bedside services and administration of medicine on the patients. A good bedside manner is typically one that reassures and comforts the patient while remaining honest about a diagnosis. Vocal tones, body language, openness, presence and concealment of attitude may all affect beside manner. Poor bedside manner leaves the patient feeling unsatisfied, worried, frightened, or alone.

http:/en.wikipedia.org/wiki/Doctor%E2%80%93patient_relationship accessed on 28.7.2014

Dominance of technology and Patient-Physician relationship: A group of seven advisers at WHO expressed their observation on ethics and health in a changing world. They pointed out that the experiences of utilization of technologies provides enough scope to realize the inability of technologies to solve all problems or to fulfill the increasing hopes and aspirations of the people of the contemporary world. There are instances of emergence of new problems or deterioration of the existing situation or shift of problems from one area to the other. Most problems are experienced due to adoption of mechanized way of solving our problems and these are surprisingly health centric. For example "grow more food in a mechanized way" or with the help of modern technologies is affecting the health of an individual, progress of medical sciences helps transplantation of human organs, diagnosis of disease quick and accurate etc. are not free from serious negative impact on the human relations. It results in most cases destruction of trust of patients on Physicians and other allied medical service providers. The group of Advisers in WHO realized very rightly that the first need is for people and societies to accept their responsibility for directing the development and use of science and technology rather than simply submitting to whatever they produce and letting them to know their own logic of expansion. They must make a critical analysis of strengths and weaknesses of them so that these can be used for the betterment of human life. Here lies the need of the consequential approach to study the utility of the modern technologies. Further, the gulf between expensive care for the few and care that is, at least in principle, affordable for all has been widened by this process and faces individuals and societies, whether rich or poor, with increasingly difficult ethical issues. Such issues and the framework of values within which they must be resolved should not be left in the hands of the medical authorities alone (*World Health Forum*, Volume 17, 1996).

To Radhakrishnan escape from decline and catastrophe depends not on scientific ideas and material forces but on the perceptions and ideas of men and women, on the moral judgement of the community. If we choose rightly, the achievements of science may lead to such a degree of material wealth and abundance of leisure as has never before been possible in human history. All this will be possible only if we achieve a revolution in the inner compulsions that control us (Radhakrishnan).

The quality of care must be evaluated on the basis of the human and therapeutic needs of the patient rather than, as too often the case, on the novelty and sophistication of technology used. The definition of these needs and quality of services required to meet them need careful consideration that goes far beyond techniques for quantifying some of the factors involved. The various economic, professional and personal interests inevitably at stake in any given case should first be clearly recognized and then prevented as far as possible from biasing the assessment (*World Health Forum*, Volume 17, 1996).

Radhakrishnan, the Indian scholar said, "I do not believe that scientific and technological studies are devoid of moral values. Science is both knowledge and power. It has interest as well as utility. It is illuminating as well as fruitful. It demands disciplined devotion to the pursuit of truth. It develops in its votaries an attitude of tolerance, open-mindedness, freedom from prejudice and hospitality to new ideas....The disproportionate emphasis on science and technology has been causing concern to thinking men all-over the world. The great crimes against civilization are committed not by primitive and uneducated but by the highly educated and the so-called civilized. One recalls the saying that the most civilized state is not farther from barbarism than the most polished steel is from rust.... Of the many problems that now face the leaders of the world, none is of graver consequence that the problem of saving the human race from extinction" (Radhakrishnan).

Again let me refer to *World Health Forum*, Volume 17, 1996 as regards the question of how society's resources should be defined and used to meet national and international health needs. Several sensitive questions and situations are raised in this context. Should the focus be on promoting equal access to healthcare for all, or on developing new technologies which require careful assessment and which in any foreseeable future will benefit only a few people ? Ethically, or even just logically, it is easy to answer that healthcare for all is the better choice, but in practice market and other forces tend to select the second option. At what point does the pursuit of technological improvement get in the way of using existing preventive and curative methods and technologies for the largest number of people possible ?

At present there is an acute shortage of opportunities for open discussion. One of WHO's functions should be to provide such opportunities, but to do so in a meaningful way it would have to assert a certain measure of courage and independence in relation to the considerable political and economic interests involved.

Dominance of economics is another issue raised by the group of advisers. The health status of population is to a very large extent determined by economic and social processes outside the medical sector, such as standards of living, nutrition, education, water supply and sanitation. A number of related factors need to be analyzed and openly discussed, such as the pressure of macro-economic policies on health policies, the increasing interventions of financial agencies in the health field, the links between health services, technology and money, the enormous weight of health expenditure in the economies of the rich countries, the effect of the aging populations on such expenditure and the need to rethink the organization and financing of health services in terms of societal choices. Neither economic thinking nor medical thinking can encompass all of life, though they often claim to.

Medical ethics used to refer to the relations between physicians and patient, but now it refers more to the relations between the medical world and society. The transition has been occasioned not only by changing attitudes but by the major role now played in care by medical institutions and socialized financing, and the growing use of sophisticated technical systems for the management of life and death.

It has highlighted that individual ethics is an inalienable part of social ethics. Social ethics is expressed and evolves within the relation between individuals. An adequate ethical system cannot consist only in a stated set of values but must have ways to manage conflicting values in concrete situation. Here emerges the evolving nature of ethical system. Human society is not static and therefore it is changeable giving scope for development which has upward trend. All changes do not bring reforms.

The role of the hospital is central to the consideration of a new system of social ethics with regard to health. Within medicine the hospital is the ultimate expression of both institutional logic and the technical management of suffering and death. More and more commonly, its financial realities rule out the possibility of including broader but less technical aspects of care, even when all the evidence suggests that such approaches would be more appropriate. Also, especially in developing countries, the hospital remains a matter of national prestige, strengthening the link between the medical profession and the political establishment.

The training of medical professionals is one of the areas in which ethical consideration is most urgently needed because this is where the attitudes and preoccupations of tomorrow's medical profession are formed. Here again, one has to give a serious thought to the fundamental values on which healthcare can be effective. Medical training has absorbed the enormous influx of new technologies, and continues to try to do so, without any pause for critical attention. It includes very little evidence of ethical thinking, and all too often it is either unaware of traditional wisdom or rejects it. Despite much protestation to the contrary, relatively little value is attached to preventive care.

These issues do not only concern the medical profession, the economic and financial departments of governments, and insurance companies. Society as a whole must be allowed to express its views on them, since they involve social and therefore political, choices.

The evaluation of health policies has to be broadened in two respects:

- Beyond the national level, because more and more variables such as the availability of drugs and technologies are determined at world level;
- Beyond the sphere of competence of ministries of health, since so many decisions vital for health are taken in other fields such as business, local government or education. Health policies must be defined in terms of the search for alliances between forces which, regardless of conflicting interests such as competition for funds, have an impact on health. *(World Health Forum,* Volume 17, 1996)

Successfulness of a doctor to cure the disease of a patient naturally widens the jurisdiction of doctor-patient relationship. It increases the reputation of the institution in which he/she serves and creates confidence in the people on the doctor. It is very rightly mentioned by Stimson that the expertness of the doctor cannot be replaced by the appreciable human relations between the two. The significant factor is that this expert knowledge has to be supplemented by all the qualities of human relations or to be guided by mutual respect, equal treatment, love, affection or sympathy needed by a human patient for strengthening his or her mental condition and it has a significant role in the process of curing the patient.

Influencing the doctor in the consultation: Patients can exert control by influencing the interaction in the face-to-face consultation with the doctor. Patient presentation—what is told or not told the doctor, what is emphasized, ordering, and so on, are all ways of exerting control. It is useful to view the outcome of the consultation as a result of negotiation or bargaining between patient and doctor, rather than as a simple product of the application of the doctor's knowledge and skills to the patient's problems.

Observations of consultations suggest that in general the overt patient behaviour tends to be passive compared to the doctor, and most frequent types of exchanges being doctor initiated information. (Stimson)

The structure, financing and organization of healthcare system affects doctor's situation and decision making strategies just as much as the patient's. While discussing doctor-patient conversation one has to take care to see the capacity differentials. The doctor has special knowledge acquired through medical education for a long period of several years which constitute the basic power or capacity of the doctor as a conversant with the patient. On the other hand, the patient, unless he is a doctor-patient, his capacity here is at the lowest level. As a layman he has imperfect understanding of the treatment, and cannot take decision in the process unless doctor explains to him in a language understandable to him. Once a patient is under treatment, it is seen that his ability to assess the efficacy of medical care he is receiving is constrained by several factors. The capacity differential is such that the doctor controls, as it were, both the demand and supply for medical care. It is the doctor who defines what is wrong with the patient and what treatment is required for its cure.

The patient conversant can come to a level of understanding provided he has no social distance with the doctor conversant. The class link helps extracting more explanations of the process and causes from the doctors.

As regards the maintenance of systematic records of medical errors it was observed:

"It is not common clinical practice to keep full systematic records of medical error. Physicians and surgeons often flinch even from identifying error in clinical practice, let alone recording it, presumably because they themselves hold the very theory of error which we are engaged in criticizing—that error arises either from their or their colleagues' ignorance or ineptitude. But without detailed records of erroneous diagnoses and prognoses of failures from effective treatment and the like, we cannot provide the empirical basis necessary for any adequate theory of the limitations upon the predicted paths of physicians. Of course there is nothing peculiar to physicians and surgeons about this lack of documentation of errors. Political scientists, economists, sociologists, for example, also do not usually keep systematic records of their own false predictions, and almost never advert to them in public utterance."

However, it may be said that accurate record keeping of individual doctor's successes or failures and release of such information to public is perhaps the best safeguard of quality healthcare. It requires cooperation between healthcare professionals, computer scientists, and behavioural scientists would probably be necessary to establish a system of recordkeeping that accurately documented doctor-patient exchanges, the diagnoses made, and the prescription or therapy recommended.

History of doctor-patient relationship reveals that in ancient India the relationship began with the full faith on the professional capacity of the doctor. The question of suspicion of the patient on the professional authority of the doctor did not arise. There were several reasons for it. Most rural people were ignorant and less mobile and agriculturalists. The number of medical service providers was also limited. The patients had no choice in selecting the doctors to approach, they generally used to go to a doctor who was easily accessible to them. They consider the position of a doctor next to God. Under that circumstances, it was quite natural to have paternalistic authority over the patients by the doctors.

In course of time, wide development of medical services and education took place in the country. Healthcare has become the minimum need of the Indians. The people also become aware of this development and as a result they started to choose the hospital/doctor for their treatment. Closely related to it is the awareness of the human rights by the Citizens due to the effort of UNO and the constitutional provisions for fundamental rights of the citizens. Gradually, issues like 'patient's autonomy, 'patient's safeguard', 'patient's informed consent' etc. emerged.

Recently, the dominating role of the science and technology in the world of medical services is influencing the relationship between a doctor and a patient. Along with it the social values have changed. Public services in India are allowing the principles commercialization and competition in delivery of service to the people.

(https://depts.washington.edu/bioethx/tpoics/physpt.html)

Change of social values causes corruption in the administration influencing medical services also. Naturally, earlier paternalistic authority of the doctor has changed. The patient himself or herself has become a part of decision making process. The patients today are conscious about the financial or otherwise benefit to be gained from a particular doctor or hospital, risks of alternative treatment etc. (Gallagher 1976)

Influencing the doctor in the consultation: Patients can exert control by influencing the interaction in the face-to-face consultation with the doctor. Patient presentation—what is told or not told the doctor, what is emphasized, ordering, and so on, are all ways of exerting control. It is useful to view the outcome of the consultation as a result of negotiation or bargaining between patient and doctor, rather than as a simple product of the application of the doctor's knowledge and skills to the patient's problems.

Observations of consultations suggest that in general the overt patient behaviour tends to be passive compared to the doctor, and most frequent types of exchanges being doctor initiated information-seeking exchanges, rather than patient-initiated information-giving exchanges.

The relative position of patient and doctor can be summed up as the idealization of ignorance. While the patient may not feel ignorant and the doctor may be aware that his knowledge is limited, ignorance and knowledge are idealized in relations between professionals and clients. Doctors and patients act towards each other as though they are personified these opposite attributes. The patient may present to the doctor in a manner suggestive of greater ignorance than is actually felt. There is an assumption that the doctor is the possessor of specialist knowledge and hence both doctor and patient collude in setting a scene in which the doctor can "act like a doctor" and patient can "act like a patient".

Another area where the patient may control is the utilization of treatment is also a means of control over the patient by a doctor. Patient may take decision about taking a drug when patients are not satisfied in consultation and doctor fails to persuade the patient to accept his perspective on the problem. He may not use the prescribed treatment as directed. The number of patients who do not obey doctor's order, whether these treatments are drugs or referral to hospital is increasing in India. Doctors cannot be aware of this aspect of patient-doctors relationship unless the patient informs the doctors. The doctors rarely know that the patients have not used the treatment.

However, it must be said that the concern to maintain autonomy involves each in attempts to control each other. From a client perspective the ability of patients to exert control over the doctor and over the medical care they receive—by not consulting, by choosing which doctor to consult, by influencing the interaction in the consultation, and by the utilization of treatment—is limited. Controls that patients do exert are small-scale, individualistic, covert, and met by counter strategies by the doctor and the staff. (Stimson)

Less satisfaction is expressed by the patients on matters like doctors did not respond to their queries, they did not give due attention to the patient, non-accessibility of doctors to patients, unwanted treatments, discouraging behaviour of doctors.

Doctors cannot force the patients to use his service and in the same way in certain cases, it is difficult for the patients not to consult doctors.

Choosing of a doctor by a patient in India is based on the opinion of the exit patients. (Gill).

Physician and Society Relationship: The Physicians have close relationship not only with the society itself. It can be realized by answering to the question, 'What is a society ?' A society is a group of individuals who exchange their ideas, interchange their opinion and where there is the clash of personalities in a given territory and participate in a common culture. While looking to what Robertson says one finds that while admitting that man is a social animal we cannot ignore that there are also animals which may also be called social animals, such as elephants, wolves etc. even many insects are social by nature, for example ants, bees etc. These non-human societies depend solely on the instinct of their members and they do not behave differently. But the human society is not under the dictates of its members' instincts. In the human society, the members themselves are the creators of social behaviour. Similarly, the 'humanity' is achieved only through social living, because an individual's behaviour and personality can be developed in the context of some society. No infant can reach maturity without the care and protection of other people and no adult can remain alive without using the values and information that have been transmitted through society.

Different social groups behave differently depending upon the geographical conditions and the values transmitted to new generation from the older one which is a continuous process since the beginning of the social life. Every society has certain fundamental requirements if it is to survive and to provide peaceful life to its members. For example, every society must have some means of replacing its members and of teaching them the culture that has been handed down over the generations. The society must also be able to protect its members against outside enemies and if possible, against domestic problems, such as, disease and food shortage. Every society must find some way of producing goods and distributing them to its members. Every society must have some system of social control—some means of ensuring that that people act in socially approved ways. Every society must have of some system shared values and of rituals to reaffirm them, so that solidarity of its members can be confirmed and enhanced. These functional needs are met by institutions.

Institutions are the stable clusters of values, norms, statuses, roles and expectations that develop around the basic needs of a society. For example, family is the primary social institution which takes care of replacement of its members and training of the young. The political and military institutions take care of the protection of the society against the outside crime and assume some responsibility for social control within the society. The economic institution organizes the production and distribution of goods and services. The religious institution provides a shared values and rituals that reaffirm them. The educational institution passes on cultural values from one generation to the next and trains the young in the more sophisticated knowledge and skills that they need in later life. (Robertson: 1980)

First Five Year Plan of India states, "On the part of the administration, efficiency and integrity are of course of the highest importance; equally, the relations between officials at different levels and the general public have an immense bearing on the response of the public. It is an essential rule in the code of a public servant, whatever his rank, to extend to every citizen courtesy and consideration and to inspire in him the confidence that so far as the law and the administration are concerned, all citizens have equal rights and claims....every unit in the administration has to discharge its duties in the understanding that major justification of its existence is the service it renders to the community and the confidence which it evokes, and that the public has a contribution to make in the fulfillment of any programme, which is no less vital than that of the administration. The approach towards public must, therefore, always be based on an attitude of close cooperation and a desire to take the utmost advantage of the people and provide for voluntary community action as large a field as may be possible." (First Five Year Plan)

With the transformation of the Indian society from traditional to modern one, political development of the country, i.e. democratization of the political process within the constitutional framework, continuous efforts of the United Nations of Organization for the protection of human rights of the people and the entrustment of responsibility to the national governments for safeguard of human rights of the citizens, the involvement of the service providers in the relationship with the society has increased. Further peoples' awareness about their rights also sensitizes the service providers about their relationship with the society in terms of responsiveness, accountability and responsibility. The Medical Ethics Manual of WMA has dealt with this social relationship.

The relationship can be characterized as a 'social contract'. The citizens of a country may be considered as taxpayers. A major portion of the public fund comes from the pockets of the citizens in the form of tax levied on them by the Governments. In the private hospitals there is the direct self-financing system for the services received by the patients is noticed. The salary including privileges and other facilities enjoyed by the service providers come from the public fund as the service providers in the government hospitals are paid by the government. The public servants are simply the trustees of public fund. In return of the salary including allowances and other facilities enjoyed by the public servants they render service to the people. Thus, it may be said that the service provided by them may be characterized as contract service.

Medicine is today, more than ever before, a social activity. It is no longer a two-way process between the physician and the patient only. It takes place in a context of government and corporate organizations and funding. It relies on public and corporate medical research and product development for its knowledge base and treatments. It requires complex healthcare institutions for many of its procedures. It treats diseases and illnesses that are as much social as biological in origin.

The Hippocratic tradition of medical ethics has little guidance to offer with regard to relationships with society to supplement the issues that arise beyond the individual patient-physician relationship and provides criteria and processes for dealing with these issues.

Physicians have various relationships with society. The areas of relationship between the physicians and the society are public health, health education, environment protection, health related laws, judicial proceedings, human rights etc.

Public health is "the science and art of preventing diseases, prolonging life and promoting health through the organized efforts and informed choices of society, organizations, public and private, communities and individuals." The dimensions of health can encompass "a state of complete physical, mental and social well-being and not merely the absence of diseases or infirmity", as defined by United Nations' World Health Organization. Public health incorporates the interdisciplinary approaches of epidemiology, biostatistics and health services, environmental health, behavioural health, health economics, public policy, insurance medicine and occupational safety and health are the important sub-fields.

The focus of public health intervention is to improve health and quality of life through the prevention and treatment of diseases and other physical and mental health conditions, through surveillance of cases and health indicators, and through the promotion of healthy behaviours. Promotion of hand washing and breastfeeding, delivery of vaccinations etc. are examples of common public health measures. But there are many other areas where the physicians and the people can meet for the improvement of public health and prevention of diseases.

Modern public health practice requires multidisciplinary teams of public health workers and professionals including physicians, medical assistants, environmental health officers/public health inspectors, pharmacists, dental hygienists, dieticians and nutritionists, veterinarians, public health engineers, public health lawyers, sociologists, community development workers, communications experts, bioethicists and others.

The focus of public health intervention is to prevent and manage diseases, injuries and other health conditions through surveillance of cases and the promotion of healthy behaviours, communities and environments. Many diseases are preventable through simple, non-medical methods. For example, hand washing with soap can prevent many contagious diseases.

There is a great disparity in access to healthcare and public health initiatives between developed nations and developing nations. In the developing world, public health infrastructure is still in the formative stage. There may not be enough trained heath workers or monetary resources to provide even a basic level of medical care and disease prevention.

The early history of public health reveals that it has early roots in antiquity. From the beginning of human civilization, it was recognized that polluted water and lack of proper waste disposal spread communicable diseases. Early religions attempted to regulate behaviour that specifically related to health from types of food eaten, to regulate certain indulgent behaviours, such as drinking alcohol or sexual relations. The leaders were responsible for the health of their subjects to ensure social stability, prosperity, and maintain order.

By Roman times, it was well understood that proper diversion of human waste was a necessary tenet of public health in urban areas. During the fourteenth century Black Death in Europe, it was believed that removing bodies of the dead would further prevent the spread of the bacterial infection. Burning parts of cities resulted in much greater benefit, since it destroyed the rodent infestations. A Cholera pandemic devastated Europe between 1829 and 1851, and was first fought by the use of what Foucault called "social medicine". Which focused on flux, circulation of air, location of cemeteries etc. All those concerns, which Foucault designated as the concept of "bio power".

As regards public health legislation it is found that the first attempts at sanitary reform and the establishment of public health institutions were made in the 1840s. Thomas Southwood Smith, physician at the London Fever Hospital, began to write papers on the importance of public health and was one of the first physicians brought into give evidence before the Poor Law Commission in the 1830s, along with Neil Arnott and James Phillips Kay.

The Poor Law Commission reported in 1838 that "the expenditures necessary to the adoption and maintenance of measures of prevention would ultimately amount to less than the cost of the disease now constantly engendered." It recommended the implementation of large-scale government engineering projects to alleviate the conditions that allowed for the propagation of disease. The Health of Town Association was formed in Exeter on 11th December, 1844 and vigorously campaigned for the development of public health in the UK.

Epidemiology: The science of epidemiology was founded by John Snow's identification of a polluted water as well as the source of an 1854 cholera outbreak in London. Dr. Snow believed in the germ theory of disease as opposed to the prevailing miasma theory. He first publicized his theory in an essay, *On the Mode of Communication of Cholera*, in 1849, followed by a more detailed treatise in 1855 incorporating the results of his investigation of the role of the water supply in the Soho epidemic of 1854.

By talking to local residents he identified the source of the outbreak as the public water pump on Broad Street. Although Snow's chemical and microscope examination of a water sample from the Broad Street pump did not conclusively prove its danger, his studies of the pattern of the disease were convincing enough to persuade the local council to disable the well pump by removing its handle.

Snow later used a dot map to illustrate the cluster of cholera cases around the pump. He also used statistics to illustrate the connection between the quality of the water sources and cholera cases. He showed that the Southward and Vauxhall Waterworks Company was taking water from sewage-polluted sections of the Thames and delivering the water to home, leading to an increased incidence of cholera. Snow's study was a major event in the history of public health and geography. It is regarded as the founding event of the science of epidemiology.

With the pioneering work in bacteriology of French chemist Louis Pasteur and German scientist Robert Koch, methods of isolating the bacteria responsible for a given disease and vaccines for remedy were developed at the turn of the twentieth century. British physician Ronald Ross identified the mosquito as the carrier of malaria and laid the foundations for combating the disease. Joseph Lister revolutionized surgery by the introduction of antiseptic surgery to eliminate infection. French epidemiologist Paul-Louis Simond proved that plague was carried by fleas on the back of rats, and the Americans Walter Reed and James Carroll demonstrated that mosquitoes carry the virus responsible for yellow fever.

In the United States, public health worker Dr. Sara Josepline Baker established many programmes to help the poor in New York City keep their infants healthy, leading teams of nurses into the crowded neighbourhoods of Hell's Kitchen and teaching mothers how to dress, feed and bathe their babies.

Dramatic increases in average life span in the late nineteenth century and twentieth century, is widely credited to public health achievements, such as vaccination programmes and control of many infectious diseases including polio, diphtheria, yellow fever and small pox; effective health safety policies such as road traffic safety and occupational safety, improved family planning, tobacco control measures, and the programmes designed to decrease non-communicable diseases by acting on known risk factors such as person's background, lifestyle and environment. Unfortunately, large parts of developing world remained plagued by largely preventable/treatable infectious diseases.

http://en.wikipedia.org/wiki/Public_ health accessed on 19.8.2014

Healthy environment is the prerequisite of protection of heath of human being. As regards environment it is said that it is a common man's knowledge that there are five basic elements needed for life: fire, water, air, earth and space. The Indian tradition also identified them as the great *Panchabhutas*. These elements are contributing to the maintenance of life, not merely in their individual and independent existence but also in their interdependence, all of them functioning together and constituting into one complex system. It is this system as a whole which is technically called Environment. (Pushparajan: 1992)

Protection of environment is of utmost necessity of the present society. Most of our environmental difficulties originate from man's ecological misbehaviour. The most alarming of man's assaults on the environment is pollution of air, earth, river and sea with dangerous and even lethal substances. This pollution is irreversible. The nature of environmental problems is different in developed and underdeveloped societies. In developed countries these problems have emerged due to the advancement of scientific and technological development, whereas the environmental problems of developing countries are in large measure those that have arisen from the lack of development. In both the towns and countryside not merely the quality of life but the life itself is endangered by poor water, housing, sanitation and nutrition and by sickness, disease and other different disasters.

In India, the environmental pollution is a multi-causal phenomenon. The principal reason of this pollution is rapidly increasing industrialization. The indiscriminate and mushrooming growth of industries in and around residential colonies has complicated the scenario. Further in several cities growth of hospitals and nursing homes and lack of carefulness in disposing of the sewages is causing air and water pollution in the country. In most cases cities and towns in India do not have sewage treatment facilities also.

It may be noted that people have been conscious about environmental problems ever since the Vedic times. It is clearly mentioned in the scriptures that nature and humankind form an inseparable part of the life support system. This system has five elements—air, water, land, flora and fauna, which are interconnected. (R.B. Jain and Kanchan Sharma: 1989)

The social customs and traditions of different communities may be understood in terms of health related issues such as, entry into kitchen is not allowed with shoe and cooking is allowed only after bathe, everyday morning house and courtyard must be cleaned so that goddess Lakshmi can come to bless the family to enhance the wealth. Thus, the traditional societies in India have number of such customs behind which protection of health rests. The most significant point is that these customs and traditions of the societies provided for self-help in taking preventive measures against disease and protection of their own health.

Gandhi's concept of *Village Swaraj* incorporates issues of public health very specifically. It is relevant even to-day basically for three reasons—first it explores simple and inexpensive ways of maintaining rural health; secondly, it involves each rural individual in the process of public healthcare activities and thirdly it helps creation of good governance in India as it involves people living even in the remote areas.

Village sanitation is of primary consideration in Gandhi's scheme of rural reconstruction. He recommended simple, inexpensive and effective remedies for tackling the problem of village insanitary condition. Those aimed at not only keeping the surroundings clean but also sought to convert the dirt into a source of wealth. So he suggested, "Lanes and streets have to be cleaned of all the rubbish, which should be classified. There are portions which can be turned into manure, portions which have simply to be buried and portions which can directly be turned into wealth. Every bone picked is valuable raw material from which useful articles can be made or which can be crushed into rich manure. Rag and waste-paper can be turned into paper, and excretes picked up are golden manure for the village field."

Again he said, "But the chief thing to remember is not the various methods of disposing of refuse, so much as the necessity of burying all refuse for the double purpose of promoting the villagers' health and their material condition. Through better yield of their crops which the manure must produce. It should be remembered that organic rubbish other than excretes must be separately buried. Attention to hygiene is undoubtedly the first step to village reconstruction."

He looked upon supply of water to villages as of glorious service fraught with incalculable benefit to the suffering humanity of India, since its neglect was responsible for many of the diseases suffered by the villages.

To him sanitation is the most effective way for dealing with diseases, since, for him, nature is the first physician, which is continuously repairing what man has damaged.

He believed that where the rules of personnel, domestic and public sanitation are strictly observed and due care is taken in the matter of diet and exercise, there should be no occasion for illness or disease.

Nature cure was a part of his plan of self-reliant society, for this kind of system of fighting diseases depends upon self-help and seeks to procure everything in the village. It relies on right and balanced diet. So to produce enough vegetables, fruits and milk in the villages is an essential part of nature cure. It is most suitable for villages because it does not depend upon costly equipment. "My nature cure', Gandhi argued, is designed solely for villagers and villages. Therefore, there is no place in it for the microscope, X-rays and similar things. Nor is there room in nature cure for medicine, such as quinine, emetine and penicillin. Personal hygiene and healthy living are primary importance.... All that can be taken and ...used. They are earth, water, ether, fire and wind...... If necessary curative herbs that grow locally, may be used". (Malhotra and Sharma: 1977)

The modern Panchayati Raj system introduced during the British rule has provided an administrative mechanism at the doorstep of the rural masses to solve their problems including rural health problems. However, the framers of the constitution made provision for the Panchayati Raj Institutions in the Directive Principles of State Policy. However, in 1992 by the 73rd Constitution Amendment has given a constitutional status to the Panchayati Raj system under Article 243 and the functions of these institutions are mentioned in the Eleventh Schedule of the Constitution. There the subjects like rural housing, drinking water, health and sanitation, including hospitals, primary health centres and dispensaries have been entrusted to these institutions. With the constitutional provision for Gram Sabha with all the residents of the village whose names are included in the voters' list. The Panchayat has become its executive body. Thus in an organized way the rural masses have been brought closer to the health service providers. Similar is the case with regard to urban local authorities.

Further, India is one of the very few countries of the world which has enshrined in its constitution a commitment to environment protection and improvement.

Article 48A of the constitution is related to protection and improvement of environment and safeguarding of forests and wildlife which states that the state shall endeavour to protect and improve the environment and to safeguard the forests and wildlife of the country. (P.M. Bakshi: 2004)

In this context, it may be mentioned that this direct reference to environment protection and its improvement was introduced with the Constitution (42nd Amendment) Act of 1976. It was perhaps the UN Conference on Human Environment held in Stockholm in 1972, which significantly influenced the government's awareness regarding the necessity of legal and organizational framework for protection of environment.

Since 1971, the Government of India has taken commendable initiatives to inject environmental considerations into the processes of planning for national development. These included comprehensive preparatory activities for India's participation in Stockholm Conference, the setting up of National Committee on Environmental Planning and Coordination (NCEPC), constitution of state environment committees, undertaking of environmental research programmes, incorporation of environment related subjects in school and college curricula, enactment of laws for environmental protection, formation in 1980, full-fledged Department of Environment at the centre etc. (R.B. Jain and Kanchan Sharma 1989).

The occupational hazard, till some time back, was a non-issue in India. Only with the growing industrialization and use of very highly toxic chemical substances, occupational hazard has become an issue amongst the communities. However, mention may be made of the Factories Act, 1948, the Mines Act, 1952, Plantation Labour Act, 1951 and *Beedi* and Cigar Workers Act, 1966 are worth mentioning in connection with the efforts of the government regarding occupational health and safety in India. (Binoy Acharya: 1989)

Relationship with Physician Colleagues, Teachers and Students: As the members of medical profession traditionally the physicians have expected to treat each other more as family members than as strangers or even as friends. The WMA Declaration in Geneva includes the pledge, "My colleagues will be my sisters and brothers." Besides the requirements to treat one's colleagues respectfully and to work cooperatively to maximize patient care, the WMA International Code of Medical Ethics contains two restrictions on physician's relationship with one another: (1) paying or receiving any fee or any other consideration solely to procure the referral of a patient; and (2) stealing patients from colleagues.

In the Hippocratic tradition of medical ethics, physicians owe special respect to their teachers. The Declaration of Geneva puts it as: "I will give to my teachers the respect and gratitude which is their due." Although present day medical education involves multiple student-teacher interactions rather the one-on-one relationship of former times, it is still dependent on the goodwill of and dedication of practicing physicians, who often receive no remuneration for their teaching activities. Medical students and other medical trainees owe a debt to their teachers, without whom medical education would be reduced to self-instruction.

For their part, teachers have an obligation to treat their students respectfully and to serve as good role models in dealing with patients. The so-called 'hidden curriculum' of medical education, i.e. the standards of behaviour exhibited by practicing physicians, is much more influential than the explicit curriculum of medical ethics, and there is a conflict between the requirements of ethics and the attitude and behaviour of the teachers, medical students are more likely to follow their teachers' example.

Teachers have a particular obligation not to require students to engage in unethical practices. Examples of such practices that have been reported in medical journals include medical students obtaining patient consent for medical treatment in situation where a fully qualified health professional should do this, performing pelvic examinations on anaesthetized or new dead patients without consent, and performing unsupervised procedures that, although minor, are considered by some students to be beyond their competence. Given the unequal power balance between teachers and students and the consequent reluctance of students to question or refuse such orders, teachers need to ensure that they are not requiring students to act unethically. In many medical schools, there are class representatives or medical students' associations that, among their other roles, may be able to raise concerns about ethical issues in medical education. Students concerned about ethical aspects of their education should have access to such mechanisms where they can raise concerns without necessarily being whistle-blower, as well as access to appropriate support if it becomes necessary to take the issue to a more formal process.

For their part, medical students are expected to exhibit high standards of ethical behaviour as appropriate for future physicians. They should treat other students as colleagues and be prepared to offer help when it is needed, including corrective advice in regard to unprofessional behaviour. They should also contribute fully to shared projects and duties such as study assignments and on-call service.

While maintaining the relationship amongst colleagues and teacher and students the problem of reporting unsafe or unethical practice has occupied a significant place. It is a sensitive issue for the colleagues to deal with and at the same time it is extremely essential in the interest of the principle that "do no harm to patient." Medicine is traditionally taken pride in its status as a self-regulating profession. In return for the privileges accorded to it by society and the trust given to its members by their patients, the medical profession has established high standards of behaviour for its members and disciplinary procedures to investigate accusations of misbehaviour and, if necessary, to punish the wrongdoers. This system of self-regulation has often failed, and in recent years step have been taken to make the profession more accountable. For example, by appointing lay members to regulatory authorities. The main requirement for self-regulation, however, is wholehearted support by physicians for its principles and their willingness to recognize and deal with unsafe and unethical practice.

Obligation to report incompetence, impairment or misconduct of one's colleagues is emphasized in the WMA International Code of Medical Ethics. For example the Code states, "A physician shall.....strive to expose those physicians deficient in character or competence, or who engage in fraud or deception." The application of this principle is seldom easy, however. On one hand, the physician may be tempted to attack the reputation of a colleague for unworthy personal motives, such as jealousy, or in retaliation for a perceived insult by the colleague. A physician may also be reluctant to report a colleague's misbehaviour because of friendship or sympathy. The consequence of such reporting can be very detrimental to the one who reports, including almost certain hostility on the part of the accused and possibly other colleagues as well.

Despite these drawbacks to reporting wrongdoing, it is a professional duty of physicians. Not only are they responsible for maintaining the good reputation of the profession, but they are often the only ones who recognize incompetence, impairment or misconduct. However, reporting colleagues to the disciplinary authorities should be the last resort after other alternatives have been tried and found wanting.

The World Medical Association. B.P.63,o1212Femey-Voltaire Codex, France, website www.wma.net

Organizational or Administrative Relationship: When two or more persons unite together to coordinate their activities with a predetermined goal need arises of organization or administration. Generally, an organization consists of three components—infrastructure, a group of personnel, rules and regulations to be followed to achieve the well-defined goal. Organization is defined differently by various scholars. Chester Barnard defines an organization as "a system of consciously coordinated personal activities or forces" or "a system of interrelated activities or forces." Ralph Davis defines it as "a group of people working under a leader to accomplish an objective."

An organization is basically a network of relationships—relationships of things, tasks, people and processes. The chief of hospital will look at the organization as a system to offer service efficiently to the satisfaction of the patients. He will always concern with work flow, end result, control, supervision, inspection, maintenance of economy, discipline, coordination etc. Here the group of personnel in the organization may be divided into two major divisions—Personnel directly linked with treatment, such as physicians and nurses and another group consisting of technicians to handle different equipment including computer man, clerical class, security personnel, cleaners, experts in finance, grievance redress personnel etc. who constitute a major part of the medical organization. The administrative chief is concerned with office lay out, execution of routine, filing or recording system, control of employees etc. In the traditional system of medicine, dominance of physician and nurses prevailed just as in an educational institution teacher and student constituted the dominating factor. Gradually with the increase in the number of patients and the students there arises the need of administrative mechanism for serving the patients and the students. It has given birth of administrative organization. In the hospital organization there emerges positions like Directors, administrative officers, departmental heads, registrars, superintendent, Public Relations Officers, clerical staff, auditors, machine men, security personnel drivers etc. whose services have become essential to achieve the primary goal of the hospital or to serve the patients efficiently by the physicians. The occupants of these positions belong to different educational and training background as required the positions. They do not have the preliminary knowledge of medicine, but their services are essential in the hospital organization. Again if we look the physicians it is found that they come to this profession with different family background, different social values inculcated in them through the process of socialization and ultimately from different medical schools of colleges. But they have to behave like family members once they join the medical services. Therefore, every interrelated group of human beings must have an ideology—that is, a conception of what is the proper way to behave and permissible pattern of relationships in the organization. To live in a group and learn correct behaviour requires social discipline. Just as in troop there must be some drill to avoid or defy enemies, in every organization also there must be some rules, regulations or codes of conduct to be observed to unite the services of different members toward the ultimate goal. This need is fulfilled by the administrative system, i.e. formal structure. Otherwise social relationships may play a negative role. Human nature is complex and changeable. The experience in India today is that behind transparency the secret inhuman relationships are appearing very starkly. For example, the nexus among corrupt persons, violators of human rights, exploiters of vulnerable, dishonest persons, criminals etc. is very strong and secret. On several occasions it is found that they are also efficient in their fields. What I feel today is that love, affection, honesty, human feeling etc. have become very fragile to keep people within an organization together whereas the greed, dishonesty, selfishness, inhuman behaviour etc. are emerging as a strong tie to keep them together. Nobody can deny that every individual has both negative and positive qualities inherited through the mechanism of birth or nurture. Everyone requires an environment or an apparatus to activate the good qualities of an individual in the greater interest of the humanity in general and in particular in the interest of the social organizations. In these organizations administrative system is the apparatus which is organically linked in the organizational behaviour. For example in the administrative process of and educational institution teachers are associated and in the similar way in a hospital system physicians are also associated. It is for the administration to create the environment to feel by each and every member of the hospital the need of ethical code effective functioning of the organization. Joan Robinson in his book, *Freedom and Necessity* stated it very interestingly as, "To regard our own feelings as rooted in a biologically determined apparatus requires a certain degree of detachment. Take the example of hunger. We think that we desire to eat because food is necessary to life, but it is by no means so simple. We desire to eat because we are endowed with an apparatus that makes us feel hungry, and we are endowed with that apparatus because a species that lacked it would not have survived". (Robinson: 1970)

The importance of efficient administration is emerging at par with that of technical expertise. This indicates the need of close relationship and ethical behaviour of the physicians towards auxiliary staff in administrative system so that the members at the lower ranks can learn it from the high ranking personnel. Under no circumstances, these low ranking employees should be engaged in unethical activities. Since these people are vulnerable from different points of view, they can be easily mobilized towards any kind of unethical and illegal activities.

In conclusion, it may be said that in any organization irrespective of its nature of functions and size integration, cooperation, dedication, commitment to the cause of the nation, sense of sacrifice, belongingness, human dignity and values etc. are the core issues to be attended by the administrative authorities of the organization. The role of the organizational leadership is an important factor in an organization. It is true that personality traits of different leaders vary from one another. However, the leader must be equipped with the traits like intelligence, communication skill and ability to assess group activities and behaviour in different situations impartially and with human approach. Then only the leader will be in a position to sustain and enhance the core values in the organization.

It is the leader who can motivate the subordinate to work hard through establishment of morale in the organization. What is Morale? The Oxford English Dictionary defines Morale as "moral condition, conduct, behaviour—especially with regard to confidence, hope, zeal, submission to discipline etc." In short "Morale is the capacity of a group of people to pull together persistently and consistently in pursuit of a common purpose" (Leighton). He goes a little ahead and said that morale thus defined depends on:

1. The confidence that individual members of the group have in the purpose of the group;
2. The confidence they have in the group;
3. The confidence they have in each other;
4. The organizational efficiency;
5. The mental, emotional and physical health of the employees. (Maheswari: 2004)

Coming to the discussion on Morale in an Organization made by A.R. Tyagi in his book, *Public Administration* one cannot deny that man does not live by bread alone. Esteem too is a powerful awakener of energetic and rightly-oriented action. Abraham Maslow in his need hierarchy list has referred about this esteem need of a man to induce a person to work. As mentioned earlier Tyagi also repeated about Morale as, "Government is a human institution and rests not only on formal arrangement, skill and principles but even more on attitudes, enthusiasms and loyalty. It must be approached as a problem of morale and personnel fully as much as a task of logic and management."

The late W.G. Wells, a critic of bureaucracy, praises, 'the tradition of honour and devotion to duty that animated the Civil service in England.' In fact it is the secret of success of the British Civil Services, because these honour and devotion to duty helps building of high morale in the services. To L.D. White, "Morale is both an index of a sound employment situation and a positive means of building up of an efficient organization." It reflects "a socio-psychological situation, a state of mind in which men and women voluntarily seek to develop and apply their full powers to the task upon which they are engaged, by reason of the intellectual or moral satisfaction which they derive from their own self-realization, their achievements in the chosen field, and their pride in the service. It is a self-stimulating incentive created within the minds and hearts of the workers. It induces them to far superior efforts in their respective fields of work than greed of money or fear of punishment does."

Morale has an individual as well as institutional aspect. The two are interactive, one sustaining and stimulating the other. In its individual form, morale is built upon "the opportunity to acquire distinction, prestige and personal power, right to be considered successful and to be respected; and an opportunity for personal development." In its latter form, it sustains on attractive personal associations, the easy adaptation of conditions in the organization to habitual methods and attitudes of employees, an opportunity for enlarged participation in the organization and a "condition of communion which is a sense of belonging to a group or an enterprise to which one is loyal and dedicated. The former gives him an incentive to efficient and honest work by satisfying his personal urge to recognition, while the latter creates in the employees of an organization an *espirit de corps* which makes them identify the aims and objectives of the organization with their own and are thus highest stimulant to superior work.

To build morale in an organization attempt has to be made for replacing old hierarchical system by cooperative effort. There may be Supervisor or Director like hierarchical system, the only difference is that instead of being commander or authoritarian leader he should be a democratic leader to get things done by the subordinates through persuasion, resourcefulness and tact. He must be a moral leader with honesty, sincerity, dedication and compassionate towards the subordinates. His interest on the employees should not confine to their official activities only. He must take care to understand his problems beyond office relationship, such about their illness, children's education and health and other family responsibilities etc.

The trust of employees in the integrity and good intent of the superiors is a very effective means of building employee morale. Where the superiors are suspected of favouritism, corruption and other malpractices, employees get demoralized and indiscipline.

It may be noted that "public servants themselves can establish high tradition of loyalty to the nation, devotion to work and a very high sense of integrity in the service". (Tyagi: 1989)

To Douglas McGregor, "behind every managerial decision or action are assumptions about human nature and human behaviour".

To O.G. Stahl, in a broad sense the inculcation of morale, of that spirit, that state of mind, which expresses itself in loyalty, enthusiasm, cooperation, pride in the service, and devotion to duty, is the end of the whole personnel system. Every aspect of the personnel programme from recruitment to retirement may be handled so that it is either an incentive or a depressant to individual and group morale. In a very real sense, this whole work is devoted to a consideration of ways of building and maintaining this most valuable asset of any organization. (Stahl: 1962)

In an organization rendering medical services to the nation family feeling amongst the members of it irrespective of their rank or position is of utmost necessity. Because it is the human being who is in driver's seat. Effective interaction in the organization helps widening path to achieve its goal with minimum hindrances.

Rensis Likert has pointed out some characteristics of an organization operating on an ideal interaction-influence system as below:

1. Each member will find his personal values, needs and goals reflected in those workgroups and organization as a whole.
2. Every member of organization would be identified with the objectives of organization and the goals of his workgroup and see the accomplishment of them as the best way to meet his own needs and personal goals.
3. Pressure for high performance goals, efficient methods and skill development come from the members themselves. The anxieties associated with hierarchical pressures in traditional organizations will be conspicuous by their absence.
4. Authentic and sensitive communication processes with and between workgroups would ensure spontaneous and accurate information flows to providing rational basis for individual and group decisions and actions at all points in the organization.
5. Every member of the organization will be able to exert his influence on decisions and actions of the organization. The amount of influence exerted by any individual will be proportionate to the significance of his ideas and contribution and not necessarily related to his position in the formal organization.
6. Cooperative motivation, communication and decision processes will enable each member in any part of the organization to exert his influence, contribute his ideas, skills, resources and improve the total capacity of the organization of problem-solving and goal-fulfillment. (Seshachalam: 2007)

Social relationship occupies a pivotal place in the medical care services. The progress of science and technology cannot do away with the human approach in these services and the culture and tradition of a county. Jawaharlal Nehru said, "in every country, in every people, there are two types of forces at work. One is what might be called continuity, continuing traditions, continuing habits, continuing structures of society, continuing beliefs and the like. That is a powerful cement which holds society together. We in India have this sense of continuity in a very powerful degree and that is what has us to function together for the last thousands years. The other force is that of change which is the reverse of continuity, and it is equally essential or more essential because anything that ceased to change completely is dead. It is only death that stops change. Everything that is living, whether an individual or social group, or a nation, if it is alive, is constantly changing." (Nehru: 1955)

Indira Gandhi, while addressing as Prime Minister of India in 1980, the Commonwealth Heads of Government at the regional meeting held in New Delhi said, "whether we like it or not, the problems of the future compel our attention, for they are already upon us. There are many aspects of the human condition which trouble thoughtful people. The crisis that we face far beyond political and economic rivalries. It is a crisis of the spirit. For the first time in the story of our world, the human species and the values of civilization, which have enabled man to rise above his circumstances, are threatened because we have lost sight of the vision of our ancient sages and are obsessed with immediate discontent."

References

Abraham, A., J. Prasad and A. Joseph and K.S. Jacob: *Confidentiality, Partner Notification and HIV Infection: Issues related to Community Health Programmes: National Medical Journal of India: Medical Ethics*; Vol. 13, No. 4, 2000.

Agarwal, R.C. (1986): *Constitutional Development of India and National Movement,* S. Chand & Co. Ltd., New Delhi.

Acharya, Binoy: *Occupational Health and Safety in India Legislations Inadequate,* IJPA; July-September Issue, 1989, Vol. XXXV, No. 3.

Bakshi, P.M.: *The Constitution of India*: 5th edition; Universal Law Publishing Co. Pvt. Ltd., 2004; New Delhi.

Bhattacharya, Mrs. Gauri (1981): Political and Social Ideas of Mahatma Gandhi: A Critique: an unpublished Ph.D. thesis submitted to Gauhati University in 1981.

Bhattacharya, Mohit: *Public Administration*, World Press Private Ltd., 1987.

Bhaskara Rao, V., Frederick Taylor; *Administrative Thinkers*, edited by D. Ravindra Prasad, V. Prasad, P. Satyanarayana and Y. Pardhrasaradhi, Sterling Publishers Pvt. Ltd., New Delhi-22.

Boorstin, Daniel J. (1974): *Democracy and Its Discontents*, Random House, New York, 1974.

Diwakar, R.R.: Trying to Understand Gandhi: *Journal of Gandhian Studies*, Vol. 14, No. 53, October 1986. Institute of Gandhian Thought & Peace Studies, Gandhi Bhawan, Allahabad University.

Gallaghar Eagene B. Ed: "Doctor-Patient Relationship in Changing Health Scene": (Conf. proceedings and papers organized in USA in 1976 by Department of Health Education and Family Welfare, Public Health Service, National Institute of Health), ed. By Eagene B. Gallagher, Professor of Medical Sociology, Professor of Behavioural Science, Kenttucky College, Medicine.

Gill, Deepak G., *Limitation upon choice and constraints over decision making in doctor-patient exchanges*: University of Missouri-Columbia Medical Center, Columbia, Missouri.

Gupta, R.C. (2006): *Great Political Thinkers*, Lakshmi Narain Agarwala, Agra.

Jain, R.B. and Kanchan Sharma: *Implementation Machinery for Environment Protection in India*, IJPA; July-September Issue, 1989, Vol. XXXV, No. 3.

Kapur, Anup Chand (1989): *Indian Political System*, S. Chand & Co., New Delhi, 1989, Kempadoo, Sri Peter Kempadoo: Sarvodaya: Gandhi's Alternative to Development Strategy for Today's World. Jan. 1983 in *Journal of Gandhian Studies*, Vol. 10, No. 37-38, Oct. 82, Institute of Gandhian Thought & Peace Studies, Gandhi Bhawan, University of Allahabad.

Kistaia, M. 2007: George Elton Mayo; *Administrative Thinkers*: edited by D. Ravindra Prasad, V.S. Prasad and P. Satyanarayana; Sterling, New Delhi, 2007.

Maheswari, Shriram: *Administrative Theory*: MacMillan India Ltd., Delhi, 2002.

Malhotra, Dr. S.L. and Dr. S.K. Sharma: *Towards Village Swaraj: Research Monograph*, Dept. of Gandhian Studies, Punjab University, Chandigarh, January 1977.

Mukhopadhyay, Lipi: *Social Conditioning and Deviant Behaviour*, IJPA, Spl Number on Social Tensions: Administration and Political Responses; July-Sept. 2002, Vol. XLVIII, No. 3.

Nehru, Jawaharlal: A Word to the Services; speech made by Nehru as Prime Minister, at Kurnool, in Andhra, on 9th December, 1955 to an audience of Public Servant, *Indian Journal of Public Administration*, Vol. 1, Oct.-Dec. 1955, No. 4.

Pushparajan, A., Environmental Challenges of Today and Gandhi—The Only Hope of the Twenty First Century; Gandhi-Jyoti, *Journal of Gandhian Thought*, 1st January, 1992-6th April, 1992.

Robertson, Ian (1980): *Sociology*; Worth Publishers, Inc, 444 Park Avenue South, New York.

Radhakrishnan, S. (1992): *The Present Crisis of Faith*, 11th Edition, Orient Paperbacks, Delhi.

Robinson, Joan (1970): *Freedom and Necessity*, George Allen & Unwin (India).

Seshachalam, P. Rensis Likert: *Administrative Thinkers*, edited by D. Ravindra Prasad, V.S. Prasad and P. Satyanarayana, Sterling, New Delhi, 2007.

Stimson, Gerry V., *Interaction Between Patients and General Practitioners in the United Kingdom*, Institute of Psychiatry, London, England.

Sinha, Jadunath, *A Manual of Ethics,* New Central Book Agency, 8/1, Chintamoni Das Lane, Kolkata-700009.

Tripathi, Anil, Gandhi's Social Philosophy: *Journal of Gandhian Studies,* Vol. 7, No. 28, July 1980, Gandhi Bhawan, University of Allahabad.

Tyagi, A.R.: *Public Administration,* Atma Ram & Sons, 1989.

Umapathy, N., Herbert Simon, *Administrative Thinkers* edited by Dr. Ravindra Prasad, V.S. Prasad, P. Satyanarayana, and Y. Paradhasaradhi, Sterling Publishers Private Ltd., New Delhi, 2010.

Six

Negligence and Error

Failure of the System

In contemporary world of medicine in India two ailments are drawing attention of the public—Negligence and Error. Media is focusing frequently the complaints of the attendants of the patients as regards the negligence of the doctors or other medical service providers and the errors committed by them. Media is focusing frequently the conflicts between the medical service providers and the patients based on mainly these two issues. Though it is not easy to ascertain the validity of the complaints, there is enough space to have doubt on the sincerity and dedication of the medical service providers in the contemporary world.

Negligence and error in administration are closely related mainly to three emerging issues in public administration in India, i.e., accountability, responsibility and secrecy. All these are again related to ethics. Medical services constitute a significant and all pervasive aspect of public administration. In ultimate analysis of any organization, it is the human being who is to make its wheel move in the right direction. When one views the relationship of the three elements, it is found that negligence is one of the factors leading to error and error induces a person to hide the error as far as possible for various reasons.

Self-control and self-regulation are the two essential principles to build a system of bureaucratic accountability which may lead to avoidance of error and to some extent negligence. The most efficient and accountable bureaucracies rest on trust between the superior and the subordinates. This trust is possible if—(a) the former believes that the latter will faithfully carry out things he has promised to do; (b) the latter believes that the former is motivated by the right objectives; (c) the two together do not join in a conspiracy to defraud the government and citizens; (d) when mistakes are committed there is always some way or mechanism of correcting them and some distinctiveness will be then to stop their recurrence (Sethi: 1983).

The concept of secrecy in administration can be envisaged as 'rationalization of the irrational' which the irrational wants to see as the rational. Whether it is depersonalization of power, or concern for feasibility, or the need of camouflaging internal conflicts and norm deviations, bureaucracy does not like itself to be presented in an un-Weberian cloak of illegitimacy. The mystique of secrecy is chosen as a necessary evil or a lesser evil for practical reasons, or for reasons of human compassion, or to discharge the obligations of primary relationships not yet fully articulated with the administrative obligations of a complex democratic society. (Sharma: 1979)

In medical sciences ethics is very close to normative accountability as the medical scientists have more autonomy than any other public servants. In support of it Carl Friedrich stated that there is need of some elasticity in the power of the administrator, some discretion to be used by him, and some inner check upon his own behaviour. Hence, he has stressed the normative and moral aspect of administrative accountability by arguing that internal 'informal' controls like professional standard, codes of ethics, social values possessed by individuals are very much necessary. Once these normative controls are strengthened, administrative accountability would increase. These serve as 'preventive' rather 'correcting' measure against malfeasance. (Mukhopadhyaya: 1983)

The Constitution of India also provides provision for reasonable restrictions on the freedom of the people to create a congenial environment for reducing the scope of enjoying the freedom arbitrarily. The limitations imposed on freedoms guaranteed by Article 19 of the constitution serve two purposes:

1. They specify that these freedoms are not absolute but are subject to regulation;
2. They put a limitation on the power of a legislature to restrict these freedoms.

Here again the problem is to determine the question as to whether a restriction imposed on any of the freedoms guaranteed by Article 19 of the Constitution, Court has to examine both substantive and procedural aspects of the restriction so imposed. There is no general standard of reasonableness applicable to all cases. Court has to decide each case on its own merit by examining if both substantive and procedural aspects of the restriction imposed or sought to be imposed are reasonable.

However, in determining the substantive reasonableness, the court has evolved certain norms. The courts have to consider the factors like the nature of the right alleged to be infringed, the underlying purpose of the restrictions imposed, the extent and urgency of the evil sought to be remedied thereby, the disproportion of the imposition and the prevailing conditions at the time.

Guidelines to determine reasonableness have been spelled out in *Pathumma* Vs *State of Kerala* case by a Constitutional-Bench of the Supreme Court had held "that Article 19 confers an absolute and unconditional right which is subject only to reasonable restrictions to be placed by Parliament or the legislature in public interest. The Court had also laid down the guidelines to determine the question of reasonableness of "restriction" as follows:

1. That, in judging the reasonableness of the restrictions imposed by clause (5) of Article 19, the Court has to bear in mind the Directive Principles of State Policy.
2. That restrictions must not be arbitrary or of an excessive nature so as to go beyond the requirement of the interest of the general public.
3. That in order to judge the quality of reasonableness no abstract or general pattern or a fixed principle can be laid down so as to be universal application and the same will vary from case to case.
4. That a just balance has to be made between the restriction imposed and social control envisaged by clause (6) of Article 19.
5. That there must be direct and proximate nexus or a reasonable connection between restriction imposed and the object which is sought to be achieved. In other words, the court has to see whether by virtue of the restriction imposed on the right of the citizen, the object of the statute is really fulfilled or frustrated.
6. That the court must see the prevailing social values whose needs are satisfied by restrictions meant to protect social welfare.
7. That so far as the nature of reasonableness is concerned it has to be viewed not only from the point of view of citizen, but the problem before legislature and the object which is sought to be achieved by the statute. (Singh: 2001)

It would be unreasonable, for example, to judge by the same criteria the conduct of a practitioner who by necessity performs an operation in a remote country district or in the patient's own house and the conduct of one who operates in a modern hospital with expert assistance and every up-to-date appliance to hand. Equally, where it is alleged that a complaint could have been successfully diagnosed with the use of particular apparatus or appliance, regard must be had to the availability of that apparatus or appliance in the particular case, in order to decide whether the failure to use it amounts to negligence. Again, where there is an urgent need for action, the practitioner will not necessarily be held negligent if in the agony of the moment he adopts a course or omits a precaution which he might not perhaps have adopted or omitted had he had time to consider the matter. His conduct must be judged in the light of emergency which existed and in the light of the facts which were known to him when circumstances compelled him to act.

Thus, it cannot be said that negligence will inevitably exist if a swab is found to have been left in a patient after an operation; for in judging the surgeon's conduct the regard must be had to such matters as the inherent difficulties of the particular operation, the condition of the patient and the risks to which he is exposed, the anxiety of the surgeon on surgical grounds to bring the operation to an end as rapidly as possible, and other similar factors.

The degree of care required varies also in proportion to the magnitude of the risks involved. More extensive precautions must be taken where treatment which involves known risks is administered than where no such risks can reasonably be anticipated.

The failure to take precautions to avoid a particular risk will amount to negligence if the risk is of a reasonably substantial character. Where the risk involved is such as would in ordinary parlance be characterized as negligible, such a failure will be quite compatible with the exercise of proper skill and care.

In many cases then negligence will consist of a failure to take sufficient precautions to guard against known risks; and by known risks are meant not simply those risks which were in fact known to the individual medical man whose conduct is in question, but risks which were known or ought to be known to the ordinarily skilled and intelligent practitioner of his class. It is scarcely necessary to emphasize that a particular course of action must be judged in the light of discoveries which may subsequently have been made.

A practitioner therefore be held negligent if he follows what is the general and approved practice in the situation with which he is faced.

"A defendant charged with negligence can clear his feet if he shows that he has acted in accord with general and approved practice". This proposition rests upon the basis that—"what is reasonable in a world... must depend on what people presumed to be reasonable constantly do."

The proposition must be regarded, however, with a certain amount of caution; for where a common practice has inherent defects which ought to have been obvious to any person giving the matter due consideration, the practice will not be any of the less negligent because it is shown to have been widely and generally adopted over a period of time.

Thus although in majority of cases a charge of negligence can be met by showing that what was done accorded with general and approved practice, it is the Court itself, not the medical profession, who decides whether negligence is established in a particular case; and the courts will not be deterred from categorizing as negligent a practice which has inherent and obvious risks, by the fact that the practice has been widely followed over a period of time.

Moreover, it may very well be negligent for a practitioner to adhere to a once approved but now outworn and discredited practice.

Negligence cannot be established, however, merely by showing that some persons or some schools of medicine disapprove of a particular practice, if nevertheless it remains a widespread and approved practice elsewhere. For where there exist two or more recognized schools of thought with regard to a particular problem, the individual practitioner is entitled to choose between rival doctrines and cannot be held negligent because he chooses one rather than the other. According to the result of the survey, 40 per cent of doctors believe that number of patients that visited them over a period of one month often exceeded safe level, 36 per cent of these doctors reported a frequency of more than once a week.

There is an ever growing problem of doctors having to take on more patients. In addition 5 per cent of the physicians reported that the heavy workload may have caused at least one death over the year.

(www.medicalnews today.com/articles/255576.php)

Scope of the Duty of Care: Where, in accordance with the principles, a person has, by assuming responsibility for the medical treatment of another, come under a duty to exercise care or skill towards him, not merely to abstain from physical action which is or may be detrimental to the patient. A medical man will of course be liable if he sets a bone negligently or if he operates without due care. But the duty extends further, so as to require the exercise of care and skill in diagnosis, in prescribing and in advising, even where the work is done gratuitously. And the duty is not even confined to cases where positive action is taken or positive advice given. For if he has once undertaken the care of a patient, even gratuitously, the medical man will be liable for sins of omission as well as for sins of commission. He will be just as much as answerable for wrongly failing to act or to give advice as for acting or advising wrongly. The National Health Service Act 1946, UK stated, "A practitioner is required to render to his patients all proper and necessary treatment"—and—"In the case of emergency the practitioner is required to render whatever services are, having regard to the circumstances, in the best interests of the patient."

Attendance: A medical man may be guilty of negligence if he fails to attend his patient with the regularity and promptitude which his patient's condition demands; but he can only be held liable civilly if his lack of attention leads to an avoidable deterioration of the patient's condition. Whether the medical man has complied with his duty to be reasonably diligent in attendance can only be decided after the fullest consideration of the circumstances of the particular case; because it is only in the light of those circumstances that it is possible to measure the extent of the duty. He may well be guilty of negligence.

It is equally impossible to lay down any exact rule with regard to the medical man's duty when summoned to attend a patient. The question whether he has failed in his duty will depend, among other things, upon the urgency of the summons, the nature of the condition communicated to him and the importance of any other commitments he may have.

Diagnosis: The diagnosis of ailments is normally the first matter with which the medical man is concerned; and there can be no doubt that he may find himself held liable in an action for negligence if he makes a wrong diagnosis and thereby causes injury or damage to the patient. In a South African case viz., *Mitchell V. Hunter* (1950) has been quoted in the book titled, *Medical Negligence* as, "*no human being is infallible; and in the present state of science even the most eminent specialist may be at fault in detecting the true nature of a diseased condition. A practitioner can only be held liable in this respect if his diagnosis is so palpably wrong as to prove negligence, that is to say, if his mistake is of such a nature as to imply an absence of reasonable skill and care on his part, regard being had to the ordinary level of skill in the profession.*"

Relationship between Surgeon and Patient: Hodgins, J.A. said in one of his judgements as, "the relationship of surgeon and patient is naturally one in which trust and confidence must be placed in the surgeon. His knowledge, skill and experience are not and cannot be known to the patient, and within proper limits it would seem to require that where an operation is contemplated or proposed a reasonably clear explanation of it and of the natural and expected outcome should be vouchsafed"—And later he stated his conclusions that—"the relationship between the defendant and the plaintiff was that of surgeon and patient and such the duty cast upon the surgeon was to deal honestly with the patient as to the probable consequences and whether success might reasonably be expected to ameliorate or remove the trouble, but that such duty does not extend to warning the patient of the dangers incident to, or possible, any operation, nor to details calculated to frighten or distress the patient."

A patient may in some cases decide to place himself unreservedly in the hands of his medical advisers and may signify his willingness to accept any decision they may make as to his treatment. In such cases, the only question is as to the extent of the medical man's duty to volunteer explanations of the proposed treatment, its probable outcome and the risks involved in it. But often it will happen that the patient makes it clear by his questions as to the nature of treatment or its consequences or risks, that he does not wish to surrender himself entirely into the hands of his medical man but desires to exercise his own judgment as to the form of treatment he is to undergo. In such a case, it is thought that ordinarily the patient is entitled to have his questions answered in a full and accurate manner and to have explained to him, if he so desires, the various factors to which consideration ought to be given in exercising a choice as to the form of treatment to be undergone. It appears, however, that the medical man may in some cases be entitled to exercise his discretion to withhold certain information from his patient or even to give false answers. The extent to which and the circumstances in which the medical man will be justified in such conduct are left in some doubt. Certainly such conduct will only be justified where the medical man is acting genuinely in the interests of the patient as he sees them. Beyond that it thus not seem possible to say more than that each case must depend upon its own circumstances; and that in judging whether in a particular case the medical man was demanded of him or in giving an untrue or inaccurate answer regard must be had to such matters as the character, health, nervous condition, intelligence and social position of the patient.

Anesthetics and Other Drugs: In a number of cases allegations of negligence have been made in connection with the administration of anesthetics and other drugs. In most cases, where untoward results have followed such treatment there is little doubt as to the existence of negligence on somebody's part; for the administering of an aesthetics or drug ought not in the ordinary course of events to produce unexpectedly deleterious effects. It must be remembered, however, that from time to time a case occurs where a patient is shown to have been adversely affected by a drug which is quite harmless when administered to the vast majority of persons; in such cases the failure to anticipate a personal idiosyncrasy on the part of the patient will not normally amount to negligence.

The hospital authority itself may be found guilty of negligence if it fails to ensure that a reasonably safe and careful system is followed in the hospital with regard to the dispensing and administration of anesthetics and other dangerous drugs. Thus, in the case where cocaine was administered by mistake for procaine; The hospital which enabled an unqualified house surgeon to obtain from pharmacist a large quantity of a dangerous drugs without being required to produce a written prescription signed by a qualified person; It was also held that the pharmacist was negligent in dispensing the solution without such prescription and in failing to verify that it was cocaine which was required. Similarly, a hospital might well be found negligent if it failed to ensure that dangerous drugs were contained only in properly labeled and readily recognizable bottles or container. It is also possible that a hospital authority may be held directly or "personally" negligent if it permits young and inexperienced persons to administer anesthetics.

Operation Theatre: Liability for negligent conduct in the course of an operation is judged upon exactly the same principles as is the liability of a general practitioner for negligence in the performance of any task he has undertaken; but the problems arising are complicated by the fact that in an operation a number of different persons take part. The operating surgeon may have another surgeon to assist him; there will almost certainly be present an anesthetist; a theatre sister and other nurses, each with important duties to perform in the course of the operation. If some mishap occurs during the operation it may well be of great importance to ascertain which of the various persons present responsible for the mishap, and to what extent, if at all, any other member of the operating team can be held legally liable for the action of that person.

The Swab case: In no case is it altogether easy to define the limits of the surgeon's personal responsibility in the operating theatre or to determine with exactitude the extent to which he is permitted to rely on the due performance by his assistants of the independent duties committed to them. The task is particularly difficult, however, in the not uncommon class of case where the complaint is that a swab has been left inside the patient at the end of an operation.

It has long been recognized by the medical profession that danger of swabs being overlooked at the end of an abdominal operation is a very real and grave one; and in the consequence extraordinary precautions are commonly taken in an attempt to reduce this risk as far as possible. The precautions naturally differ in detail from hospital to hospital and from country to country. A common device, however, is to have a long tape attached to one corner of every packing swab used in an abdominal operation, to which it is the duty of one of the nursing staff to fix a pair of forceps before the swab is handed to the surgeon for the purpose of operation. The forceps attached in this manner to the tape are then left outside the wound by the surgeon and act as a flag or signal indicating the presence of a swab inside the wound.

Even the precaution of tapes and forceps, however, has been found to be fallible. It is not impossible, for example, that in the stress of the operation a swab may inadvertently be handed to and received by the surgeon without its forceps having been attached; nor can the possibility that during the operation a pair of forceps may without being noticed become detached from its swab be entirely excluded. Hence, it has become an almost universal practice to assign to one or more of the nursing staff present at the operation the duty of counting of swabs inserted by the surgeon and checking that the correct number are removed. This duty is commonly assigned to the nursing staff and not undertaken by the surgeon because it is generally recognized that the surgeon, beset as he is by the other cares of the operation, cannot reasonably be expected to assume the additional burden of keeping a mental tally of the swabs he uses. Indeed, it is reasonably clear from the cases that for the surgeon to entrust this task to the nursing staff will be regarded as proper and reasonable course to adopt; and that the surgeon could not be found negligent on the ground that he himself did not count the swabs. It is true that this is really a question of fact to be decided upon the circumstances of each particular case, after consideration of any expert evidence which has been tendered as to the accepted practice in the matter, and further that the court is not bound to accept the views of medical experts as to the reasonableness or otherwise of the practice. Nevertheless, it is thought that the practice of entrusting the duty of counting swabs to the nursing staff is so widely adopted and so universally approved that it can be stated with confidence that for a surgeon to follow the practice will not amount to negligence.

It has been seen that a nurse entrusted with the duty of counting the swabs is regarded, not as a servant of the surgeon, but as an independent collaborator performing a wholly independent; and for that reason, the surgeon cannot be held responsible for negligent counting by the nurse. The problem is therefore to define the extent of the surgeon's responsibility with regard to the removal of swabs and to discover how far his responsibility is affected by the fact that an independent count is being made.

That there is a personal duty upon the surgeon cannot be doubted. For just as it is his task to put the swabs in, so it is his task to take them out; so much is made abundantly clear that surgeon's duty with regard to the removal of swabs is not an absolute one. His only duty is to take reasonable precautions to ensure that none are left behind; and when a swab is found to have been left inside the patient the proper question for consideration by the judge or jury, if there is one, is whether the surgeon has taken such precautions by way of search or otherwise as were reasonable and necessary in the circumstances. The courts however, have uniformly refused to lay down any rigid rules in the matter. The point was put thus by Innes, C.J., in the leading South African case of *V an Wyk* vs. *Lewis* as: "*Medical practitioners are required in their professional work to exercise reasonable skill and care. In regard to the removal of swabs at the conclusion of an operation, therefore, they are bound to make such search and take such precautions as are reasonable under the circumstances. In view of the consequences involved the search must be careful and the operation and the precaution strict; anything less would not be reasonable. But it is undesirable to endeavour to define the steps which should be taken or the care which should be observed, even if it were possible for a court of law to do so. These would vary with circumstances, for diligence, like negligence, can never be disentangled from the facts.*" (Nathan:1957)

What is negligence ? In legal context "negligence means more than heedless or careless conduct: whether in omission or commission: it properly connotes the complex of duty, breach and damage, thereby suffered from the person to whom the duty was owing.

In the general law of negligence the standard is that of "reasonable man". In this context, the meaning goes like this, "negligence is the omission to do something which a reasonable man, guided upon those considerations which ordinarily regulate the conduct of human affairs, would do; or doing something which a prudent or reasonable man would not do."

In many cases no doubt there will exist some specific negligence on the part of a servant or servants for which the institution will be vicariously responsible. An organization cannot discharge its obligations otherwise by means of its servants or personnel; but it cannot escape liability for the breach of an obligation because a servant or agent has been employed to discharge the obligation.

It has long been recognized that the unqualified person who practices medicine is as much liable to an action for negligence as the qualified person. The quack cannot escape liability by protesting that he did not have the qualifications necessary to entitle him to practice; nor can the chemist who exceeds his proper spheres and prescribes for his customer evade liability if he fails to use due care. And even a lay man who neither has nor professes to have any special skill or knowledge may find himself under a liability if he assumes the responsibility of the medical care of another.

A medical man who holds himself out as being a specialist in a particular field, whether it is in the treatment of certain conditions or in the use of certain apparatus or in any other way, will necessarily be judged by higher standards than the ordinary practitioner who does not possess any such specialized skill. Here again, the specialist will be required to attain not to the highest degree of skill and competence but to the ordinary level of obtaining amongst those who specialize in the same subject.

The medical man must therefore exercise reasonable skill and care, measured by the standard of what is reasonably to be expected from the ordinarily competent practitioner of his class. If he does so he will have discharged his duty and cannot be held answerable even if the treatment has untoward results. For the medical man is not an insurer; he does not warrant that his treatment will succeed or that he will perform a cure.

Thus, in order to decide whether negligence is established in any particular case the act of omission or course of conduct complained of must be judged, not by ideal standards nor in the abstract, but against in the background of the circumstances in which the treatment in question was given. This is not to say that the standard of skill and care required varies with the circumstances of each case; the standard is always the same, the conduct of the ordinarily competent and careful practitioner, but the degree of care required varies with the circumstances of the case. It is the degree of care which varies not the standard.

(www.medicalnews today.com/articles/255576.php)

Negligence is also considered as failure to exercise the care that a reasonably prudent person would exercise in like circumstances.

According to Jay M. Feinman of Rutgers University of School Law, the core idea of negligence is that people should exercise reasonable care when they act by taking account of the potential harm that they might foreseeably cause harm to others.

Legal Services Commission of South Australia defines negligence as "a failure to take reasonable care to avoid causing injury or loss to another person. There are four steps in proving negligence. The plaintiff must prove:

(i) That there is a duty in the circumstances to take care of *duty of care;*
(ii) That the behaviour or inaction of the defendant in the circumstances did not meet the standard of care which a reasonable person would meet in the circumstances (*breach of duty);*
(iii) That the plaintiff has suffered injury or loss which a reasonable person in the circumstances could have been expected to foresee (*damage*);
(iv) That the damage was caused by the breach of duty (*causation*).

The standard of care for a health is that expected of the reasonably competent practitioner of that profession. The actions of the health professional will be compared with the standard. The court, not the professional, sets the standard, so even if a particular practice is common or accepted by other practitioners, it may still be negligent. Negligence may occur in any aspect of professional practice, whether history taking, advice, examination, testing or failing to test, reporting and acting on results of tests, or treatment. The standard is one of reasonable care, not of perfection. The court will decide having regard to all the circumstances whether the health professional has been negligent. Negligence is different from mistake or *error of judgment*. The fact that a risk of treatment eventuated, or that a desired medical outcome was not achieved, does not necessarily establish negligence."

(http:/www.law/handbooksa,gov,au/ch29s051.phpS.)

V. Joga Rao in his article, 'Medical Negligence Liability under the Consumer Protection Act: A Review of Judicial Perspective' has referred the concept of negligence as, simply, 'the failure to exercise due care'. It contains three ingredients as below:

1. The defendant owes a duty of care to the plaintiff;

2. The defendant has breached this duty of care; and
3. The plaintiff has suffered an injury due to this breach.

The medical negligence is not different from the negligence in other services. It is only that in a medical negligence case, most often, the doctor is the defendant. Every doctor owes a duty to the patient who approaches him or her for treatment on two conditions mainly, the patient's treatment falls within the jurisdiction of the doctor's expertise; and the doctor concerned must agree to undertake the task of taking care of patient. As Rao mentioned, the duty may be contractual or a duty arising out of tort law. There may also be an occasion to undertake this task beyond this relationship. He highlighted the *Paramananda Kataria* vs. *Union of India* case, in which Supreme Court of India said, "every doctor, at the governmental hospital or elsewhere, has a professional obligation to extend his services with due expertise for protecting life. These cases are however, clearly restricted to situations where there is danger to life of the person. From this one can come to the conclusion that in other situations it is not applicable.

The Supreme Court also clarified the concept of 'duty owed' in the case of *Laxman* vs. *Trimback* as, 'it is to bring to his task a reasonable degree of skill and knowledge and to exercise a reasonable degree of care and competence in the light of the circumstance. A patient may be cured or may not be cured, but the doctor has to ensure that reasonable care has been offered to the patient. Reasonable degree of care means that a doctor exercises his skill and competence which he has in taking care of the patient in the circumstances. A distinction is also made between the standard of care and the degree of care. The standard of care is consistent in all cases. The conduct of doctor must be reasonable and the consideration of highest degree of care and lowest degree of care does not come to the picture in this situation. However, the degree of care may vary depending upon the nature of situation. Again one has to determine the reasonableness of care to the patients.

Reference was also made of the knowledge expected from a doctor to take care of patient. A doctor has to be equipped with reasonable knowledge. The knowledge acquired at the time of entry into service is not enough to justify the reasonableness of knowledge. There is the need of updating the knowledge of a doctor to meet the standard of care expected from him or her.

The most significant point raised by Rao is that the liability of doctor arises not when the patient has suffered any injury, but when the injury has resulted due to conduct of doctor, which has fallen below that of reasonableness.

(*http/www.ncbi*.nim,nih.govt/pmc/articles/PMC2779962/7/7/2014)

Negligence is a failure to exercise the care that a reasonably prudent person would exercise in like circumstances. The area of tort law known as negligence involves harm caused by carelessness, not intentional harm. According to Jay M. Feinman of the Rutgers University School of Law, "The core idea of negligence is that people should exercise reasonable care when they act by taking account of the potential harm that they might foresee ably cause harm to other people."

Through civil litigation, if an injured person proves that another person acted negligently to cause their injury, they can recover damages to compensate for their harm. Proving a case for negligence can potentially entitle the injured plaintiff to compensation for harm to their body, property, mental well-being, financial status, or intimate relationships. However, because of negligence cases are very fact-specific, this general definition does not fully explain the concept of when the law will require one person to compensate another for losses caused by accidental injury. Further, the law of negligence at common law is only one aspect of the law of liability. Although resulting damages must be proven in order to recover compensation in a negligence action, the nature and extent of those damages are not the primary focus of negligence cases.

In England a more recent case of *Caparo* vs. *Dickman* (1990) introduced a 'threefold test' for a duty of care. Harm must be: (1) reasonably foreseeable; (2) there must be a relationship of proximity between the plaintiff and defendant; and (3) it must be 'fair, just and reasonable' to impose liability. However, these act as guidelines for the courts in establishing a duty of care; much of the principle is still at the discretion of judges.

Breach of duty is not limited to professionals or persons under written or oral contract; all members of society have a duty to exercise reasonable care toward others and their property. A person who engages in activities that pose an unreasonable risk toward others and their property that actually results in harm, breaches their duty of reasonable care. An example is shown in the facts of *Bolton* vs. *Stone*, a 1951 legal case decided by the House of Lords which established that a defendant is not negligent if the damage to the plaintiff was not reasonably foreseeable consequence of his conduct. In the case, a Miss Stone was struck on the head by a cricket ball while standing outside the house. Cricket balls were not normally hit a far enough distance to pose a danger to people standing as far away as was Miss Stone. Although she was injured, the court held that she did not have legitimate claim because the danger was not sufficiently foreseeable. As stated in the opinion, 'Reasonable risk' cannot be judged with the benefit of hindsight. (*en.wikipedia.org/wiki/ Negligence*).

Jurisprudence rejects any precise definition of negligence. While defining negligence it may be treated as tort. Under this, "Negligence is the breach of a duty caused by the omission to do something which a reasonable man, guided by those considerations which ordinarily regulate the conduct of human affairs would do, or doing something which a prudent and reasonable man would not do. Actionable negligence consists in the neglect of the use of ordinary care or skill towards a person to whom the defendant owes the duty of observing ordinary care or skill by which neglect the plaintiff has suffered injury to his person or property. This definition involves three constituents of negligence: (1) A legal duty to exercise due care on the part of the party complained of towards the party complaining the former's conduct within the scope of the duty; (2) Breach of the said duty; and (3) Consequential damage. Here the cause of action for negligence arises only when damage occurs. Damage is necessary as it is an ingredient of this tort". (Kumar: 2008)

Charlesworth and Percy identified three meanings of negligence: (i) a state of mind, in which it is opposed to intention; (ii) Careless conduct; (iii) the breach of duty to take care as imposed by either common or statute law. All three meanings are applicable in different circumstances. But all the three are related to have full meaning of negligence. The essential components of negligence, as recognized, are three—duty, breach and resulting damage:

- *Duty*: existence of a duty to take care, which is owed by the defendant to the complainant;
- *Breach*: failure to attain that standard of care, prescribed by the law, thereby committing a breach of such duty; and
- *Damage*: it is both casually connected with such breach and recognized by the law, has been suffered by the complainant.

If the claimant satisfies the court on the evidence that these ingredients are made out, the defendant should be held liable in negligence.

Negligence may be viewed as a crime. The term negligence is used for the purpose of fastening the defendant with liability not only under civil law, but also under criminal law. Jurisprudentially no distinction can be made between negligence under civil law and negligence under criminal law. The submission so made cannot be countenanced in as much as it is based upon a total departure from the established terrain of thought running ever since the beginning of the emergence of the concept of negligence up to the modern times. Generally, it is the amount of damages incurred which is determinative of the extent of liability in tort; but in criminal law it is not the amount of damages, but the amount and degree of negligence that is determinative of liability. To fasten liability in criminal law, the degree of negligence has to be higher than that of negligence enough to fasten liability under civil law. Referring to the opinion of Lord Diplock in a bench of five it has been highlighted by Kumar in the book as regards the concept of Recklessness as, "Recklessness on the part of the doer of an act does presupposes that there is something in the circumstances that would have drawn the attention of an ordinary prudent individual to the possibility that his act was capable of causing the kind of serious harmful consequences that the section which creates the offence was intended to prevent, and that the risk of those harmful consequences occurring was not so slight that an ordinary prudent individual would feel justified in treating them as negligible. It is only when this is so the doer of the act is acting 'recklessly' if, before doing the act, he either fails to give any thought to the possibility of there being any such risk or, having recognized that there was such risk, he nevertheless goes on to do it."

The moral culpability of recklessness is not located in a desire to cause harm. It resides in the proximity of the reckless state of mind present when there is an intention to cause harm. There is, in other words, a disregard for the possible consequences. The consequences entailed in the risk may not be wanted, and indeed, the actor may hope that they do not occur, but this hope nevertheless fails to inhibit the taking of the risk. Certain types of violation, called optimizing violations, may be motivated by thrill-seeking. These are clearly reckless.

In order to hold the existence of criminal rashness or criminal negligence it shall have to be found out that rashness was of such a degree as to amount to taking a hazard knowing that the hazard was of such a degree that injury was most likely imminent. The element of criminality is introduced by the accused having run the risk of doing such an act with recklessness and indifference to the consequences. Lord Atkin in his speech in *Andrews* vs. *Director of Public Prosecutions* (1937) AC576 stated, "Simple Lack of Care such as will constitute civil liability is not enough; for purpose of criminal law there are degrees of negligence; and very high degree of negligence is required to be proved before the felony is established."

Negligence by Professionals: In the law of negligence, such as lawyers, doctors, architects and others are included in the category of persons professing some special skill or skilled persons generally. Any task which is required to be performed with a special skill would generally be admitted or undertaken to be performed only if the person possesses the requisite skill for performing that task. Any reasonable man entering into a profession which requires a particular level of learning to be called a professional of that branch, impliedly assures the person dealing with him that the skill which he professes to possess shall be exercised and exercised with reasonable degree of care and caution. He does not assure his client of the result. A lawyer does not tell his client that the client shall win the case in all circumstances. A physician would not assure the patient of full recovery in every case. A surgeon cannot and does not guarantee that the result of surgery would invariably be beneficial, much less to the extent of 100 per cent for the person operated on. The only assurance which such a professional can give or can be understood to have given by implication is that he is possessed of the requisite skill in that branch of profession which he is practicing and while undertaking the performance of the task entrusted to him he would be exercising his skill with reasonable competence. This is all what the person approaching the professional can expect. Judged by this standard, a professional may be held liable for negligence on two findings: either he was not possessed of the requisite skill which he professed to have possess, or, he did not exercise with reasonable competence in the given case, the skill he did possess. The standard to be applied for judging, whether the person charged has been negligent or not, would be that of ordinary competent person exercising ordinary skill in that profession. It is not necessary for every professional to possess the highest level of expertise in that branch which he practices.

With no data on incidence of medical errors and no authority tracking cases of medical negligence, one might be forgiven for imagining that over 8-lakh registered doctors in India are perfect professional who never make any mistakes.

Recently, the parliamentary committee on health and family welfare expressed concern over the fact that there is negligible prosecution of medical negligence cases in India. But the committee's observation draws attention to an even more shocking fact—that there is no centralized collection of data on negligence cases filed in India or their outcome.

Since developed countries track such data meticulously, there are constant efforts to bring down the incidence and curb the consequences of medical errors.

In response to repeated questions in Parliament regarding data on medical negligence cases, health minister Ghulam Nabi Azad came up with a rather lame reason—health being the state subject no such information was maintained centrally and no data was available on deaths caused by medical errors in the country.

State Medical Councils and the Medical Council of India (MCI) are supposed to maintain registers of all complaints filed against doctors, their status and the outcome of such complaints. But till to-day the MCI has not bothered to put together regional data to build a central database for the nation. This means that the magnitude of the problem of medical negligence remains ignored in India.

The parliamentary committee's recently submitted 73rd report on the Indian Medical Council (Amendment) Bill, 2013 has drawn the attention to the increasing incidents of negligence on the part of doctors "All members of the MCI are medical professionals and whenever any complaint of negligence or violation of code of ethics is brought before the council, such cases are decided by the medical professionals themselves. There are reports that the medical professionals probing into the allegations of medical negligence are very lenient towards their colleagues guilty of negligence and none of them is willing to testify another doctor as negligent", stated the report adding that the impact of this arrangement was that the prosecution in medical negligence cases by the MCI is dismal.

In many state medical councils, the disciplinary committee bearing complaints against doctors does include members from the lay public as is the case in Delhi Medical Council (DMC). However, a closer look at the composition and working of the committee shows how easily this safeguard is subverted. The disciplinary committee comprises three doctors including the chairperson of DMC and one expert in the field of medicine related to the complainant and three-non-doctors—a lawyer nominated by the state assembly speaker, and one eminent person nominated by the Delhi government. In the case of DMC eminent person nominated by the government is Dr. Prem Aggarwal, yet another doctor. DMC secretary Dr. Girish Tyagi admits that the MLA, being very busy, hardly attend any disciplinary hearings. The quorum required for the hearings is just three. Hence, complaints against doctors end up being "State Medical Councils mostly comprise doctors and most are not even functioning properly. The ones that function do not reveal any data on the complaints or their outcome", says, Dr. Amar Jesani, editor, *Indian Journal of Medical Ethics*. In Maharashtra, the medical council was not properly functional for two decades. From 1990 till 2011, it remained mired in controversies regarding malpractices in the election of council members.

"We had tough time trying to get data from the different state medical councils. Even with RTI, they give vague information. There is no price to be paid when council members shield doctors in cases that come before them as the public will never know what happens", says Dr. Saha. (Nagarjan: 2013)

Causes of Negligence: While looking into the causes of negligence, it is noticed that there are common factors contributing to an act of negligence and error committed by an individual. Sometimes negligence may also be a cause of error. In addition, an individual may neglect his or her duty due to lack of command over the work and failure of the authority to provide effective motivating devices with the changing situation. Referring to motivation Alexander H. Leighton said, "The striking thing about this new science of human relations is not the vast areas of what is unknown—which many are fond of emphasizing—but the degree to which what is known is not used." (Leighton: 1949)

Reform Measures: The ethical approach to remedial measures is very well analyzed by Aristotle. To him this approach begins with the enquiry into the ultimate goal of every action of man. This goal can be identified with happiness. His writing, titled *Nichomachean Ethics* is after the name of his son Nichomachus, published in fourth century B.C. may be considered as stimulating introduction to moral philosophy, as stated by M.G. Gupta, in his book, *History of Political Thought*. "In every pursuit and art", he says, "the chief good is that for the sake of which all that we do is done; this in medicine is health, in war victory, in house building the house. Happiness according to Aristotle is the ultimate end of human effort and aspiration. (Include Non-medics in probing medical negligence cases, *The Times of India*, 10th December, 2013)

Neo-Human Relations theory is the advent of the behavioural scientists. The prominent among them are Likert, Argyris, Maslow, Mc.Gregor and Herzberg. Each one of them discussed different aspects of human behaviour in an organization. For example, Likert emphasized on management, Argyris on employees' well-being, Herzberg on job enrichment, Maslow on human needs and Mc. Gregor on employee motivation. Psychology, Social psychology, Sociology and partially

Political Science may be identified as behavioural sciences. Psychology deals with the study of mind and its relationship with behaviour, Social Psychology with behaviour of an individual as influenced by a group, Sociology with evolution, forms and functioning of group.

According to this theory, one of the characteristics of human being is the dislike for work. While accepting this, it is also difficult to disagree that man cannot live without work. However, there are some works which are generally avoided by human being, such as—very hard work; non-profitable work, especially in terms of money and reputation; the works tagged with risks of various kinds. How to motivate a man or woman to work? A group of personnel in any organization may be compared with a cricket team in which the ultimate goal of the team is to win the game. In order to achieve it provision is made to encourage or motivate each and every player through reward or recognition of individual performance in all the three departments—fielding, batting and balling. The efficient performance of each individual is directed towards the ultimate goal of the team. Similarly, every service provider to humanity must be motivated to render efficient service through recognition and reward without being biased. In every personnel system state of mind of an individual is expressed through loyalty, enthusiasm, cooperation, pride in the work, devotion to work. The inner factor in every service or work is morale along with expertness. Both must go together. O.G. Stahl referred in his book, "Public Personnel Administration" the concept of Morale as defined by an authority, 'Morale is the capacity of a group of people to pull together persistently and consistently in pursuit of a common purpose.' Further explanation of it highlights important aspects of the concept as below. It is dependent on:

1. Confidence that individual members of the group have in the common purpose;
2. Confidence they have in its leadership;
3. Mutual confidence amongst the members of the group;
4. Organizational efficiency of the group, both formally or over a cup of tea; and
5. The mental, emotional and physical health of the individuals. (Stahl: 1983)

Here two theories of human motivation may be discussed—Need Hierarchy theory as advocated by Abraham Maslow and X and Y theory as envisaged by Douglas McGregor.

Need Hierarchy Theory: Human behaviour is directed by the aims or aspirations (whether covert or overt) of an individual. Analysis of human behaviour through human needs is a new approach to the study of social psychology. The advocate of this need hierarchy theory is Abraham Maslow, an American Sociologist. Maslow identified five categories of human needs on the basis of hierarchy—physiological, security, belongingness, esteem and self-actualization needs.

Physiological Needs: The physiological needs include hunger, thirst, sex etc. These are very strong devices to direct human behaviour in an authoritative way and work as motivating factor unless these are satisfied by an individual. Once these are fulfilled they become defunct as motivating factor to make a man work. Because man is a wanting animal.

Security Needs: Security of life, financial security, social security etc. also work as motivating factors to an individual. In short, human security is also a strong motivating factor to liberate the will to work.

Belongingness Needs: Man is basically a social animal. Mutual dependence of individuals of a family or in a society is a common need. Childhood, old age and sickness man needs help, love or affection from parents and family members or neighbours. Discontinuation of affectionate or sympathetic relationship amongst families in a locality and members in a family creates feeling of loneliness and being neglected causing frustration to the individual. It may stand as a hindrance to have the will to work. It is the love, affection and human approach which work as very significant motivating factor to all categories of people.

Esteem Needs: Man is sensitive to his self-respect and self-esteem. He never forgets any humiliation by others in any situation, though all men do not have revengeful attitude towards the humiliator. Self-esteem needs have basically two dimensions—achievement and recognition needs. The achievement is closely connected to self-confidence, assertion and independence. Anybody who wants to achieve something must acquire these qualities. He or she has also to be physically and mentally strong enough to be the possessor of them. We, as human beings have strong desire to be respected and recognized by others for our achievement or success. It is a source of inspiration to undertake new task or to activate our sense of creativity. Non-satisfaction of these esteem needs may cause inferiority complex, mental weakness, frustration and helplessness. Maslow termed these four categories as "Deficit Needs."

Self-Actualization Needs: The term self-actualization was first coined by Kurt Goldstein, the German Neurologist and Psychiatrist. The will to self-fulfillment and living a meaningful life is found in this category of needs. (Prasad: 2011)

***Theory X and Theory Y*:** The chief advocate of these two theories was Douglas McGregor. He is remembered for his significant contribution to management. He made an attempt to remove misconceptions from the path of control of human behaviour. To him control is nothing but selective adaptation. It is need-based according to changing situation in the workplace due exposure to the outside world and the growth of the members in age, experience and their family related duties and responsibilities along with the growth of the Organization itself. Further the entry of young men also requires the management or the higher authority to watch their behaviour and attitude to provide them necessary guidelines. It is difficult to deny that every new entry brings with it new attitude, behaviour and belief which require to be filtered in the perspective of organizational goals and challenges faced by it during the development of the organization. Any attempt to control the personnel without dynamism in adjustment keeping the ultimate goals on firm footing may go against human nature, because of this management may fail to achieve its desired goals. With this assumption in mind McGregor advocated theory X and theory Y. The theory X is tradition based theory and is also known as "Carrot and Stick theory". Under theory "Coercive Compulsions" take place in the process of management it assumes:

1. The average human being has inherent dislike for work and avoids it whenever opportunity arises;
2. Most people must be corrected, directed, controlled and threatened to get things done by them to achieve the ultimate goals of an organization; and
3. Average human being waits for direction, avoids responsibility and is in search of security.

The theory Y: The theory Y moves in the opposite to the theory X. This theory may be termed as "Non-coercive compulsions theory". This theory assumes the human nature as—

1. Desire of man for work is as natural as play or rest;
2. Commitment of man to a particular goal makes him self-controlled and self-directed;
3. The average human being learns willingly to accept and carry out responsibility in a congenial environment;

4. The capacity to exercise high degree of creativity, imagination and ingenuity in solution of organizational problems widely spread over the whole population; and
5. In the industrial era intellectual potentialities of average human being are not fully used.

To McGregor theory Y is an appeal to innovation. However, he did not root out the need of managerial authority. He suggested limited use of managerial authority so that new ideas flourish from the all categories members of the organization. He realized the value of practical experience which works as very significant source innovative ideas. McGregor correlate the acceptance of responsibility with commitment to the objective of the organization. Learning by experience can provide deep rooted impression in the mind of a person than learning from book or instructions. Thus, he has underlined long standing tradition of human civilization which can never be erased by modern management technique. The integration and self-control are the two basic requirements of the human society which are applicable in all organizations that are in existence in the society—whether traditional or modern. These are the two common languages to be taken care of. P.D. Sharma, in his article, "Douglas McGregor" has rightly pointed out that it is quite relevant to line-staff relationship, which often results in waste of human resources, friction, costly protective mechanism, low commitment to organizational objectives. It not only strengthens the superior and subordinate relationship but also democratize the social relationship. (Sharma: 2011)

Coming to the healthcare services, it is interesting to note that as regards the question that only health professionals can inquire into cases of medical negligence, a parliamentary panel is of the opinion that the experts from various fields, including social activists and representatives of patients may also look into such complaints.

The committee headed by Brajesh Pathak in its report on the Indian Medical Council (Amendment) Bill 2013, which was tabled in the Lok Sabha also objected to the bill giving 'sweeping powers' to the centre to influence functioning of the Council and interference with day-to-day working.

It said medical professionals probing into allegations reportedly "very lenient" towards their colleagues guilty of medical negligence. "The immediate impact of this arrangement is that the percentage of prosecution in the medical cases by MCI is almost negligible", the committee said in its recommendation. It said in other countries non-doctors like patients and social workers are mandatorily made members of the medical council and they are known as "lay members" and on occasions they may even lead the council as was the case with UK's General Medical Council.

"The Committee therefore, recommends that all such cases of medical negligence should be inquired into by a committee of experts drawn from various fields and experience including social activists, patient's representatives etc....the committee said." (Include Non-medics in probing medical negligence cases, *The Times of India,* 10th December, 2013)

Remedial Measures: Several remedial measures have been forwarded by different doctors:

1. Apart from stricter laws to penalize offending surgeons and heavy compensation for patients, hospitals need to streamline operation procedures.
2. The MCI must blacklist quacks and derecognize such surgeons; patients need to be empowered with information on safety standards.
3. Apart from criminal action against rogue surgeons and hospitals, the MCI should cancel license of the doctors involved. Upgradation of checks is also needed.
4. Make it mandatory for hospitals to install hi-tech monitoring devices, like the bispectral index, that enable doctors to know the depth of consciousness in a patient during an operation.

(http/indiatoday.in/story/10+most+common+medical+mistakes/1/27376.html accessed on 22.5.2014)

Medical Errors: Media in India focuses various kinds of medical mistakes making people aware of the consequences of them. Such as, patient suffers from paralysis after surgery, occurrence of death during chemotherapy after being injected in the spine instead of vein, declaration of baby as dead found alive etc.

Of the 110 cases brought to Delhi High Medical Association between January 2007 and April 2008, negligence was proved in just 34 cases. The most common medical blunder in India are—scissors, gauze, towels, screws, forceps, metal clamps—the list of objects the surgeons leave behind inside the patients.

It is also alleged that inappropriate doses of Botox injection that cause expressionless faces; cheaper breast implants that rupture or leak; excessive skin stretching during facelifts, giving a too-tight look; large volume liposuctions done in ill-equipped clinics that lead to fluid overload in the body and serious heart-lung complications; aggressive removal of nose cartilage, giving a pinched appearance. Besides removing of wrong parts is also another kind of serious medical mistake.

Waking during surgery and feeling pain without being able to cry out is found in the hospitals of the country. Many surgeons mention that they have faced this in the OT. Several studies have found "anesthesia awareness" to be a 1-in-1000 occurrence, with an estimated of 20,000 to 40,000 patients waking up from general anesthesia each year and one-fourth reporting pain. Anesthesia typically consists of three medications: a paralytic to ensure the patient does not move; a hypnotic to induce unconsciousness and a narcotic to numb pain. "It is the combination of these drugs in their various doses that determines the depth of unconsciousness", says Dr. G.P. Dureja, anesthesiologist and head of the Delhi Pain Management Centre. Apart from faulty drug doses, breakdown or misuse of equipment, patient health status and lack of expensive monitoring technology can also cause anaesthesia to fail, he explains.

(http/indiatoday.in/story/10+most+common+medical+mistakes/1/27376.html accessed on 22.5.2014)

Valid knowledge is distinguished from doubt and erroneous knowledge, where the ideas do not lead to successful action. Illusions and hallucinations fail to realize their ends. We become conscious of error when the demands of our ideal past are not met by the present. We see a white object and take it to be silver, pick it up and find it to be a piece of shell. The new experience of the shell contradicts the expectations of silver. According to the *Nyaya*, all error is subjective. Vatsyayana says, "What is set aside by true knowledge is the wrong apprehension, not the object." Uddyotakara observes, "the object all the while remains what it actually is. In regard to the flickering rays of the sun, when there arises the cognition of water, there is no error in the object; it is not that the rays are not rays, nor that the flickering is not flickering: the error lies in the cognition: as it is the cognition that which instead of appearing as the cognition of a thing as something which it is not. The rays are the cause of illusion. All erroneous cognition has some basis in reality. Vatsyayana says, "No wrong apprehension is entirely baseless". Error is the apprehension of an object as other than what it is. (Radhakrishnan: 2013)

In the US, the full magnitude and impact of errors in healthcare was not appreciated until the 1990s, when several reports brought attention to this issue. In 1999, the Institute of Medicine (IOM) of the National Academy of Sciences released a report, "To Err is Human: Building a

Safer Health System." Marshall Allen in the article, titled, *How Many Die From Medical Mistakes In U.S. Hospitals* ? stated that in 1999, the Institute of Medicine published the famous "To Err is human" report, which mentioned that up to 98,000 people a year die because of mistakes in hospitals. Though the number was initially disputed, later on accepted by doctors and hospital officials.

In 2010, the Office of Inspector General for the Department of Health and Human Services said that bad hospital care contributed to the deaths of 180,00 patients in Medicare alone in a given year.

The new estimates were developed by John T. James, a toxicologist at NASA's space center in Houston who runs an advocacy organization called Patient Safety America. James has also written a book about the death of his 19-year old son after what James maintains was negligent hospital care.

James based his estimates on the findings of four recent studies that identified preventable harm suffered by patients—known as "adverse events" in the medical vernacular.

Dr. Lucian Leape, a Harvard pediatrician who is referred to the "father of patient safety", was on the committee that wrote the "To err is Human" report. He expressed confidence in the four studies and the estimate by James.

Dr. David Classen, one of the leading developers of the Global Trigger Tool, said the James study is a sound use of the tool and a great contribution.

Dr. Marty Makary, a surgeon at Johns Hopkins Hospital whose book *Unaccountable* calls for greater transparency in healthcare, said the James estimate shows that eliminating medical errors must become a national priority. He said it is also important to increase the awareness of the potential of unintended consequences when doctors perform procedure and tests. The risk of harm needs to be factored into conversations with patients.

(www.npr.org/blogs/health/2013/09/20/224507654/how-many-die-from-medical-mistakes-in-u-s-hospitals)

It may be called as deviation from the accepted norms and standard. A medical error is a preventable adverse effect of care, whether or not it is evident or harmful to the patient. This might include an inaccurate or incomplete diagnosis or treatment of a disease, injury, syndrome, behaviour, infection, or other ailment. Similarly, an error in any service or profession may be said as preventable one. Therefore, utmost care has to be taken to do things without committing mistakes. This is very essential in the case of medical service providers as they deal with the affairs which have direct impact on the survival and suffering of the patients.

However, it cannot be denied that man has his own weakness and makes mistakes. To Radhakrishnan "Error is not crime, it is only youth, immaturity."

Causes of Healthcare Errors: The simplest definition of healthcare error is a preventable adverse effect of care, whether or not it is evident or harmful to the patient. Errors take place for variety of reasons. Errors have been in part attributed to–

- *Human Factors*: variations in healthcare provider training and experience, fatigue, depression and burnout.
- *Diverse Patients, unfamiliar settings, time pressure*;
- *Failure to acknowledge the prevalence and seriousness of medical errors.*
- *Medical complexity* like complicated technologies, powerful drugs, intensive care, prolonged hospital stay.
- *System failures*: poor communication, unclear lines of authorities of physicians, nurses and other care providers etc.

Infrastructure Failure: According to WHO 50 per cent of medical equipment in developing countries is only partly useable due to lack of skilled operators or parts.

(en.wikipedia.org/wiki/patient-safety. Accessed in August 2013)

Knowledge deficiency in the field: It is a human factor. The Physician with knowledge deficiency is an immature physician. There is every possibility of committing errors by them while rendering service to the patients. Enough scope has to be provided for in-service learning or education to be equipped with updated knowledge in one's own field of work. Entry into the medical colleges of an aspirant for being medical scientist must be on the basis of merit in the perspective of the medical world. After entry into the medical colleges due education must be imparted not only on the medical syllabi but also for full development of human personality. In India provision for reservation of seats in the educational institution is adopted in the midst of controversy. While appreciating this policy in the interest of involvement of candidates belonging to backward classes in the services one should not neglect to see that utmost care is taken to see that the students of this category do not suffer from knowledge deficiency. Because this is a service to humanity and in the process very costly error may take place, even the taking away the life of a patient who is the victim of it. Allegations are also heard very frequently about various forms of corruption in the process of admission into the institutions of medical education. These have to be avoided in order to make physicians free from knowledge deficiency to reduce errors in the service.

Plato, perhaps, was the first person to talk of education, exclusively provided by the state. Anything of crucial importance should not be left to private initiative. Of the value of education, Plato says that without education, the individual will make no progress any more than a patient who thinks to cure himself by some medicine. Without education he can have no power of self-control. It touches the evil at its source. It alters the whole outlook on life. It is a mental medicine to mental malady. It keeps the soul in an environment in which it would develop itself fully. It initiates a citizen into the spiritual life of the state. It is the means by which the principle of justice is maintained. It enables a person to discharge his duties in the light of knowledge and not by the rule of thumb.

Education has also other positive values. It imparts intelligence which is better than ten thousand eyes. Plato is convinced that vice arises chiefly from ignorance and may be cured by education. The educator should, however, remember the fact that his aim is not to put into mind knowledge that is not there but to turn the eye of soul towards the light that is in the mind so that it can see for itself. His business is not to impose thoughts on the pupils' head but to make them to think for themselves. The aim of Platonic education is not to banish individualism, abolish amateur incompetence and establish the rule of efficient.

While talking about the Ideal State in Republic, Plato said that for the realization of Ideal State it must be ruled by a man of vision. To Plato society can never be rightly ordered until Philosophers are Kings or Kings are Philosophers. The rule by Philosopher does not mean the imposition of the will of the few. Rather it is a government that embodies the real will of the many. The Philosopher Kings are those who are able to articulate and express what all desire. There is nothing arbitrary and oppressive in such a rule. The qualifications of the Philosopher Kings are:

1. He must have a definite knowledge of the principles by which he is guided.
2. He must have boundless curiosity for new experience.
3. He must have passion for truthfulness.
4. He must have courage. (Rao: 1980)

The physicians who rule the patient must have clarity of thought and definite knowledge while taking a decision on the process of treatment and must have passion and curiosity to have the comprehensive knowledge about the disease of the patient.

Fatigue: Another cause of error is fatigue. Free Encyclopedia refers fatigue as a subjective feeling or tiredness which is distinct from general weakness and has a gradual onset. Unlike weakness, fatigue may be alleviated by rest. Fatigue may occur due to both physical and mental causes. Physical fatigue is the transient inability of a muscle to maintain optimal physical performance, and is made more severe by intense physical exercise. Mental fatigue is a transient decrease in maximal cognitive performance from cognitive activity. It can manifest as somnolence, lethargy, or directed attention fatigue.

Physical fatigue, or muscle fatigue, is the temporary physical inability of a muscle to perform optimally. The onset of muscle fatigue during physical activity is gradual, and depends upon an individual's level of physical fitness, and also upon other factors, such as sleep deprivation and overall health. It can be reversed by rest. Physical fatigue can be caused by a lack of energy in the muscle, by a decrease of the efficiency of the neuromuscular nervous system. Mental fatigue is also caused by similar factors.

Fatigue is a normal result of working, mental stress, over stimulation and underestimation, jet lag or active reaction, depression, and also boredom, disease and lack of sleep. In any big hospital with heavy rush of patients physicians are loaded with heavy work and deprived of rest. In this situation mistakes are made by them.

(http://en.wikipedia.org/wiki/Fatigue_%28medical %29 6.1.2015)

Diversity: India is well known for its diversity in language, culture and religion. The patients belong to different languages, regions, culture, religion etc. The diseases from which the patients suffer may be due to different factors—habit, environment, food, water, customs etc. Further, the effectiveness of communication between the patient and the physician depends upon the understanding of the language of the patient by the physician and *vice-versa*. In many cases, the patients hide information due to various reasons. These may also be considered as sources of medical errors.

Excessive Work Load: In any hospital entertaining large number of patients with limited number of medical service providers time constraint is a common hindrance to do things correctly. Sometimes, the physicians have no time to receive due information from the patients as he/she has to attend large number of patients waiting in the queue in OPD. Excessive workload causes errors to the physician.

(www.telegraph.co.UK./health news/9905742/overworked-doctors-pose-alarming-threat to-safety-html)

The British Medical Association said that Junior doctors were under "intolerable pressure". Despite the European Working Time Directive which brought an average 48 hour working week, many Junior doctors are working for longer hours as their working time is "averaged out" over the month, the survey found.

One Junior doctor from Scotland told the surveyors, "My average working week may have compiled but on occasions, especially at nights, I would have worked over 100 hours in one week which was not safe in the end."

A Chairman of the BMA's Junior Doctors Committee said, It is of great concern that Junior doctors are being forced to work excessive hours and are often under intolerance pressure in order to ensure patient safety. The Keogh Review highlighted that despite the lack of support and value placed on Junior doctors, they remain the best champions of their patients and this must not be lost to the growing sense of frustration they feel.

(www.telegraph.co.UK./health news/9905742/overworked-doctors-pose-alarming-threat to-safety-html).This kind of allegation is found in medical services in India also)

Ignorance of consequences of Error: Till recently the issue of medical error did not occupy a prominent place in the medical world of the country nor among the common people. The physicians could command parental control over the patients and patients too had deep faith on the physicians. Neither patients nor physicians paid much attention to the worst consequences of medical error. To-day situation changes in India like any other country of the world. The conflicts between the physician and the attendant of the patients appear in media very frequently drawing attention of the people to the medical errors and medical negligence. There are occasions when the compensation for medical errors is demanded even through the court from the physicians for doing serious harm to the patients resulting even death due to medical errors. Sometimes, correction is made by the concerned physicians after having known about the error through the patients, wherever possible to do so.

It is not that in earlier days medical errors were not committed. Errors were committed both in indigenous treatment and modern medical services. The patients were not aware of them. Further, the people were not aware of their rights also. They did not have any suspicious look to the capacity of the physicians. Today with the spread of education, increase of the number of ailing population and hospitals, health awareness campaign by governmental and non-governmental agencies and also exposure to the outside world due to progress of Information Technology, the common people are no longer illiterate about preliminaries of health services to be provided by the hospitals or dispensaries and their rights.

While realizing to err is human it is also noticed by the medical fraternity the urgent need of reducing the scope of committing medical errors in the interest of the safety of the patients. At the South Asian Conference and CME on Synergy in Healthcare (SASHCON-2008) at the All India Institute of Medical Sciences (AIIMS) on Planning and Designing of Speciality Healthcare Facilities, Safe Hospitals and Patient Safety threadbare discussion was made. In fact, AIIMS is India's first government hospital to have implemented a patient safety programme at its Cardio Thoracic and Vascular Surgery (CTVS) centre.

Several Studies reveal that due to medical errors the provision has to be made for additional stay of the patients in the hospitals at a very heavy cost in UK and USA in the west huge amount of money has been spent medical negligence to be one of the leading causes of death in USA and UK. Similarly, a report by the Institute of Medicine (IOM) of the National Academy of Sciences shows nearly 98,000 preventable deaths occur annually due to medical error and 7,000 preventable deaths related to medication errors alone. The Institute of Medicine is an American non-profit, non-governmental organization. It provides unbiased and authoritarian advice to decision-makers and public. It is a health arm of National Academy of Sciences, which was chartered under President of Abraham Lincoln in 1863 itself. Nearly 150 years later, the National Academy has expanded into what is collectively known as the National Academies consisting of the National Academy of Sciences, the National Academy of Engineering, the National Research Council and the Institute of Medicine.

In 1990s, the medical community realized the seriousness of the problem, following reports on medical error from various countries. But the irony is that there is no such system in place in India.

"There is an urgent need to ensure patient safety. There is a need to keep record for all wrong surgeries, over-medication, timely checking of patient's medical parameters etc. Unlike US and UK, which have a rough estimate of deaths due to medical negligence, we do not know where we stand," said Dr. Shakti Gupta, head of the department of hospital administration, AIIMS and the organizing chairman of SASHCON2008.

Earlier this year, St. Stephen's Hospital participated in the pilot project on patient safety under WHO, Dr. Sudhir Joseph, medical director, St. Stephen's hospital said, "We had studied 1,000 patients before and after surgery. A check-list was prepared for all patients who underwent a surgery and we monitored all the parameters both before and after surgery. We monitored the dose of medicine given to the patient, patient care post-surgery among other things. This helps in reducing the scope of error."

Inspired by the project, AIIMS implemented a similar programme at the CTVS unit. The findings of the project were presented at SASHCON-2008. It is estimated that one in 10 people receiving healthcare in developing countries suffers preventable harm. "In developing countries, the incidence of medical negligence is much higher. There is a dire need to implement patient care", Gupta said.

(timesofindia.indiatimes.com/city/delhi/AIIMS-first-to-implement-patient-safety-programme/articleshow/3678599.cms.)

Unhealthy Social Relationship: All organizations whether medical or non-medical in nature may be considered as social organizations. Because in ultimate analysis of every organization there remain human beings constituting the in-house society. They belong to different ranks, different specializations, different families, but within the organization they are the members of one family with common ultimate goals in front of each one of them. Social relationship amongst the colleagues, between seniors and juniors and other allied service providers within the organization may also contribute to medical errors, provided social relationship is not healthy.

In an organization there occur interaction, contact, exchange of ideas, interchange of opinions or in short social relationship. These relations may be friendly or hostile. These contacts are informal. The informal relationship may influence to a great extent the functioning of the organization. Friendly relationship creates homely atmosphere having social control of behaviour, habits and attitude of the members of the organization. It makes a member free from tension, anger, feeling of alienation, depression etc. But if the relationship is in the other way round then the whole organization may become defunct. This kind of social relationship is very harmful not only to the recipients of the services from such organization but to the organization itself. In medical services, the situation may be worst as it has direct impact on the life of the individual. Here mention may also be made of the Hawthorne experiment carried out by Elton Mayo in the General Electric Company of the United States in the late 1920s and 1930s. The attention of the Hawthorne experiment was drawn by the human and social factors. The researchers found that human and social factors were very significant variables needed for effective functioning of an organization. In other words, the Hawthorne experiment provided enough scope to be convinced that every organization is a social system based on human relationships and group attitudes. They are the strong wheels of an organization. Therefore any kind of unhealthy social situation may cause affect effective functioning of an organization. Here lies the significance of ethical principles to be followed for developing regards for human life and dignity. (Maheswari:1994) Human relations are very fragile and in most cases controlled by hidden interest. James C. Worthy rightly pointed out, "There is no easy way to improve employee relations. Basically, the problem is moral and ethical." (Worthy: 1959)

Failure of the System

- Medical complexity like complicated technologies, powerful drugs, intensive care, prolonged hospital stay.
- System failures: poor communication, unclear lines of authorities of physicians, nurses and other care providers; complications increase as patient to nurse staffing ratio increases; disconnected reporting system.orgs names that look alike or sound alike.
- The impression that action is being taken by other groups within the institution.
- Reliance on automatic system to prevent errors.
- Inadequate systems to share information about errors hamper analysis of contributory causes and improvement strategies.
- Environment and design factors.

Infrastructure Failure: According to WHO 50 per cent of medical equipment in developing countries is only partly useable due to lack of skilled operators or parts.

(en.wikipedia.org/wiki/patient-safety. Accessed in August 2013)

Lack of Communication skill: The bad conversation between the physician and the patient and physician and nurses may cause problems. In India generally a large section of patient population suffer from language constraint. Further a patient may not be mentally strong to afford to give concentration to understand the advice of the physician. Because the credibility of the conversation is closely bound up with understandability. Lack of understanding by a patient may lead to errors committed not only by the physicians but also by any service provider in the field. This conversation is quite different from gossip as it has specific aim and urgency in the nature.

(www.ncbi.nlm.ger/pmc/articles/pmc2078554)

Effective communication may be considered as the primary requirement for the safety and correct decision for the treatment of a patient. There are no doubt hindrances in the conversation between patient/ attendants and physicians, such as language, culture and lack of healthcare awareness etc., the clinicians have to collect data about the family history, nature of suffering including duration of it, any other health problems besides the problem for which the patient approaches the hospital etc. through conversation. The data which collected through conversation are transformed into information which are recorded in the file and are disseminated among the concerned persons. These different stages comprise management of information.

In the process of medical care information management occupies wide space considering treatment team as delivery agent and the patient and attendants as receivers of information. The process of treatment begins with the conversation and therefore due attention or care has to be given to it so that accuracy and comprehensiveness of patient-specific data can be maintained. It is the determinant for involving patient in the treatment planning, eliciting informed consent, providing explanations, instructions and education to the patient and the attendant. Here lies the communication skill. Every word must be simple, communication and familiar as far as possible to the patient and attendant, so that they need not make extra effort to understand the instruction, counseling, explanation provided by the treatment team. Then only the conversation between both the parties will be effective, absence of which may give birth to medical errors exposing the patient to the risk of life.

(www.ncbi.nlm.ger/pmc/articles/pmc2078554)

Lack of Patience to listen: Generally, it is noticed that the political leaders in India are not good listeners to the people whom they represent or whom they are to rule. Similar behaviour is also noticed in the case of most physicians in the country. The reasons may be different in each case. So far as political leaders are concerned they may be constrained by heavy responsibility to take decisions in different fronts for fulfilling the wishes and aspirations of people, challenges faced for redressing the grievances of the people, failure to get things done by the administration as they desire, involvement of unethical or corrupt practices, heavy rush of the visitors etc. Similarly, in the case of physicians there is always constraint of rush of patients, especially in the Out Patient Department (OPD), tension caused by conflicts of interest, unwelcome behaviour of the superior authority, problems of handling excited/depressed attendants, constraint of time etc. may not permit the physicians to be good listeners.

(en.wikipedia.org/wiki/patient Safety 2007)

Adverse events: When adverse events occur, physican has a responsibility to be open and honest in the process of communication with the patient, to review what has occurred and to report appropriately. When something goes wrong, good medical practice involves:

1. Recognizing what has happened.
2. Acting immediately to rectify the problem, if possible, including seeking any necessary help and advice.
3. Explaining to the patient as promptly and fully as possible what has happened and anticipated short-term and long-term consequences.
4. Acknowledging any patient distress and providing appropriate support.
5. Complying with any relevant policies, procedures and reporting requirements, subject to advice from your medical indemnity insurer.
6. Reviewing adverse events and implementing changes to reduce the risk of recurrence.
7. Reporting adverse events to the relevant authority, as necessary.
8. Ensuring patients have access to information about the processes for complaint making.

(www.healthandkarma.com/2011/03/3-reasons-why-government-hospitals-in-html)

Alcoholism and Drug Addiction: Alcoholism and Drug Addiction is a serious ailment penetrated to a great extent to the youth generation of the country. It is not surfacing so far to draw the attention of the people in India as major factor for committing errors in the medical services. However, due care has to be taken to see that it cannot enter into the list of factors to make mistakes by the medical service providers.

Transparency and Medical Errors: Disclosure of error is a part of responsibility and accountability of a person or group of persons who commit the error. The universal truth is that to err is human. It is also said that forgiveness is a divine act. However, it is also noticed that various attempts have been made to minimize errors, such as training, healthy work environment, supervision, regulation of working condition etc. All these measures are adopted from outside or these are external measures to prevent errors. Disclosure of errors is a recently adopted device to minimize errors. In medical sciences it is a recent attempt toward this end.

Disclosure of errors appears to be simple but in practice it is a very complex task. It may invite multifaceted problems to the service providers and the people as a whole. In medical service it is extremely sensitive and complex issue. To disclose the error affecting a patient requires first of all moral strength of the physician. This cannot be injected in him from outside. The physician may face multiple challenges, such as, the risk of losing job, other punishments, facing the court case instituted by the patient, immediate unpleasant situation created by the patient's attendants and others. In India such kind of violent situations are coming to light in recent times.

The repairable damages caused by medical errors can help the physicians or service providers to get back reputation or confidence of the patients. But in the case of unrepairable damages caused by error is a serious matter to handle.

There are occasions demanding disclosure of medical records. Legal cases, Police enquiry regarding criminal cases, health safety measures, medical errors, medical negligence etc. require transparency in the medical services. The Government of India passed the Right to Information Act under which disclosure of information is mandatory. There is also the need of disclosure of information to the higher authorities, Insurance for security.

However, there is no general guidance on the use of medical records. The disclosure of medical records generally is necessary in the interest of the patients as well as public interest. Here the delicate question is, *Can the disclosure of medical records to the patients help cure of their diseases* ? In some cases, when the knowledge of the problem may help the patient to regain mental strength to overcome the fear complex or darkness about the nature of the problem. But, there are also instances about cases of getting nervous or deterioration of mental condition of the patient after coming to know about the seriousness of the problem. Therefore, it is not an easy task for a doctor to decide whether the record is to be disclosed to the patient and if so to what extent it should be done? Further all patients may not be in a position to listen or may not understand the medical language. In India, may be in other countries also the general practice is to disclose the record to the relatives or the attendants of the patients. Once the recorded information are disclosed to the attendants or relatives, the medical authority loses control over the principle of secrecy to be maintained on the medical record. Similarly, the record on a patient which is kept under the custody of medical authority cannot be controlled by the patient. Once the patient is released from the hospital, the question of taking consent of the exit patient for disclosing the medical record to others does not arise. Or it has also become irrelevant to the patient after being recovery of his health. Sometimes, the patient himself or herself discloses to others with proud by narrating the difficult time of suffering from serious diseases and the process of treatment by a doctor. In the case of the death of a patient, the relatives do not bother about the maintenance of secrecy of the medical record.

The information about the patient does not remain either under the custody of the doctor nor under his own custody. Further once these computerized the computerizers, if they are not honest may disclose them to others. These information may require for undertaking medical research or improvement of medical treatment in future course of action which demand disclosure to researchers and other doctors. This dilemma is arising due to the fact that a doctor, as a professional is bound by the obligation of professional secrecy and on the other hand as a citizen he must take care of the public or nation's interest. He has the responsibility to contribute to the health security of the citizens. (Philips:1985)

(Melanie Phillips and John Dawson; book: *Doctors' Dilemmas: Medical Ethics and Contemporary Science*, published by Harvester Press, 1985)

Confession of Medical Errors: One of the effective ways to reduce medical errors is the confession of it at least to the higher authorities in the organization. It helps exploration of the roots of errors and therefore precautionary measures become easy to be identified. Trust in Medical service providers by the patients can also be ensured through it. Generally, non-confession of errors is grounded on two basic reasons—fear of being punished and loss of public confidence. To avoid punishment and gain public confidence, the confession of errors is essential. Error is not a crime, it is immaturity as Radhakrishnan has said. So, it is not punishable and but corrective through learning process. However, one cannot deny that repetition of similar error is the indication of habit and refusal to learn. Therefore, it deserves punishment.

Punishment and corrective measures may be considered as immediate solution to the problems caused by errors in the case of those who are already in the service. However, it must be admitted that education may also help to a great extent to make a service provider careful to do the work without committing mistakes. V.R. Krishna Iyer has rightly said "education begins with heart, with human sympathy without which dignity, equality and fraternity—those vital values which make the life and liberty worthwhile—make no sense....Intellect is amoral.... The point is that excellence is not intellectual elitism or attainment but skill in action guided by humanism.... Pursuit of excellence means possession of character.... Pursuit of excellence means possession of character. If character makes a man, and it does—we need its basic components. They are courage, honesty, compassion, perspective of perfection. Courage is the seat of all virtues and cowardice is the graveyard of all good traits. That is why Vivekananda exalted *abhaya*, as the great need of man. Gandhi was like granite. Though frail in figure, he was strong in determination. So was Socrates, Christ, Prahlad, Meera—why Bertrand Russell himself. Fear of physical infliction or pain or prison never deters the man of character. (Iyer: 1988)

References

Dubhasi, P.R. (1983): Accountability and Ethics, *Indian Journal of Public Administration*, Vol. XXIX, No. 3, July-Sept.

Dwivedi, O.P. (1983): Ethics and Administrative Accountability; *Indian Journal of Public Administration*, Vol. XXIX, No. 3, July-Sept.

Dwivedi, O.P. (1987-88): (Presidential Address of O.P. Dwivedi on "Moral Dimensions of Statecraft: A Plea for an Administrative Theology" delivered in June 1987 to the Canadian Political Science Association, Hamilton, which is being recorded from *Canadian Journal of Political Science*, Vol. XX, No. 4. December 1987 published in the *Indian Journal of Public Administration*; October-December 1988; Vol. XXXIV, No. 4).

Iyengar, N.K.N. (1979): Personal Privacy in the United States: (review Article) *Indian Journal of Public Administration*, October-December, Vol. XXV, No. 4.

Iyer V.R. Krishna (1988). *Justice and Beyond*: Deep & Deep Publications, New Delhi.

Jain, R.B. (1979): The Right to Privacy and Freedom of Information: The Search for a Balance, *Indian Journal of Public Administration*, October-December 1979 Vol. XXV, No. 4.

Kumar, Dr. Vipul (2008): Legal Solutions for Medical Profession: published St. Matthew's Scientific Research Foundation; 2010; (Here reference is made of the Law of Torts, Ratanlal & Dhirajlal (twenty fourth Edition 2002, edited by Justice G.P. Singh).

Lambert Commission: In March 1979, Royal Commission on Financial Management and Accountability (also known as Lambert Commission) submitted its final report to Government of Canada. Published in IJPA, Special number on *Administrative Accountability*, July-September, 1983, Vol. XXIX, No. 3.

Leighton, Alexander H. (1956): Preventive Psychiatry in Industry; Management News, January 28, 1949, as referred in the book titled, "*Public Personnel Administration*" by O.G. Stahl; fifth edition of earlier work of William E. Mosher, J. Donald Kingsley and O. Glenn Stahl, published by Oxford & IBH Publishing Co., New Delhi.

Maheswari, S.R. (1994): *Theories and Concepts of Public Administration*, Allied Publishers Ltd., New Delhi.

Maheswari, S.R. (1983): Article: Accountability in Public Administration: A Conceptual Analysis: published in the *IJPA*; July-Sept., 1983, Vol. XXIX, No. 3.

Mallay, N.N: Public Enterprises in India (1971): *The Control and Accountability*; Delhi; National.

Melanie Phillips and John Dawson (1985): *Doctors' Dilemmas: Medical Ethics and Contemporary Science*; Haevester Press.

Minocha, O.P. (1983): 'Accountability in Public Sector Enterprises', *IJPA*; July-Sept., Vol. XXIX, No. 3.

Mukhopadhyay, Ashok (1983): *Administrative Accountability: A Conceptual Analysis*; *IJPA*; July-Sept., Vol. XXIX, No. 3.

Nagarjan, Rema: *The Times of India*, 15th December, 2013: Clean Slate for Doctors on Medical Negligence?

Nathan, Lord (1957): in Collaboration of Anthony R. Barrowclough: *Medical Negligence*, Butterworth & Co. Ltd.

Palkhivala, Nani (1997): *We, The People*, UBS Publishers' Distributor Ltd., New Delhi.

Phillips, Melanie and John Dawson, Doctors (1985). *Dilemmas: Medical Ethics and Contemporary Science,* Harvester Press.

Prasad, D. Ravindra: Abraham Maslow (2011): *Administrative Thinkers*, edited by D. Ravindra Prasad, V.S. Prasad, P. Satyanarayana and Y. Pardhasaradhi, Sterling Publisher, New Delhi.

Radhakrishnan, S. (1992): *The Present Crisis of Faith*, Orient Paperbacks, New Delhi.

Radhakrishnan, S. (2013): *Indian Philosophy*, Vol. 2; Oxford University Press, Ninth Impression.

Raj, Dr. Hans (2001): *Principles of Public Administration*, Surjeet Publication, Delhi.

Rao V.V. (1980): *A History of Political Thought*, S. Chand & Co. Ltd., New Delhi.

Sharma, S.R. (1965): *The Soul of Indian History*: Bhratiya Vidya Bhawan.

Sharma, P.D., Doughlas McGregor (2011): *Administrative Thinkers*, edited by D. Ravindra Prasad, V.S. Prasad, P. Satyanarayana and Y. Paradhasaradhi, Sterling Publishers, New Delhi.

Stahl, O.G. (1983): Administrative Accountability, *Indian Journal of Public Administration*, Vol. XXIX, No. 3, July-Sept..

Sethi, J.D. (1983), Bureaucracy and Accountability, *Indian Journal of Public Administration*, Vol. XXIX, No. 3, July-Sept.

Sharma, P.D. (1979): Secrecy needs in Public Administration, *Indian Journal of Public Administration*, October-December, 1979, Vol. XXV, No. 4.

Singh, M. Ibohal (2001): *Human Rights in India*, Vibhav Law Publications.

Seven
Accountability

Accountability is an essential part of every act of a man, especially when he or she does it in public capacity or as service provider to the people. A public servant is a trustee of public fund, a major part of which is constituted by the taxes paid by the citizens. The citizens may also be called as taxpayers. Every act of a public servant has not only financial implication but also moral implication. A public servant exercises the authority entrusted to the position of which he or she is an incumbent. However, the incumbent must exercise the authority in the interest of the taxpayers. Even the salary may be said as compensation, as it is paid for the services rendered by a public servant to the people. Therefore, the public servants must be accountable or answerable for their activities to the public. In a modern democracy various devices are adopted to ensure accountability of the public servants. But the sense of accountability must be rooted in the heart of a person to make the external devices effective. Significantly, it is cultivated at the family and is gradually strengthened in the environment created by educational institutions and later in the service career of an individual.

A physician is also a public servant and therefore accountability is an inalienable part of his or her activities. Here it may be mentioned that it is very difficult to distinguish a public physician from a private physician as regards their responsibility. But there are differences between the two on administrative aspect. A physician in a government sector is paid from the public fund and has to carry out his or her duties within the framework of the laws of the country. On the other hand, physician in the private or corporate sector is paid from the fund constituted within the organization, a major part of which is contributed mainly by the patients only. This system may be called as self-financed system on the ground that only those who pay are the recipients of the service. Nobody is compelled to pay for the services by which an individual is not benefitted. Further there is no financial control of the private medical care system from outside. Here heavy amount of money is to be paid by the patient in lieu of the services received from the physicians in particular and organization in general. These organizations cannot be free from commercial flavour. In the public medical care system financial control is made from outside. The people as tax-payers may pay taxes towards public fund and it the government which has to distribute to different services. The public servants are the trustees of public fund and therefore they have to be very careful while formulating any policy and implementing a policy so that there is no misuse or waste of public money. They must be ready to give account of their activities to the public on the floor of the legislature. However, it is found that the physicians have to carry out similar responsibility to cure the disease of a patient with their counterparts in the public sector. There may be differences in the nature of facilities and official formalities and the financial background of the patients in both the hospitals, the accountability aspect of the physician cannot be divorced from the act of any service provider in the private sector also.

Let me quote what the Lambert Commission, Canada stated in its report of 1979:

"The Government of Canada has announced new initiatives related to the management of resources and has taken some potentially significant steps designed to reduce expenditures. There are also widely publicized reports from the auditor general, the public accounts committee of the House of Commons, and the standing committee on national finance.

From these initiatives and report, it has become apparent that the management of the Government requires great attention from parliament, minister and public servants than it has been given in the recent past. Programmes and activities must not be approved without more carefully defined goals and objectives, and a realistic forecast of costs. Parliament should pursue more vigorously its role of holding the government to account. The cabinet and individual ministers should provide more leadership and direction to officials to ensure that they administer their operation with economy, efficiency and effectiveness and should be more directly involved in holding them to account for carrying out their assigned tasks.

In addition, the unsustainable rate of growth of government and its complexity and size make it increasingly obvious that there needs to be greater care in the use of the resources that have been entrusted to government. Not only is waste to be avoided, but in the context of today's fiscal situation and the pervasiveness of government activity, managers in the public services are being challenges to rediscover a sense of frugality and commitment to the careful husbanding of resources.

In framing out recommendations, we have been mindful of how governments and bureaucracies react to proposals for change. New requirements must not be massive as to overwhelm or immobilize the public services; nor must they deter the public service from its fundamental role of serving people. We recognize that the circumstances in which we are working are not like that those led Dean Acheson, the former U.S. secretary of state, to write that "carrying out administrative reforms in the state department is like operating for an appendectomy on a man carrying a piano upstairs". What we recommend, therefore, must not add new complications. We have been conscious throughout our work of the danger that processes and structures at the level of parliament, the government, and the departments and agencies can become overloaded and thereby frustrate the best intentions for involvement. Similarly, proposals to strengthen management should not foster a new growth industry in the bureaucracy.

As we stated in the progress report, that patient cannot be returned to good health by poultices alone. Any cure that will work must look to the fundamental diagnosis of the alignment, and take into account the economic cost of the cure and any adverse side effects of the treatment. There is a price for any reforms which must be judged, like any other cost, in term of foreseeable benefits. But it is surely not beyond our will and wit to prescribe for the disease without crippling the patient.

We have been struck by the great pressures facing those who now exercise leadership in the public services, and by the need to reinforce the self-image and public image of those being a good job. Great dedication and competence are often frustrated by the force of public demands and by weakness in the system of the government itself. There is, in many public servants, a high degree of commitment to sound management. This commitment must be nurtured if we are to halt the decline in the image, morals and effectiveness of the Canadian public services. Without the reinforcement of the values of integrity, competence, and dedication it is not likely that the esteem and confidence will be restored. Indeed, this is critical, because the regard in which the public servant is held by those he serves both the government and the people is in the final analysis, the standard by which he measures the value of his contribution to society. That the challenge is a great and continuing one was stated with force and eloquence almost a decade ago in the memories of the late Arnold Heeney, one of the great architects of the Canadian public service.

In a complex society which makes ever increasing demands on government, a large and complicated public service is inevitable. Great size and complexity carry with them terrible dangers, chiefly of course the dangers commonly associated with the word 'bureaucracy'. "Individual civil servants may lose or may never acquire the sense of vocation which is so important to the quality of human achievement. They may well feel themselves to be without purpose in a massive government machine. Should this happen, able men and women will not be persuaded to enter the public service. To prevent this happening should be the continual care, not only of government, but of all Canadians."

As human being and a citizen of a country naturally a physician is entitled to the rights guaranteed by its Constitution to the citizens. In addition, due to the nature of work he or she enjoys certain privileges. A privilege is a special entitlement to immunity granted by the state or another authority to a restricted group, either by birth or on a conditional basis. It can be revoked in certain circumstances. In a modern democratic state, a privilege is conditional and granted only after birth. By contrast, a right is an inherent, irrevocable entitlement held by all citizens or all human beings from the moment of birth. Etymologically, a privilege means private law or rule relating to a specific individual or institution. (*en.wikipedia.org/wiki/privilege_(legal ethics*)

In traditional society of India the physicians occupied a privileged position. High prestige was attached to this profession. People had deep faith on them. They enjoyed parental command over the patients. Naturally, the autonomy of the physicians was a significant privilege in the traditional Indian society.

In a modern democracy accountability is a strong device to secure people's active cooperation for the success of administration to serve the human society. People are familiar and more concern with the financial accountability only. We are yet to underline ethical accountability in the public service, though it constitutes a significant part of democratic administration. We are yet to give a serious thought to the issue that the main root cause of financial irregularities is ethical vacuity.

Now let us look into the origin of the concept of accountability. The word 'Accountable' was used in English language for the first time in 1583 in the financial context. Surprisingly enough, the financial context is still remaining as a dominating part of accountability in the administration. In the modern democracy, it occupies a very significant position due to increase of the volume of workload of the state, adoption of indirect method of democracy. The status of the citizens as taxpayers and recipient of the service make the service providers as trustees of public fund. The state cannot exploit the citizens nor its own servants.

The concept is a comprehensive one embracing almost each and every act of an organization, whether public or private. Shorter Oxford English Dictionary defines 'accountable' as 'liable' to be called to account, responsible to some authority for one's work. A correct perspective of accountability may be gained with a much sharper focus when a public functionary so socializes himself as to look at his official work strictly from the viewpoint of an ordinary citizen or, to be more apt, the '*daridranarayana*', i.e. poorest of the poor, as Mahatma Gandhi stated. All these have become very significant with the expansion and modernization of the activities of a modern democracy.

The Royal Commission on Financial Management and Accountability, 1979 defined accountability as, "Accountability, like electricity, is difficult to define, but possesses qualities that make its presence in a system immediately detectable. To touch a live wire in a circuit is enough to establish the presence of electricity without further need of definition. The shock of recognition that attends the presence of accountability in a system of government may not be quite as direct, but it is nonetheless detectable. We see accountability as the activation, but fragile, element permeating a complex network connection the government upward to parliament and downward and outward to a geographically dispersed bureaucracy grouped in a bewildering array of departments, corporations, boards, and commissions. Accountability moves through this network like the current in a circuit but always in some sort of relation to the control centre, the cabinet. The dispersal and structural complexity of the bureaucracy make the control centre vulnerable to stoppages and short-circuits or overloading. The control centre, the government, although ultimately responsible for answering to the legislature, may find itself out of touch with what is happening, or failing to happen, at the other end of the network. Similarly, a signal from the centre may never reach the departmental unit or agency concerned or may reach it in so confused a state that judgments as to performance become impossible to make.

In short, accountability relies on a system of connecting links—a two-way circuit involving a flow of information that is relevant and timely, not only for managers but for those who must scrutinize the decisions and deeds of managers. We gauge its presence when we observe that a certain 'discipline' has been imposed upon those who are assigned roles and duties in the system. In simple terms, "accountability is that quality of a system that oblige the participants 'to pay attention' to their respective assigned and accepted responsibilities, to understand that it does matter". (Lambert Commission: 1979)

Need of Accountability: Accountability is an inalienable aspect of any service rendered to a society, group of people or to any individual. What a man does, particularly in the official capacity must be prepared to be accountable for it. It helps maintaining efficiency, reducing errors, strengthening social relationship amongst the persons within an organization and also between an organization and public and enhancing the reputation of the organization. A reputed organization itself is a strong motivating factor to make its members work hard and to command confidence of the client.

The concepts like, 'development', 'public interest', 'welfare', 'democracy' are evolving and have comprehensive concepts. To translate the ideals behind these concepts one requires autonomy or discretionary power. The traditional administrative hierarchical system or Weberian model of bureaucratic authority may not work effectively as the administration becomes complicated day by day demanding expertness or specialization in each field.

Ethical accountability in the public services relates issue of specialization. Not only in the medical services, in almost every service emphasis is given on specialization. Today old method of learning by trial and error method has become irrelevant. Only a child learns through trial and error method. Various theories of learning, training provisions through counselling and other audio-visual means have been invented in the place of the traditional method of learning. In medical services, specialization is most welcome as it deals with the issue of life and death of a person demanding quick and expert decision for treating a patient. Unless a doctor has the expert knowledge in his field he may not be in a position to appreciate the urgency and the way render a service to the patient suffering an ailment of his area. It is a strong tool to safeguard or relieve the patient from ailment. But at the same time, the specialist must realize that his human approach to the patient or consideration of ethical principles will certainly make his expert decision more effective and people-friendly. O.G. Stahl stresses, "there must be care not to confuse one's professional viewpoint, functional preoccupation, or personal prejudices with the public interest."

The notable point here is that the identification of the jurisdiction of corruption is a complex affair. It is not confining to financial province only. It penetrates to lying, stealing, incompetence, violation of human rights and scarce of public resources also.

Naturally, the administrators at the higher level must be innovators, must have discretionary power. Development administration is different from regular administration which is to a great extent possible within the framework of rules and regulation. What is required under this circumstances is the honest and moral leadership to implement new policies and programmes. Because proneness towards corruption and abuse of power in different positions in the modern administration is very high. An intelligent man who is corrupt, selfish and cruel may adopt all devices (misinterpretation of public interest and laws, involvement in unnecessary debate, non-disclosure of the fact, avoidance of responsibility etc.) to hide his corrupt intention, selfish motive and cruel attitude or behaviour towards the client. These will result lack of confidence of the people on the administration, emergence of unethical activities and most dangerous result is the exploitation of citizens who are the taxpayers, because every act of a civil servant has financial involvement. Here is the need of ethical accountability on the part of the service providers in a modern state. One must act at the dictate of his conscience and it will make him accountable first to his own conscience. It is the main reason why education is insisted upon on the candidates to enter into public service. Lord Macaulay in 1850s itself, while asserting on the need of introduction of merit system for recruitment to the civil service pointed out that an educated man is a moral man or in other words education makes a man moral. However, the very concept of education has been degenerated and becomes very fragile to enhance inner power of the individuals.

Ashok Mukhopadhaya, in his article, titled, *Administrative Accountability: A Conceptual Analysis* published in the *IJPA* stated the expanding concept of accountability. In a democracy, accountability is essential not only to maintain efficiency but also in the interest of the taxpayers. Public officials have been found to be guilty of non-feasance, malfeasance and overfeasance. By non-feasance is meant that they have not done what law or custom requires them to do due to laziness, ignorance, or want of care for their charges, or corrupt influence; malfeasance means a duty is carried out with waste and damage because of ignorance, negligence and technical incompetence; and overfeasnace occurs when a duty is undertaken beyond what law and custom oblige or empower—it may occur out of dictatorial temper, vanity and ambition of an official or his genuine, sincere, public-spirited zeal. The public official must be held accountable for any of these three activities. (Mukhopadhayaya: 1983)

Accountability is not just in the negative sense of holding public servants responsible for their lapses. It has a positive connotation. They have the responsibility to discharge duties which are of great public significance. (Dubhasi: 1983)

Moral responsibility is the status of morally deserving praise, blame, reward or punishment for an act of a man. People who have moral responsibility for an action are called moral agents.

(En.wikipedia.org/Moral responsibility: accessed on 17.6.2014)

If we think of the need of ethical accountability in the medical services it is difficult to deny the need of it in these services. The medical service is the only service which can contribute directly to the human security. Besides, the doctors and nurses particularly, have to render serious services to mankind in an environment in which their eyes are always on the wounds of the patients, and always they have to alert and equipped mentally to serve the patients according to the requirement or demand of the ailments. Negligence, inefficiency, error on the part of the service providers may cause serious consequences. The patients or ailing people are vulnerable and depend mainly on their service for relief. They face emotional challenges at every moment from the attendants and close relatives of the patients. But they must take decision on their expertness with the sole aim of curing the disease of the patients, to take preventive measures to maintain the health of the people. Therefore, ethical accountability in the medical services is a significant one in the face of emergence of modern sophisticated equipment, high degree of awareness of human rights, increased ailing population in India, control, mobilization and distribution of public resources, adoption of rule of law, emergence of humanitarian laws.

Accountability *vs.* Autonomy

The importance that Aristotle attaches to the individual will always carry universal appeal. It is because of it Aristotle may be regarded as the father of modern individualism. His ideas on family and property as natural and necessary institutions for the development of individuality, received wide support. His statement that 'state comes into existence for the sake of life but continues to exist for good life' was a very significant declaration supporting the cause of the individual and indicating the duties of the state. Although he admitted that a man has personal value only as a member of the state, the state is not an end in itself. Because the fullest development of man's personality is not possible through a complete control of man by the state. The state has to allow individual to lead a complete life through exercise of freedom. (Ebenstein) The law of truth, according to Gandhi does not merely refer to truth of speech, it also refers to truth in action and truth in thought. Truth has reference to all spheres of life of a man. If he fails to practice this principle, he departs from the path of truth, denies the soul in himself. Truth rules out prejudices, evasion, secrecy and deception as well as exaggeration, suppression or modification of reality. Truth helps mutual toleration and avoidance of dogmatism and bitterness. Gandhi also advocated that while speaking the truth one should take care that it is not bitter. Truth must be accompanied by non-violence. However, non-violent truth does not mean hypocrisy, even every harsh truth can be communicated courteously and gently.

Like truth, non-violence is also omnipotent, infinite and synonymous with God. Non-violence means avoiding injury to anything on earth in thought, word and deed. *Ahimsa* is often mistaken for a negative doctrine. To Gandhi it is a positive and dynamic force. In its active and positive form non-violence means goodwill towards all life, love for every soul—even for the evil doer. It seeks to conquer violence by good. In short, *Ahimsa* means allowing others maximum of convenience even at the cost of inconvenience of us. (Deep Dogra: 1980)

Loyalty: One dimension of Gandhiji's *Satyagraha* is loyalty to truth. To Gandhi loyalty is the supreme principle of morality. His concept of duty is based on loyalty. What is loyalty ? It is nothing, but devotion of a person to a cause. Loyalty demands first of all a cause. In medical services, the cause is service to humanity. Loyalty of a person is expressed in deeds and it is a supreme ethical principle. Gandhiji respected loyalty in all men open heartedly. Gandhiji's loyalty is based on *Swabhava* and *Swadharma* and it means one's own duty with one's own nature. His concept of loyalty is evolutionary in nature. Justice, charity, industry, wisdom, spirituality may be defined in terms of loyalty in the contemporary social set-up.

Non-violence: Compromise with non-violence is not allowed. The key of non-violence is love. There is no place for bargaining, fear, rivalry, humiliation in non-violence. It always preserves self-respect of every person including his opponent.

John Ruskin said, "Humility is the solid foundation of all the Virtues.' Gandhiji's greatness lies in his humility. Further, he learned to be punctual from Western culture. Another principle which Gandhi adopted was secularism for which he gave his life. By secularism he meant neither irreligion nor indifference to religion but equal respect for all religions.

A very significant thought of Gandhi is that he never believed that a man can be wholly wicked and ignoble. He formulated the Ashram Vows on this strong faith in inherent goodness of man. His concept of human nature is the basis of his entire socio-political and economic life. Man is both means and end. Behind every success of science there remains the human brain and in the similar way every success of science has to be directed to the progress of humanity only by human being.

Truth: Truth is the function of reason, not the function of passion. Science is providing us comfort and increases facilities to serve the humanity. The progress of science is towards but Gandhi's Ashram Vows is a progress within. Without the progress of inner faculties mere progress of science remains incomplete. It is not only incomplete, it is a threat to humanity. The facilities and comforts provided by the science must be directed towards service to humanity stepping carefully on the constructive path and it is possible only to a man equipped with human qualities or whose inner qualities are fully developed. Otherwise there will be moral turbulence bringing rapid degradation to humanity. Every moment one has to be aware of his or her self, every moment one has to be ready for acquiring self-knowledge for correction or purification of mind just as a physically sick person search for medicine to cure his/her diseases. If any person is involved in act of exploitation, unfair practices, misuse of authority etc. are manifestations of untruth and to cover up these acts the doer has to take the help of unwelcome and socially unacceptable methods.

Gandhi's vows may not be pleasant but these are always good for health and character. What are those vows? 1. Non-violence, 2. Truth, 3. Non-stealing, 4. *Brahmacharya* (control of senses), 5. Non-possession, 6. Bread-labour, 7. Non-palate, 8. Fearlessness, 9. Equal respect for all religions, 10. *Swdeshi,* and 11. Removal of untouchability. (Gopalakrishnan: 1985)

Medical Service is a significant component of governance. This service like all other services has both legal and moral responsibilities. So, far as legal responsibility is concerned it is not difficult to ensure or to entrust it either to an individual or an organization. There exists specific legal framework within which each service is to function. As the government of a modern state consists of three components—Executive, Judiciary and Legislature and each component has its specific jurisdiction and functions. It is not difficult to ascertain their authorities and responsibilities. Further, it is closely linked to freedom or autonomy of an individual. It is the inner force of an individual. The moral responsibility one must say it is all pervasive encompassing each and every act of the statecraft. Further, it is not an exterior part of state machinery. It is not only the interior element of statecraft its presence is felt in each and every individual irrespective of his or her position in the state mechanism. It is manifested in the attitude, behaviour and application to the work undertaken by a person. To Hegel, legal act of state has its root in the moral and ethical principles.

While looking back to the traditional society of India, especially to traditional Assam one can realize that people were very sensitive to the moral principles. In traditional Assam there prevailed the custom of mutual help amongst the neighbours, taking care of family members, especially elderly members, entertainment of guest to the family, doing no harm to any creature, offering of cloths to the naked and food to the hungry. These customs were adopted by them out of moral compulsion. The people had immense faith on the village elders and religious leaders. They had firm belief on the indigenous doctors that they would never do harm to the patient. To them any act against social customs and traditions was sin. Gradually, the people started stepping in the escalation of modernization. Unfortunately, they failed to carry with them the customs and traditions which were rooted in the moral principles and human values required for the establishment of the peaceful and democratic society.

Today's administration of India is not confining to the functions of the Police State of the nineteenth century. It is entering into all aspects of the life of an individual in the perspective of progress and welfare of the nation competing with other nations of the world and honouring the global compulsions. Naturally administration has become a very complex affair. To be specific it may be mentioned that the growth of population with new aspirations and fresh problems of different communities, easy exposure of the nation to the rest of the world through e-media, emergence of the concepts of globalization, privatization and commercialization affecting government administration, activism of Non-Governmental Organizations, the role of United Nations of Organization in the field of protection of human rights of the individuals, adoption of different developmental strategies, emergence of complicated and sensitive issues arising from neigbouring countries, democratic deficiency, prevalence of hypocrisy amongst educated people, adoption of multi-standard of life, politicization of administration and criminalization of politics etc. are some of the causes demanding assertion on the need of accountability in almost every sphere of the public services of the country.

The common ailments in the public services may be classified in the language of Ashok Mukhopadhyay who said that public officials have been found guilty of non-feasance, mal-feasance and over-feasance. By 'non-feasance' is meant that they have not done what law or custom requires them to do owing to laziness, ignorance, non-caring for their duty, and corruption. Mal-feasance means that the duty is carried out with waste and damage due to technical incompetence and over-feasance means undertaken of a duty beyond what law and custom oblige or empower—it may be due to dictatorial temper, vanity and ambition of an official or his genuine, sincere, public spirited zeal.

Accountability is of different kinds—legislative, judicial, political, informal and normative accountability. Carl Friedrich stressed on the normative accountability, which is ethical accountability. It is a device to have internal controls like the professional standard, codes of ethics, social values adhered by individuals, respect for human dignity etc. All these constitute a very significant part of administrative accountability. These norms as and when developed and internalized by the administrator become an effective preventive measure rather than corrective measure against mal-feasance.

This does not mean non-recognition of variation of ethical obligations in the face of professional differences. For example, doctors working in Government hospitals owe primary allegiance to the norms of the medical profession and may justifiably protest against laws and rules which conflict with his professional and ethical relationship with patients. This may not be applicable to a nuclear scientist working for a government department, who can hardly afford to act accordance with his professional norms under the Government. (Ashok Mukhopadhyay: 1983)

O.G. Stahl in his article '*Administrative Accountability in USA*' said that greatest moral attention centres round the occupations having more autonomy or discretionary power. In these occupations the state of ethical accountability must be very high in the interest of the people. The high ranking administrative officials, experts with super-speciality, decision makers etc. fall within this category of occupants with more autonomy.

Referring to unethical aspect of specialization he said that high level specialization may concentrate on narrow objectives with single track techniques, which may become source of undetectable source of corruption or unethical behaviour. It may provide scope for insidious evil. Its remedy cannot be reached by arbitrary restraints or punishment. It may be treated by wise personnel policy which may broaden perspective of specialists. The continuous training exposure, periodic professional meetings, diversification of experience through new assignments, rotation, and teamwork.

Generally, it is noticed that blatant, overt corruption involving money matters are considered as unethical practices. This view does not address many other unethical behaviours of public servants which are not directly related to money. It is found that even educated and experienced persons are succumbed to their prejudices, ideologies and narrow perspective. Further extra care of their wealth and children, outside income or additional sources of income of these officials affect the innocent and deserving people of the services of the state.

According to William J. Siffin, the depravity of corruption is not limited to lying, stealing and mayhem. It extends to the violation of the principles of not wasting scarce resources.... Under this principle, it is corrupt to engage incompetent personnel in any system.

O.G. Stahl is very close to Gandhi in solving human problems when he said that the constructive ways to develop a sense of responsibility or accountability to a great extent on the caliber of the management that recruits candidates on merit and supervision that develops ways to motivate personnel to be committed to the goal of the service. The positive connotation of accountability reminds us that India needs durably competent, ethical and accountable civil servants. The most suitable way to achieve it is through serious attention to the best precepts of personnel management rather than through disparagement of public employment and absurd, unworkable prohibitions or punitive measures. However, he did not rule out the need of negative restraints even punishment in ensuring accountability. (Stahl: 1983)

Public accountability is a matter of attitude of public servants towards public. P.R. Dubhasi pointed out that public administration should be efficient, but it is more important that it should be ethical. (Dubhasi: 1983)

In India another common administrative problem is the abuse of power by the civil servants. There is more danger to the society from immoral, improper and illegal actions committed in the name of the state than from a few cases of unethical cases by public servants. The abuse of power in public sector can undermine public confidence and trust in government, reduce the capacity of the government to carry out its functions effectively, subvert ethical responsiveness to the citizenry, and impose unnecessary financial burden on taxpayers. The capacity of a political system to prevent, detect, punish and control such abuses will have direct bearing on its legitimacy, and will strengthen the moral basis of its authority. The abuse of power not only relates to the commission of a crime as defined by statute but also to the omission of the use of power or non-enforcement of the law where an official on duty is duty bound to act but does not do so either because of refusal, incompetence, or ignorance. Under these circumstances, it is very essential that there should be code of ethics to guide them whenever they are in dilemma. (Dwivedi: 1983)

In medical sciences ethics is very close to normative accountability as the medical scientists have more autonomy than any other public servants. In support of it, Carl Friedrich stated that there is need of some elasticity in the power of the administrator, some discretion to be used by him, and some inner check upon his own behaviour. Hence, he has stressed the normative and moral aspect of administrative accountability by arguing that internal 'informal' controls like professional standard, codes of ethics, social values possessed by individuals are very much necessary. Once these normative controls are strengthened, administrative accountability would increase. These serve as 'preventive' rather 'correcting' measure against malfeasance. (Mukhopadhayaya: 1983).

O.G. Stahl, the American scholar has said that to many people ethical performance in public service means simply avoidance of blatant, overt corruption involving money—such as the acceptance of bribes in return of dispensing some favour or for exemption from some governmental imposition or the taking of actions that advance one's own financial interests. Concentration on this type of unethical behaviour has three flaws—it is a negative and limited view of ethics in public services; it focuses upon the relatively rare, the crudest and often the least important violations of acceptable performance; and it misses the common, subtle and serious breaches of truly ethical action. This elementary view, so often stressed in laws intended to induce good behaviour, completely overlooks that men and women are more likely to succumb to their prejudices, ideologies, and limited perspectives than they are to the prospect of monetary gain. Preoccupation with official's financial status—their wealth, their outside income, or their investments—fails to stress the really important conditions that might affect their acting for or against the public interest.

A similar omission lies in the failure to recognize that incompetence is itself a form of corruption. William J. Siffin stated that the depravity of corruption is not limited to lying, stealing, and mayhem. It extends to the violation of the principle of not wasting scarce resources. Under this principle, the corruption of incompetence is usually excluded from the concerns of corruption fighters (Stahl: 1983).

O.P. Dwivedi has added that the abuse of power in the public sector can undermine public confidence and trust in government, reduce the capacity of government to fulfill its functions effectively, subvert ethical responsiveness to citizenry and impose unnecessary financial burden on taxpayers. The abuse of power relates not only to the commission because of a crime as defined by statute but also to the omission of the use of power or non-enforcement of the law where an official is duty-bound to act but does not do so either because of refusal, incompetence or negligence. (Dwivedi: 1980) P. Minocha in the article, 'Accountability in Public Sector Enterprises' defined accountability as, "a means to give an account of one's action and to report on the achievements and failures together with explanation of declared objectives." It helps measuring of duties in terms of standard, adherence of ethical principles, understanding of pre-determined objectives of the organization. (Minocha: 1983)

The concepts like 'responsibility', 'control', 'supervision', 'direction' etc. are maintaining very close relationship to 'accountability'. Responsibility is the obligation to stand by and answer for and own the consequences of one's act. It makes a physician or an administrator to offer best performance to achieve the goal, to choose the best means and best materials towards the end. Interestingly, the concept of responsibility not only motivate a person to act, it may also dissuade a person to act. A great French statesman and administrator said, "Responsibility frightens men much more than the danger of cannon." However, it cannot be denied that the fear of the consequences of responsibility may lead to efficiency. It obliges a man who has the sense of responsibility to acquire all the information that may be necessary to weigh the arguments for and against any suggested action, to think and reflect on the possible consequences of a proposed action or to view it from all possible directions. The sense of responsibility makes a man to study, think and to have deliberations before undertaking the task. Even during the course of action he will be watchful of the consequences of each step of action. (Ruthnaswamy: 1972) As regards the concept of Control, N.N. Mallay defines it as directing, restraining, stimulating a person or an organization while in action to achieve the goals. (Mallay: 1971)

Coming to the concept of supervision one may say that it is nothing but direction accompanied by authority and is more than inspection and investigation. Because the act of supervision includes teaching the employees to be supervised as to how the work has to be done efficiently. Supervision is a specialized job. According to Pfiffner, a supervisor must have—(a) expert knowledge of the job at his disposal; (b) integrity and ability to communicate his ideas to the employees; (c) have the capacity to make the employees understand the philosophy of management; (d) love and willing to inspire others; (e) ability to take quick decision and courage to own failures and faults; (f) free from vices; (g) knowledge of administrative techniques, and (h) possess intellectual alertness and have willingness to acquire new knowledge.

To G.D. Halsey a good supervisor should be thorough in his work and take of every care of every necessary detail. He should have the sense of justice and be very much considerate towards his workers. He must have courage, self-confidence and decision making capacity. He must have the capacity to win loyalty from others. (Raj: 2001)

Morale

Professor B.S. Khanna, Indian Institute of Public Administration, New Delhi stated that in many progressive countries also it is realized that efficiency of public administration depends not only upon the effectiveness of the organizational arrangements and administrative procedures or upon the skill of the personnel but also upon the level of morale which exists among the employees.

Morale may be defined as the readiness of a group of persons to work enthusiastically and persistently for furthering the purpose and for achieving the objectives of the organization. Morale depends upon the physical, mental, and emotional health of the employees, upon their active consciousness, and confidence in the purpose and the objectives of the organization in which they are working, and upon their trust not only in each other but also on the leadership. (Khanna: 1959)

It is generally recognized to-day that there is no such thing as a fixed human nature good or bad, competitive or co-operative or aggressive or submissive, which determines human behaviour in a specific manner. There is no evidence that men always act on self-interest nor that material or monetary gains are the most important incentives to the worker, in industry or elsewhere. Improvement in the physical, or biological environment of the worker (in lighting, ventilation, noise, heating, humidity etc.) does not necessarily mean satisfactory conditions of work much less that it makes the workers happy. Individuals do not function as isolated units but relationships. The social norms and values of a culture steer individual or group behaviour and operate like a 'psychic gyroscope' to keep it in a straight course.

A proper understanding of the behaviour of an individual would imply the appreciation of the complex conditions in which it occurs. The problem of morale in a modern civil administration as in an industrial system is largely the study of the worker, his adjustment problems, his motivational system, his relationship with his supervisor, to the group to which he belongs, his feeling pride in the job, the degree of his participation and his emotional attitude, not only towards the members of his group and towards the hierarchy to which he belongs but in general to his family adjustment, his sources of satisfaction etc. The problem is basically the problem of personality adjustment, motivation and group-dynamics.

Following may help to understand morale:

1. Morale refers to a condition of physical and emotional well-being in the individual or in the group that make it possible for him (or group) to function with energy, confidence and enthusiasm. Today in India educated and in some cases uneducated persons also aware of the health with differentiation in degree of awareness. In most cases, the patients exercise their choice of hospital and physicians for their treatment. Generally, it is noticed that in this case generally exit patients act as confidence builder for the patient decision-maker. This confidence becomes the source of their enthusiasm and energy. Suspicion on the physician's expertness remains extremely fragile here.
2. Morale refers to the condition of a group where there are clear and fixed group goals and purposes that are felt to be important and that are integrated with individual goals. There must also be confidence in the attainment of these goals, confidence in the means of attainment, i.e. in the leaders, associations and finally in oneself.
3. Morale is a function of the integration and cooperation among the members of the group. Here aggression and hostility, if they occur, are expressed against forces frustrating the group rather than towards the individual within the group.
4. Morale also implies the degree of participation in the determination of the goals or objectives of the work.
5. Prestige and recognition are invariably related to morale.
6. The feeling of security and anxiety directly determine high or low morale.
7. Adequate leadership is an important factor in building morale.

8. Group-belongingness.
9. Personality of the individual and patterns of his adjustment in response to various situations of stress would determine his morale.
10. Morale is adversely affected by authoritarian leadership or atmosphere.

Opportunities for development and improvement in status and position inevitably raise morale. There is no such thing as a fixed human nature good or bad, competitive or co-operative or aggressive or submissive, which determines human behaviour in a specific manner. There is no evidence that men always act on self-interest nor that material or monetary gains are the most important incentives to the worker, in industry or elsewhere. Improvement in the physical, or biological environment of the worker (in lighting, ventilation, noise, heating, humidity etc.) does not necessarily mean satisfactory conditions of work much less that it makes the workers happy. Individuals do not function as isolated units but relationships. The social norms and values of a culture steer individual or group behaviour and operate like a 'psychic gyroscope' to keep it in a straight course.

The prevailing idea that money is the strongest incentive is quite misleading. Further, there is no one ideal incentive for all; one person may value money whereas another may consider leisure, security or pride in the job or recognition of achievement. (Prasad: 1959)

India won freedom on 15th August, 1947 after a long and hard struggle against the British rulers. The process of the struggle for independence of India may be traced with the efforts of Mahatma Gandhi to fight for human rights in South Africa. Throughout the long struggle he devoted to the cause of the human rights of the Indians through *Satyagraha* and Non-violence. He could mobilize even the Indian women to come out of the four walls of their habitation to participate in the movement at a time when the Indian society was in dark about the ways of development and rights. Thus, Mahatma Gandhi could mobilize not only the men folk but also the ignorant and uneducated women to come forward and to take active part in the freedom struggle of the country. The non-cooperation movement which was a major tool of the freedom struggle could embrace even the young students of the country.

The leaders of freedom struggle like Dadabhai Naoroji, Gopal Krishna Gokhale, Lokamanya Bal Gangadhar Tilak, Lala Lajpat Rai, Bipin Chandra Pal, Surenda Nath Banerjee, Pandit Madan Mohan Malaviya,

Motilal Nehru, Sardar Vallabhbhai Patel, Maulana Abul Kalam Azad, Dr. Rajendra Prasad, Jawaharlal Nehru etc. were men of eminence and strong personality. In the beginning of the twentieth century, the great freedom fighter Balgangadhar Tilak gave voice, "Swaraj is my birthright and I shall have it". Ultimately, the British went away and we gained independence on 15th August, 1947.

When India gained Independence it was found that the British left India leaving severe negative impact on the country. However, they also left scope to pick up some positive impact on us. Here mention may be made of Lord William Bentinck (1828-35) for his humane prohibition of *Sati* (self-immolation of widows on the dead husband's pyre) in which he was heartily assisted by Raja Ram Mohun Roy—the Morning Star of modern India. He also took bold step to reverse the anti-native policy of Cornwallis in respect of Government employment in responsible offices. Among the pioneers of this liberal policy were also British civilians like Sir Thomas Munro, Sir Charles Metcalfe and Sir John Malcolm. Lord Dalhousie (1848-56), the last Governor General of India under the Company's regime had as great a flair for administrative advancement as he had for territorial annexations. There was not a sphere of activity, in which he did not leave the impress of his personality. Another person to be remembered is Lord Ripon, an Irish and Catholic, the only non-English-or-non-Protestant, to rule India (1880-84). Ripon's constructive measures for extension of local self-government, "What I want to secure by extension of local self-government", Ripon explained, "is ....gradual training of the best, most intelligent, and most influential men in the community to take an interest and an active part in the management of their local affairs.... What I am trying to do is not to impose an English system on India, but to revive and extend the indigenous system of the country. That indigenous system we have done a great deal to destroy, but the remnants of it exist to a greater or lesser extent in most parts of the country, and it is upon those remnants that I hope to build up the edifice of local self-government."

Mahatma Gandhi, leader of the movement stated clearly that *Swaraj* is to be gained by educating the masses to a sense of their capacity to regulate and control authority. Albert Einstein summed up Gandhi's life-work and position in the world as, "The veneration in which Gandhi has been held throughout the world rests on the recognition, for the most part unconscious, that in our age of moral decay he was the only statesman who represented that higher conception of human relations in the political sphere to which we must aspire with all our powers. We must learn the difficult lesson that the future of mankind will only be tolerable when our course in world affairs, as in all other matters, is based upon justice and law rather than the threat of naked power." (Palkhiwala).

Jawaharlal Nehru also gave tremendous value to individual freedom. The purpose of a democratic society was essentially to provide necessary conditions of creative development. Explaining the reasons for accepting the democratic process in India, Nehru observed: "It is not enough for us merely to produce the material goods of the world. We do want high standard of living, but not at the cost of man's creative spirit, his creative energy, his spirit of adventure, not at the cost of all fine things of life which have ennobled man throughout the ages. Democracy is not merely a question of elections."

Nehru also insisted that a scientific approach to be accepted as the guiding principle of life and as a process of thinking regarding our problems. Nehru seems to have a profound sense of history and deep respect for India's heritage. He wanted the Indian people to be free from the shackles of the past. At the same time he urged them to recondition their mind equipping themselves with the problems of the present and perspective on the future. This is possible through humanism and scientific spirit. Despite an apparent conflict between the two, there was a growing synthesis between humanism and scientific spirit, resulting in a kind of scientific humanism. Nehru expressed his mind very clearly in the last chapter of *The Discovery of India* as, " The modern mind, that is to say, the better type of the modern mind, is practical and pragmatic, ethical and social, altruistic and humanitarian.... It has discarded to a large extent the philosophic approach of the ancients, their search for ultimate reality, as well as the devotionalism and mysticism of the medieval period. Humanity is its god and social service, its religion."

In the language of Radhakrishnan gaining independence has been a simpler task compared with the one of administering the country in a clean, decent way. This seems to be more formidable task. For it we require selfless leadership, an honest and competent civil service. We require a disciplined military and police force. We require expert industrial managers and skilled workers and good agricultural peasants. Our ordinary citizens should have civic sense and national feeling. Here lies the basic truth of the contemporary ailments of the political world of the country. Because the political leadership gradually deviating from the qualities of moral leadership, either they could not realize the ideals of constitution of the country which have been enshrined in it by the eminent Indians in the beginning of the political march of Independent India or they have failed to emancipate their inner person from the bondage of irrational elements of mind. Or they are unable to realize the energy, time and scholarly thought of the members of the Constituent Assembly which they put in the task of framing the Constitution. Or they fail to understand the significance of the Constitution itself.

The Constituent Assembly, constituted on its first meeting elected Dr. Rajendra Prasad as its chairman on 11th December, 1946 for the purpose of administering independent India. Dr. B.R. Ambedkar was the chairman of the Drafting Committee of the Constitution. Independent India was given a Constitution after threadbare discussion and study of different social, political, administrative and economic issues.

Radhakrishnan said that all these things cannot be had in a day. What we are attempting to do to our best of our power is to take some steps towards developing a sound administration, a stable government and a healthy nation. We cannot say that we are satisfied with what we have done. There are things happening in different parts of the country which make us feel sad, depressed and ashamed of ourselves. What is necessary is the strong sense of patriotism. It is true that we developed a negative kind of patriotism when we struggled to rid of the country of foreign rule. (What we do not want: Foreign rule) But a positive patriotism, a dynamic fellow-feeling, a sense of belonging to this country, of being proud to belong to it, these things yet to come. We have to build these in the minds and hearts of men.

We fought for independence with a desire to develop a democratic set in the society. Democracy has three basic dimensions—political, economic and social. Political and economic democracy are rooted in social democracy. Social democracy has been said by Mahatma Gandhi as a way of life. It is not merely a way of life but an ethical way of life. Nobody could deny it and the Indian scholars have started discussing about good governance in the country. The government did not make any explicit pronouncement of it nor the course of actions of the government reflects it till recently. Only the government led by Narenda Modi as Prime Minister made explicit pronouncement of it when it said, "Minimum Government and maximum governance". Here lies the need of ethical way of life. As Radhakrishnan said, "Democracy is a faith. It is a faith on human power as well as intellectual power. The concept of maximum governance also demands freedom which means restraints. Once a man restraints himself from encroaching upon other's freedom there emerges humility of man which is the core element of good governance. Good governance is nothing but democratic or self-governance." (Radhakrishnan)

Corruption

Corruption is an immoral act which annihilates human personality of an individual tempting him to be involved in all kinds of inhuman, illegal and unethical activities. It also pushes an individual to take the shelter of superfluous vanity, false arguments, utmost secrecy in behaviour and manipulative social environment/social relationships. It reduces the mental or moral strength of an individual. However, it is defined differently by the scholars. J.S. Nye, in the article, *Corruption and Political Development* published in the American Review in 1967 defined corruption as, "behaviour which deviates from the formal duties of a public role because of private-regarding (personal, close family, private clique) pecuniary or status gains; or violates rules against exercise of certain types of private-regarding influence." (Tyagi: 1989) Stephen D. Morris, a Professor of Politics, defines corruption as the illegitimate use of public power to benefit private interest.

The term 'corrupt' when used as an adjective liberally means 'utterly broken'. The term was first used by Aristotle and later by Cicero who added the terms bribe and abandonment of good habits.

In philosophical, theological or moral discussions, corruption is the abuse of bestowed power or position to acquire personal benefit. Corruption may include many activities including embezzlement.

(http://en.wikipedia.org/wiki/corruption accessed on 29th Apl.2015)

The concept of corruption has a close relationship to the terms, misconduct and unethical activities. Misconduct may be said as the behaviour not conforming to prevailing standards of laws; impropriety; an act of adultery; dishonest or bad management, especially by persons entrusted or engaged to act on behalf of others; deliberate wrong doings. It may be said that misconduct refers to an action, rather than neglecting to take action, or inaction which could be referred to as poor performance.

The unethical activities indicate lack of moral principles; unwillingness to adhere to proper rules of conduct.

(http://www.thefreedictionary.com/misconduct, accessed 29th Apl. 2015)

A.R. Tyagi, in his book, "*Public Administration*" highlighted the definitions found in the Indian Penal Code and the Prevention of Corruption Act 1947 as below:

As per Indian Penal Code, Section 161,

> "Whoever being or expecting to be a public servant, accepts or obtains, or agrees to accept, or attempt to obtain from any person,

for himself or any other person, any gratification whatever, other than legal remuneration, as a motive or reward for doing or forbearing to do any official act or for showing or forbearing to show, in the exercise of his official functions, favour or disfavour to any person, or for rendering or attempting to render any service or disservice to any person, with the Central or State Government or Parliament or the Legislature of any State or with any local authority, Corporation or Government Company referred to in section 21, or with any public servant, as such shall be punished."

The Prevention of Corruption Act 1947 in the section 5 (1) stated, "A public servant is said to commit the offence of criminal misconduct–

(a) If he habitually accepts or obtains or agrees to accept or attempts to obtain from any person for himself or for any other person, any gratification (other than legal remuneration) as a motive or reward as mentioned in the Indian Penal Code;
(b) If he habitually accepts or obtains or agrees to accept or attempts to obtain from any person for himself or for any other person, any valuable thing without consideration or for a consideration which knows to be inadequate, from any person whom he knows to have been, or to be, or about to be transacted by him, or having any connection with the official functions of himself or of any public servant, to whom he is subordinate, or from any person whom he knows to be interested in or related to the person so concerned; or
(c) If he dishonestly or fraudulently misappropriates or otherwise converts for his own use any property entrusted to him or under his control as a public servant or allows any other person to do so; or
(d) If he or any person on his behalf is in possession or has, at any time during the period of his office, been in possession, for which the public servant cannot satisfactorily account, of pecuniary resources or property disproportionate to his known sources of income."

Corruption also indicates ethical vacuity in any institution. Referring to the concept of corruption, the Second Administrative Reforms Commission said corruption is an important manifestation of the failure of ethics. The word 'corrupt' is derived from the Latin word 'corruptus', meaning 'to break or destroy'. The word 'ethics' is from the original Greek term ethikos, meaning 'arising from habit'. It is unfortunate that corruption has, for many, become a matter of habit, ranging from grand corruption involving persons in high places to retail corruption touching the everyday life of common people.

However, it cannot be denied that these definitions are not enough to address new areas and techniques adopted by the persons engaged in public services in different capacities.

Causes of Corruption: The causes of corruption may be discussed under three major heads, such as Political environment, Economic environment and Social environment.

Political Environment: India, like most newly liberated countries of Asia and Africa faced political and administrative challenges. The Political system was the choice of ours but the administrative set up was the creation of the British. However, it has to be admitted that the British provided the basic structure of the public service, especially the recruitment to the public services on the basis of merit, All India Service, salary, promotion systems etc. were developed during the British rule. At the initial stage of administration, the Indian nation was united together very tightly by the spirit of freedom struggle and the political leadership was in the hands of eminent personalities of the country, they had very rich experience of freedom struggle of India. They were the immediate sufferers of the adverse effect of colonial rule. Gradually, the strength of that tie has become fragile. Under the constitution of India, the Indians started enjoying freedom within the framework of parliamentary democracy. The concept of democracy is very wide and hard realization. Further, the success of democracy depends on human values, human power, non-violence etc. It requires perseverance, dedication and enough mental strength. This was realized by then scholars, political leaders, social reformers etc. and expressed it through their writings, speeches and the ways of life. In course of time, the frailness of the power of freedom struggle as a tie of unity has become prominent with the assertion of the rights of different communities and the socio-economic inconveniences for their development. The Governments have initiated developmental programmes in the face of backwardness of different communities, underlining economic development. Development is a dynamic concept and it invites changes in the policies and programmes. Further, it requires application of technical knowledge and discretionary power of the public servants.

Coming to the concept of political democracy gradually it has been narrowed down to a large extent to the system of election only. In the election also there emerged the perverted form of 'public opinion'. Money and emotion have become the main tools to be used by the candidates in the elections to the legislatures. The criminalization of politics has come to surface.

In the administration it has become the open secret of the emergence 'spoils system' and 'selling of post' to the candidates, selling of service to people at the lower strata of the administrative system, complexity in the administrative procedure such as tax and licensing systems etc. are the root causes of corruption. Politicization of the grassroots level democracy is a serious threat to Indian democracy. Because Indian democracy must acquire power from the grassroots level of it, otherwise naturally it will be withering away because of weak base. The Panchayati Raj Institutions are nothing but the democratic power generating systems. Unfortunately, these were the most neglecting areas of Indian democracy for a long time. Since 1990s, though their status has been strengthened, politicization of these Institutions has become a threat to democracy. In this situation corruption takes shelter in every walk of our life.

Closely connected to political leadership is policies of the government. As a conscious choice, the Indian state in the early decades after Independence chose a set of policies whose unintended consequence was to put the citizen at the mercy of the State. Overregulation, severe restrictions on economic activity, excessive state control, near-monopoly of the government in many sectors and an economy of scarcity all created conditions conducive to unbridled corruption. In addition, many state subsidies and beneficiary-oriented programmes in a situation of asymmetry of power converted the public servant into patron and master and reduced most citizens into mendicants. This at once enhanced opportunities to indulge in corruption and reduced the citizens' capacity to resist extraordinary demands. These are referred in the report of the Second Administrative Reforms Commission. In addition it stated that perhaps the most important determinant of the integrity of a society or the prevalence of corruption is the quality of politics. If politics attracts and rewards men and women of integrity, competence and passion for public good, then the society is safe and integrity is maintained. But if honesty is incompatible with survival in politics, and if public life attracts undesirable and corrupt elements seeking private gain, then abuse of authority and corruption become the norm. In such a political culture and climate, desirable initiatives will not yield.

Economic and Administrative Environment: India has to undertake developmental policies in almost every sector of administration. Since these programmes are generally innovative programmes there arises the scope of corruption, as every developmental programme has heavy financial implication and development administration is not only changeable but also complicated in nature. It is different from regulatory administration. Another cause of corruption in this field is the unemployment problems. With the increase of educational facilities or spread of education Government efforts are not enough to utilize youth power in the positive way resulting unemployment, overemployment and underemployment problems. The exposure to the development of high technology for leading a comfortable life provokes the temptation not only of youths, but also of others—whether poor or rich. In other words, it creates 'Man of Greed' and a greedy man will be a corrupt man.

In the words of Rajagopalachari, "the system of permits, licenses, allocation of transport routes, quotas and similar attempts to administer the economy of a big and busy nation from the Secretariat instead leaving such things to the consumer and competition in the market, is at the root of corruption.... The contact between the official and party bosses on the one side, and the very clever, far too clever, businessman on the other, with a tremendous lot of money expected in the business, produces the national malady we call corruption...... Unless we minimize official intervention and ministerial power, making or marring the fortunes of business and industrialists, unless we reduce controls up to the level called for by international trade and exchange pressures and bravely decide to knock out the rest and try out the consequences, we are bound to suffer this newly-introduced and wide spread malady of corruption at the ministerial and secretariat level".

Social Environment: The social environment may appear as a very wide and deep rooted source of corruption in a country. Because the administrative and political cultures are the sub-cultures of social culture. Family, religion, customs and tradition of a society play a significant role in the creation of social culture. The education of a child begins at home. The child picks up habits, values etc. from the family environment created by the parents and other members of the family. In the traditional joint family all the brothers and their families lived under the same roof and the social control was very strong over the behaviours and thought process or development of child's personality. Religion and social customs played a significant role allowing the moral principles to influence the life of an individual in the formative stage. The habits an individual forms at the childhood, the values adhered at home by the children, the pattern of social relationship to which a child becomes familiar are reflected in his future life or when starts rendering service to the nation from any profession. This is added by the knowledge acquired by the children in the educational institutions. These are reflected in the service life of an individual.

With transformation of the society from traditional to modernity changes are taking place in the structure and functioning of the family as a socializing agency. The fundamental rights of the citizens and other laws formulated by the Governments, developmental programmes undertaken in the country since independence are causing tremendous change in the family life. The most significant change is noticed in the role of the family as a socializing agency. In the traditional Indian society mother was the key person to inculcate values to her child, besides other members. Gradually both mother and father of a child become the earners who have to remain outside the family for longer time. Further, the position of a teacher was next to parents in the process of socialization till recently, but now the status of the teachers is deteriorating due to various reasons.

Unfortunately, there emerges widespread corruption in almost every field of state administration, the power of higher education becomes fragile, ethical principles almost disappeared from social life, violation of human rights or inhuman treatment in all possible forms (cheating, exploitation, thefts, dacoits, human trafficking) has become the common sight, the process of criminalization of politics and politicization of bureaucracy is reaching the culminating point. The intellectuals, politicians, social welfare workers and public service providers maintain multi-standard of life providing comfortable space to hypocrisy in social life. Money power of the state is misused instead of using it for public service. Jobs in government services, seats for admission into medical colleges are sold at all levels, natural public opinion is disregarded by the political leaders and they started manufacturing public opinion according to their own convenience either with the help of money or muscle power. To-day it appears that man can do everything with money except making a man human. Recently, the political world of India is clouded by the controversy, 'Political Party *Vs.* State' on the issue of supremacy. (Radhakrishnan: 1992)

The Second Administrative Reforms Commission pointed out certain factors of corruption and abuse of office, such as, there is a colonial legacy of unchallenged authority and propensity to exercise power arbitrarily. In a society which worships power, it is easy for public officials to deviate from ethical conduct. There is enormous asymmetry of power in our society. Nearly 90 per cent of our people are in the unorganized sector. Quite a number of them lead a precarious existence, depending on subsistence wages with no job security. And nearly 70 per cent of the organized workers with job security and regular monthly wage are employed by the state directly or through public sector undertakings. Almost all these employees are 'educated' in a largely illiterate and semi-literate society and economically even the lowliest of public servants are better off than most people in the country. What is more, their employment in government comes with all the trappings of power. Such asymmetry of power reduces societal pressure to conform to ethical behaviour and makes it easy to indulge in corruption. (ARC: 2007)

Corruption is a global phenomenon and has also become a serious global concern. The United Nations Convention against Corruption was adopted by the UN General Assembly in October 2003, providing an international instrument against corruption. The ADB-OECD Anti-Corruption Action Plan, which has been signed by the Government of India, is a broad understanding to further the cause of inter-regional cooperation in the matter of prevention of corruption. The World Bank has also declared war against corruption by refusing to fund projects whose implementation is tainted by corrupt practices. At the annual meeting of the International Monetary Fund and the World Bank Group in Singapore in 2006, a joint statement was issued with major multilateral financial institutions agreeing on a framework for preventing and combating fraud and corruption in the activities and operations of their institutions.

Remedial Measures

During Second World War (1939-45) administrative corruption became a public concern for the first time. Sardar Vallabh Bhai Patel, the Home Member while piloting the Delhi Special Police Establishment Bill of 1946 in Central Legislative Assembly, observed in his speech: "You cannot stop bribery and corruption so long as there are many controls and licenses which control all branches of our life, public life and private life and necessities of life." (Patel: 1946) The Act set up an administrative machinery for investigation of cases in public services. The Santhanam Committee on Prevention of Corruption recommended for establishment of Central Bureau of Investigation (CBI).

Later an Administrative Reforms Commission was set up in 1966 under the chairmanship of Morarji Desai, later K. Hanumantaiya emphasized the need of redress of grievances and recommended for establishment of Lokpal and Lokayukta as grievance redress machinery.

Recently people of the country protested against the accumulation of black money in the foreign bank by the leaders of our Welfare State under the leadership of Yoga Guru Ramdev. It has been followed by hunger strike under the leadership of Anna Hazare for passing of the Lok Pal Bill which is being defeated on several occasions on the floor of parliament. These movements are against corruption in the government. To be successful in making the country free from corruption each and every citizen must make an effort to discipline his and her on self through moral power or to strengthen the moral qualities. Let's us hope that this movement against corruption will be a turning point in the history of India to regain the human power to reduce the social ailments, especially immoral behaviour of men and women.

The idea of the institution of Lokpal is borrowed from that of Ombudsman. Ombudsman is a Scandinavian institution originated in 1809 itself. This institution was in dark for a long time due to various reasons. Only after 1950s, it could draw the attention of the nations of the world as grievance redress machinery. Now, let us have a look to the background of this institution.

Definition: The word "OMBUDSMAN" is derived from the word "OMBUD" Swedish word. It did not refer to Complains Handling Mechanism in the beginning. It indicated a spokesman or representative of another person or group of person. Various efforts were made by some institutions and eminent persons to maintain uniformity in the usages of the term. Of these the most important is the Ombudsman Committee of the International Bar Association. This committee suggested that the terms refers to the grievance handling mechanism which comes within the scope of the following definition:

> "An Ombudsman institution is an office provided for, by the Constitution or by the action of the Legislature or Parliament and headed by the independent, high level public official who receives complains from aggrieved persons against Government agencies, officials, and employees or who acts on his own motion and who has the power to investigate, recommend corrective action and the issue reports".

The Swedish Ombudsman for the civil affairs was created in 1809 by the Constitution. In creating this office the Constitutional Committee was influenced by the theory of separation of powers.

The executive had already the Attorney General to look after the administration of justice. It was felt necessary to arm the legislature with similar supervisory powers. The result was the Procurator ship. In the beginning there was only one Procurator supervising the civil as well as military administration. But in 1915 another Ombudsman was appointed with jurisdiction in the military field. The Justice Ombudsman (JO) was to exercise general supervision over courts and civil servants to ensure obedience of the law. He was to investigate charges of illegality and negligence or gross disregards of interests of their services in the performances of the official duties. The Justice Ombudsman (JO) would prosecute those who had committed unlawful acts through partiality, favouritism or any such reasons or had neglected to perform their official duties properly. He has to be appointed by the parliament. Since 1941 he was selected for a period of four years. He could be re-elected for any number of terms. The election board consisted of representatives of all the parties represented in the parliament. His election was above party politics and was almost unanimous. It required that he had and his duties should be of citizens known legal abilities and outstanding integrity. Parliament had the power of discerning the Prosecutor and his deputy form the office even before the expiry of the term provided the members lose confidence in him.

Procedure of work: Both the JO in two ways, investigated complaints and sent reports to their offices. They also undertook tours and carried on enquiry in to the working of than state officials. The complaints to be investigated by the Prosecutor must be supported by evidence. Otherwise he may refuse to investigate the complaints. The complaints if accepted, were forwarded to the office or official whose action being challenged, the office concerned sent back the complaints with its comments. The JO's Office forwarded the complaints to the appropriate authority. The complaints covered the whole range of administration.

The Ombudsman had considerable amount of discretionary power in the matter of proceedings against the officials. He was unwilling to prosecute the official concerned before the ordinary courts unless the offence was serious and he had left with no alternative. On an average, ten cases per year involved prosecution in Sweden. The JO had to obtain permission of the Parliament before proceeding against the minister.

Origin: the Swedish Constitution created the office of Ombusdman in 1809 itself as the watch-dog of the Parliament against the royal officers. It remained as unique feature of Swedish administration. It was adopted by another Scandinavian country—Finland in 1919, a country with close historical ties with Sweden. Norway became another Scandinavian country to set up an Ombudsman scheme to deal with military affairs in 1952. The institution found its third and historically most important adoption by Denmark. Norway appointed Ombudsman for civil affairs in 1962, the same year New Zealand become the first Commonwealth country to adopt the Ombudsman institution. Since 1962, a large number of the countries set-up similar types of investigations. For instance, Australia, Canada, Fiji, France, Great Britain, Guyana, India, Israel, Northern Ireland and Switzerland. In the U.S. there were Ombudsman officials in the States of Hawaii, Nebraska Iowa, New York and Washington. By 1977, Ombudsman or ombudsman like institutions existed in as many as twenty five countries. Besides, in the countries like Bangladesh, Philippines and Greece, provisions pertaining to the establishment of Ombudsman-like institutions have been incorporated in their respective Constitutions.

The all-round response evoked by the ombudsman institution during the last two decades and a half was probably unmatched and unparallel by any other administrative institutions during the entire spectrum of the twentieth century. Surprisingly enough, in spite of all kinds of social, economic, legal, constitutional, political, administrative, demographic and ecological diversities prevalent all countries favoured the Ombudsman institution.

No single factor or reason could amount for the worldwide spread of this idea in the post-second World War era in general and post-1962 period in particular. A few reasons may however, be stated as some of the significant factors that account for the world widespread of the Ombudsman idea in the last century.

Change in socio-political environment: The socio-political environment of the world in the post-Second World War period has changed mainly due to two reasons—

First, a large number of countries accepted the welfare Concept ideal. Second, an equally large number of countries achieved liberation from the colonial rule. The unprecedented increase in the volume of the functions of the state following the acceptance of the welfare state ideal and the consequent growth in its structure, powers and discretion, all traditionally available means of control over its operations and personal proved ineffective. As power corrupts and absolute power corrupts absolutely and "where there is the discretion there is room for arbitrariness", necessity to search for an effective means for exercising control over the vast power and discretion enjoyed by the functionaries.

Greater Awareness about Protection of Citizen's Rights: The gradual culmination of the ideal of Welfare state into the reality of what ultimately came to be known as the administrative state soon lead to the realization of its possible danger for the enjoyment of fundamental democratic rights by the citizens. Thus, time and again, a growing concern was expressed both by the established as well as the newly born democratic states for providing effective safeguards against the infringements of democratic rights and freedoms of the citizens. However, it was not until the passage of two decades after Second World War that the Ombudsman institution came to be identified as an effective measure for the protection of such rights against the ever-expending state horizons.

Efforts of Professor Hurwitz: The rapid spread of the ombudsman idea in the Post-Second World War era, owes itself to a certain extent to the efforts of Prof. Hurwitz, the first Danish Ombudsman. Prof. Hurwitz, after his appointment in 1955, devoted much energy to promote the plan. He wrote articles for European and International Journals and travelled as far as possible to several places to speak about it. He also willingly interrupted his busy schedule to give information to visitors or enquiries from other countries. The early discussion of the plan and its adoption in New Zealand owe much to his ability and willingness to write and speak in English. He prepared a long pamphlet in English on his office and wrote articles for British and American journals. He also spoke to academic audiences and appeared on television in Britain. One of the indications of its strength of his impact are that after his return, he began to receive letters of complaint against British administration.

Lastly, Judge Baxelium—a Swedish Ombudsman and Guy Powels, the Chief Ombudsman of New Zealand, contributed in no less significant measures to the prorogation of the idea through their writings and speech—making foreign tours.

***Role of UN Conferences and International Commission of Jurists*:** The spread of the idea of Ombudsman has also been stimulated by the activities of the UN and International Commission of Jurists. Both have taken a very active interest of the Ombudsman institution and organized periodic Conferences on Human Rights in the various parts of the world where the idea has been a subject of discussion. These Conferences have induced key officials from most of the countries in the areas concerned. The International Commission of Jurists, in addition to the influential report prepared by its British section in Bulletin. Among the efforts of UN in propagating the idea, the 1967 UN Seminar in Jamaica for Central and South America with Swedish Ombudsman, Baxelius as a great expert is noteworthy.

***The Ombudsman Committee of the International Bar Association*:**

The chief motto of the Ombudsman Committee of International Bar Association, headed by Barnard Frank, was the diffusion of the idea of Ombudsman throughout the world. The contribution made by the Committee is very significant towards the adoption of the Ombudsman institution by many countries of the world. They furnish the nations with information of latest developments regarding these institutions through newsletters, survey reports etc.

Role of Jurists: It would be no exaggeration to say that the contribution made by the intellectuals in these fields is no way less than that of others. The names of Professor D.C. Rowatt, Professor Walter Gelhon, Professor W.A. Robson, Professor Anderson, Professor Davis, Professor Brian Chapman and Professor Hill, through their writings, research works and institution has become familiar among the nations.

Why OMBUDSMAN? The citizens of a democratic country in the modern world have realized the necessity of effective handling of their grievances by the Government. Mere enumeration of Human Rights in the Constitution, the Charter, the declaration and the Laws cannot protect the Human Rights. They can be ably protected by the effective machineries which implement the Constitution, Charter, Laws and Declarations. The ombudsman is one of the institution essential to a democratic society. Barnard Frank identifies the reasons for the desirability of the Ombudsman institution as follows:

First, the modern state is a Welfare State. The functions of the Welfare State are unlimited. It covers each and every aspect of human life. It has extensive powers and discretion in the formulation of policies affecting a man from birth to death. Extensive powers and discretion have been granted to the Government Departments and their allied agencies. As a consequence, there is a wide scope of friction between the citizens and the officials. Protection of the individuals has become the fundamental requirement against the executive and administrative mistake and abuse of powers. This has became a great concern of the citizens of both developed and developing countries.

Second, the activities of bureaucracy are not only increasing in number but also becoming more complex and comprehensive in nature. The trend compels people to reemphasize their legal rights which invites additional protection.

Third, one important function of the legislature is supervision of the administration. Extensive delegation of the power to the bureaucracy makes legislative supervision inadequate. This inadequacy can be made up with the introduction of Ombudsman institution.

Fourth, the complaint-handling role is played by the legislators also. One of the earliest scholarly references to this may found in the work of political anthropologist F.G Bailey. Prof. Baily wrote an article and published in the *European Journal of Sociology*, "the electors see their M.L.A. not as 'legislators' but as their representatives who will intercede for them with the administration." He must be noted that the legislator has no direct access to file and information. (Rowatt: 1964)

What is required to-day is moral political leadership or ethical political environment as the primary instrument to reduce corruption in public services. This is indicated by the Second Administrative Reforms Commission also. If politics attracts and rewards men and women of integrity, competence and passion for public good, then the society is safe and integrity is maintained. But if honesty is incompatible with survival in politics, and if public life attracts undesirable and corrupt elements seeking private gain, then abuse of authority and corruption become the norm. In such a political culture and climate, desirable initiatives will not yield.

Ethics cannot be divorced from the notion of responsibility and accountability. In democracy each and every public servant is accountable to people. The accountability is ensured through various devices in a modern democracy such as laws and rules and regulations, judiciary etc. The fundamental principle in a democracy is that all persons holding authority derive it from the people; in other words, all public functionaries are trustees of the people. With the expansion of the role of government, public functionaries exercise considerable influence over the lives of people. The trusteeship relationship between the public and the officials requires that the authority entrusted to the officials be exercised in the best interest of the people or in 'public interest'.

The public service expresses high moral values. Any framework of ethical behaviour must include the following elements:

1. *Selflessness*: Holders of public office should take decisions solely in terms of public interest.
2. *Integrity*: Holders of public office should not place themselves under any financial or other obligation to outside individuals or organizations that might influence them in the performance of their official duties.
3. *Objectivity*: In carrying out public business, including making public appointments, awarding contracts or recommending

individuals for rewards and benefits, holders of public office should make choices on merit.

4. *Accountability*: Holders of public office are accountable for their decisions and actions to the public and must submit themselves to whatever scrutiny is appropriate to their office.
5. *Openness*: Holders of public office should be as open as possible about all the decisions and actions they take. They should give reasons for their decisions and restrict information only when the wider public interest clearly demands.
6. *Honesty*: Holders of public office have a duty to declare any private interests relating to their public duties and to take steps to resolve any conflicts arising in a way that protects the public interest.
7. *Leadership*: Holders of public office should promote and support these principles by leadership and example.

These principles of public life are of general applicability in every democracy. Arising out of such ethical principles a set of guidelines of public behaviour in the nature of a code of conduct becomes essential for public functionaries. Indeed any person who is privileged to guide the destiny of the people must not only be ethical but must be seen to practice these ethical values. Although all citizens are subject to the laws of the land, in the case of public servants there must be standards of behaviour more stringent than those for an ordinary citizen. It is at the interface of public action and private interest that the need arises for establishing not just a code of ethics but a code of conduct. A code of ethics would cover broad guiding principles of good behaviour and governance while a more specific code of conduct should, in a precise and unambiguous manner, stipulate a list of acceptable and unacceptable behaviour and action. (ARC: 2007)

Nani A. Palkhivala, said, "Civilization is an act of spirit. Ancient India was far more civilized than modern India with its satellites in space." Education has been called the technique of transmitting civilization. In order that it may transmit civilization, it has to perform two major functions: it must enlighten the understanding, and it must enrich the character.

We are as careless about public property as we are careful about our own property. Those who would not allow any trespass on their private estate are willing to contemplate, with total equanimity, encroachments of public property and destruction of public amenities. (Palkhivala: 1997)

Under the above circumstances, medical service providers cannot be expected to be strong enough to protect their human power from the influence of the polluted socio-political environment. Because any scientist if he is to be successful to render service to humanity must develop qualities of disciplined devotion and disinterestedness. He must possess tolerance, open-mindedness, freedom from prejudices and hospitality to new ideas. (Radhakrishnan: 1992) The Second Administrative Reforms Commission in the preface of the report very rightly expressed that the problem of corruption may be effectively dealt with ethical approach or by changing the heart of man not merely by rules and regulations. In any human society, it is ethics which is a set of standards for its functioning influencing the social behaviour and actions. It requires cultivation of the culture of integrity to be reflected in the day to day way of social life. The preface goes as:

"As human beings, our greatness lies not so much in being able to remake the world—that is the myth of the atomic age—as in being able to remake ourselves."

The Mahatma's vision of a strong and prosperous India—*Purna Swaraj*—can never become a reality if we do not address the issue of the stranglehold of corruption on our polity, economy and society in general.

Governance is admittedly the weak link in our quest for prosperity and equity. Elimination of corruption is not only a moral imperative but an economic necessity for a nation aspiring to catch up with the rest of the world. Improved governance in the form of non-expropriation, contract enforcement, and decrease in bureaucratic delays and corruption can raise the GDP growth rate significantly. The six perceived governance quality measures, each an aggregate of a number of sub-measures, are: voice and accountability; absence of political instability and violence; government effectiveness; reasonableness of the regulatory burden; the rule of law; and the absence of graft. Of these, the last two are the most directly significant in the context of ethical governance. 'Rule of law' measures whether crime is properly punished or not; enforceability of contracts; extent of black market; enforceable rights of property; extent of tax evasion; judiciary's independence; ability of business and people to challenge government action in courts etc. 'Absence of graft' measures relative absence of corruption among government, political and bureaucratic officials; of bribes related to securing of permits and licenses; of corruption in the judiciary; of corruption that scares off foreign investors.

There is a perception that the public services have remained largely exempt from the imposition of penalties due to the complicated procedures that have arisen out of the Constitutional guarantee against arbitrary and vindictive action. Those Constitutional safeguards have in practice shielded the guilty against the swift and certain punishment for abuse of public office for private gain. A major corollary has been the erosion of accountability. The huge body of jurisprudential precedents has crowded out the real intent of Article 311, and created a heap of roadblocks in reducing corruption. Such a provision is not available in any of the democratic countries including the UK. While the honest have to be protected, the dishonest seem to corner the full benefit of Article 311. Hence, there is need for a comprehensive examination of the entire corpus of administrative jurisprudence to rationalize and simplify the procedures. One of the indicators of lax enforcement is delay in sanctioning prosecution of a delinquent by the competent authority. Reference may be made to the Annual Report of the Central Vigilance Commission for the year 2004. Out of 153 cases for sanction, 21 cases were pending for more than 3 years, 26 cases between 2-3 years, 25 between 1-2 years. The departmental enquiries are soft-pedaled either out of patronage or misplaced compassion.

> "You must be the change you wish to see in the world," Mahatma Gandhi.

Integrity is much more than financial honesty. Public office should be treated as a trust. There are two facets to corruption: (1) the institution which is highly corrupt; (2) individuals who are highly corrupt. There is a need to work on public profiteering and also value to be attributed to the services rendered by officers. Interlocking accountability is a process by which evaluation could be done easily and accountability ensured.

Building trust and confidence requires an environment where there is a premium on transparency, openness, boldness, fairness and justice. We should encourage this.

Clearly, the absence of rules is not the problem. One cannot mandate honesty. The rule of law can only defeat the perverse mind. However, it cannot defeat the perversity of the heart. In the words of Aleksandr Solzhenitsyn: "The line separating good and evil passes not between states nor between classes… but through the middle of every human heart". We have no destinies other than those we forge ourselves. He who administers government by means of his virtues may be compared to the Pole star which keeps its place and all other stars turn towards it. When the ruler himself is right, the people naturally follow him in his right course. If governance is by men who are derelict, the governed will suffer. We have to keep in mind Plato's injunction:

"The punishment suffered by the wise who refuse to take part in government, is to suffer under the government of bad men".

Good governance must be founded on moral virtues ensuring stability and harmony. Confucius described righteousness as the foundation of good governance and peace. The art of good governance simply lies in making things right and putting them in their right place. Confucius's prescription for good governance is ideally suited for a country like India where many of our present-day players in governance do not adhere to any principle and ensure only their own interests.

Confucius emphasizes the righteousness for life and character building. This is in conformity with *Dharma* or righteousness as taught by all religions in the world and preached in Buddhism very predominantly in its fourth noble truth. He also emphasizes that man himself must become righteous and then only there shall be righteousness in the world. This is comparable with what Gandhiji said, "Be the change you wish to see in the world".

So, in the ultimate analysis, it is a question of ethics. Ethics is a set of standards that helps guide conduct. One of the problems is that the present codes of conduct are not direct and to the point. They are full of vague sermons that rarely indicate prohibitions directly. For formulating a code of ethics, it would be useful to keep in mind the advice of Napoleon who said, 'Law should be so succinct that it can be carried in the pocket of the coat and it should be so simple that it can be understood by a peasant'.

While it may not always be possible to establish the criminal offence of misappropriation in a court of law, the Government servant can still be removed from service for causing serious monetary loss to the State. An engineer may have deliberately permitted the construction of a defective irrigation dam or building. It may not be possible to get him convicted in court on charges of corruption but he could be removed from service on grounds of incompetence. A tax official may have connived to allow the leakage of revenue for return favours in the future. Such conduct may not provide the ingredients of a criminal offence but can lead to his exit from service.

The standard for probity in public life should be not only conviction in a criminal court but propriety as determined by suitable independent institutions specifically constituted for the purpose. We have broadly copied the British model of governance. Ministers in Tony Blair's government have had to resign on such minor improprieties as a telephone call to the concerned person to fast track the issue of a visa for the 'nanny' of the Minister's child or the grant of British citizenship to a generous contributor to a cause supported by the Government. Such principles were upheld and pronounced by Jawaharlal Nehru in the Mudgal case in which the said Lok Sabha Member was expelled by Parliament on 24th September, 1951 even when the Member volunteered to resign. The Mudgal case is often cited as the noblest example of the early leadership's efforts at setting high standards of conduct in parliamentary life.

We need to reverse the slide by prescribing stringent standards of probity in public life instead of providing shelter to public figures of suspect integrity behind the argument of their not having been convicted in a court. The standard should be one of not only the conduct of Caesar's wife but of Caesar himself.

The solution to the problem of corruption has to be more systemic than any other issue of governance. Merely shrinking the economic role of the state by resorting to deregulation, liberalization and privatization is not necessarily the solution to addressing the problem. Prevalent institutional arrangements have to be reviewed and changes made where those vested with power are made accountable, their functioning made more transparent and subjected to social audit with a view to minimize discretionary decisions. All procedures, laws and regulations that breed corruption and come in the way of efficient delivery system will have to be eliminated. The perverse system of incentives in public life, which makes corruption a high return low risk activity, need to be addressed. In this context, public example has to be made out of people convicted on corruption charge and the legal process in such cases has to be expedited. This hopefully, will also address the growing permissiveness in the society, in the more recent times, to the phenomenon of corruption. In addition, with changes in economic policy regime, regulatory bodies that guide and monitor the functioning of the relevant economic agents, lay down the rules of conduct in the interest of consumers and devise such practices that help in efficient functioning of the system, will have to be established in many sectors of the economy that are now being opened up. At the same time, social monitoring through empowered autonomous and credible structures will have to be established even for the highest of the public offices. Right to information has to be the starting point for some of these changes.

The focus should be on e-governance and systemic change. An honest system of governance will displace dishonest persons. As Gladstone so aptly said, "The purpose of a government is to make it easy for people to do good and difficult to do evil".

We always find alibi for our lapses by quoting trespass from other democratic institutions, by resorting to a blame game. The executive/ civil services blame interference by the political executive or legislatures and *vice versa*; legislators blame the judiciary and *vice versa*—the main problem lies in each one leaving space for others to occupy. If any of the democratic institutions leaves space, the mafia or extra-constitutional authority occupies that space. Realization of its own authority and discharging its sphere of responsibility, developing accountability and responsiveness are the real solutions to the conflicting situations of eroding democratic polity. I conclude by quoting an ancient *subhashit* (good message)—

> "Rivers do not drink their waters themselves, nor do trees eat their fruit, nor do the clouds eat the grains raised by them. The wealth of the noble is used solely for the benefit of others."

Ethics is a set of standards that society places on itself and which helps guide behaviour, choices and actions. The Commission is painfully aware that standards do not, by themselves, ensure ethical behaviour; that requires a robust culture of integrity. The crux of ethical behaviour does not lie in bold words and expressions enshrined as standards, but in their adoption in action, in sanctions against their violations, in putting in place competent disciplinary bodies to investigate allegations of violations and impose sanctions quickly and in promoting a culture of integrity. (ARC: 2007)

The Constitution and the laws and regulations formulated after independence of India provide enough devices to ensure accountability of the public servants. But what is necessary is the moral strength of a person to make these laws effective to achieve the goals of the nation. These are in addition to India's past cultural heritage and the ideals behind the long freedom struggle of the country under the leadership of Mahatma Gandhi. It is really surprising to experience that all these have failed to motivate our leaders at all levels and fronts to strengthen inner power or moral qualities in them. To-day it is noticed that nobody bothers to give a serious thought to the consequences of the appearance of moral-crisis in the country. The modern Indian is falling to have effective control over money power by human power. Instead of being accountable to the people, who are the taxpayers, the most service providers enter into debate by giving arguments in favour of their unethical activities, which shows the lack of sense of accountability on the part of the service providers to the human society. Dysfunctions of the social and educational institutions are also responsible to a great extent for this state of affairs.

References

Administrative Reforms Commission: Government of India constituted the Second Administrative Reforms Commission in August 2005 to prepare a detailed blueprint for revamping the public administration system. It consisted of the following members:

(i) Shri Veerappa Moily – Chairperson
(ii) Shri V. Ramachandran – Member
(iii) Dr. A.P. Mukherjee – Member
(iv) Dr. A.H. Kalro – Member
(v) Dr. Jayaprakash Narayan – Member
(vi) Smt. Vineeta Rai – Member-Secretary.

The Commission was asked to suggest measures to achieve a proactive, responsive, accountable, sustainable and efficient administration for the country at all levels of the government. The most significant aspect is 'ethics in governance'.

Deep Dogra, Km. Sandhya: 1980: Mahatma Gandhiji's Social Philosophy, *Journal of Gandhian Studies*: Vol. 7. No. 28, July, 1980; Institute of Gandhian Thought and Peace Studies, University of Allahabad.

Dubhasi, P.R.: *Public Accountability and Ethics*, *IJPA*; July-Sept; 1983, Vol. XXIX, No. 3.

Dwivedi, O.P. Presidential Address of O.P. Dwivedi on "Moral Dimensions of Statecraft: A Plea for an Administrative Theology" delivered in June 1987 to the Canadian Political Science Association, Hamilton, which is being recorded from *Canadian Journal of Political Science*, Vol. XX, No. 4. December 1987 published in the *Indian Journal of Public Administration*, October-December 1988; Vol. XXXIV, No. 4.

Dwivedi, O.P.: *Ethics and Accountability, IJPA*, July-Sept; 1983, Vol. XXIX, No. 3.

Ebenstein, W.: *Introduction to Political Philosophy.*

Iyer, V.R. Krishna. *Justice and Beyond*, Deep & Deep Publications, New Delhi, 1988.

Khanna, Dr. B.S., Asstt. Prof., IIPA, New Delhi, Morale in Public Services presented in the Conference on Morale in Public Services, held on 3-4 January 1959.

Prasad, Prof. Kali Paper; Morale in the Public services: A Social Psychological Analysis; *Ibid.*

Lambert Commission: In March 1979, Royal Commission on Financial Management and Accountability (also known as Lambert Commission) submitted its final report to Government of Canada. Published in *IJPA*, Special number on *Administrative Accountability*, July-September, 1983, Vol. XXIX, No. 3.

Raj, Dr. Hans (2001), *Principles of Public Administration*, Surjeet Publication; Delhi.

Maheswari, S.R., *Accountability in Public Administration: A Conceptual Analysis, IJPA*; July-Sept; 1983, Vol. XXIX, No. 3.

Mallay, N.N., Public Enterprises in India (1971): *The Control and Accountability*, Delhi: National.

Minocha, O.P., 'Accountability in Public Sector Enterprises', *IJPA*; July-Sept; 1983, Vol. XXIX, No. 3.

Mukhopadhyay, Ashok; *Administrative Accountability: A Conceptual Analysis*; *IJPA*; July-Sept. 1983, Vol. XXIX, No. 3.

Rowatt, D.C.: Ombudsman, 1964.

Ruthnaswamy, M. 1972, *Principles and Practice of Public Administration*: Central Book Depot, Allahabad.

EIGHT
Challenges to Medical Sciences

The healthcare system in India is making significant progress since independence. While appreciating the efforts made by the governments for improvement of healthcare system one cannot deny the role of the private healthcare system also in providing services to the ailing population in the country. At the same time it is felt that healthcare is increasingly unaffordable to average people in the country due to various reasons—high cost of treatment in the private sector, heavy rush in the public sector hospitals, shortage of service providers in rural areas, changes of values in the society and impact of globalization and privatization on the healthcare systems. India's Draft Sixth Plan (1978-83) pointed out some serious weaknesses of the healthcare system in India: (a) it has been borrowed from industrially advanced and consumer oriented societies; (b) it is divorced from social, economic and ecological factors, conditions of work, social stratification, etc.; (c) it is unrelated to such other issues as nutrition, water supply, dietary requirements and habits, food preservation practices etc.; (d) its health services have been concentrated mostly in urban areas and here too these services have been largely used by the affluent classes; (e) it is largely concentrated at one end, i.e. doctors and hospitals; (f) it is based on the medical education system which prepared doctors not for care of the health of the people but instead for medical practice that is unrelated to anything except disease and the technology dealing with it; (g) it has seriously undermined and at places destroyed whatever traditional methods of healthcare system that existed for centuries in this country; (h) it is based on the growing use of drugs instead of their avoidance by improving physical conditions of living and hence is largely influenced by the interests and the philosophy of the drug industry; (i) its educational base is divorced from the rest of the education system, particularly informal education etc. (Sethi: 1980)

In India emerging problems are air and water pollution, food security, lack of awareness about sanitation system, deforestation, lack of awareness of cooperation of the people to maintain cleanliness of the public places and civic sense. For example, a report of the Water Aid, an international organization working for water sanitation and hygiene based on the data from the Ministry of Urban Development (2013), census 2011 Pollution Control Board estimates that 75-80 per cent water pollution by volume is from domestic sewage, while untreated sewage flowing into water bodies including rivers have almost doubled in recent years. This in turn is leading to increasing burden of vector borne diseases, cholera, jaundice and diarrhea etc. Water pollution is found to be a major cause for nutritional standards and development in children also.

Indian social customs and traditions demand cleanliness of the household and the surroundings of the house since long. They used to filter water in their own traditional way. Keeping the kitchen clean and not to allow entry into it without clean cloths, not to enter the kitchen without bath etc. were common practices in the traditional societies. Nobody was allowed to enter into it with shoe and other things which are not clean. Thus the traditional way of preventing preventable harm to health was maintained at a cheapest cost and interestingly these were rooted in the social customs and tradition. Mahatma Gandhi repeatedly asserted to maintain cleanliness by adopting simple and cheap devices. What is needed to keep the house and the surrounding clean at a low cost without having financial burden is the development of habit and commitment to the social cause. Indian culture is also flooded with customs and traditions with cleanliness orientation even in the name of God and Goddesses. These are taught in the family itself by the elderly members through 'should' and 'should not' without explaining the reasons for it. To-day we are asserting it in different forms or in modified form with the explanation of the reasons behind it.

Religious leaders also advocate simple ways of maintaining cleanliness and several health related activities like restriction of movement of ailing persons from the household premises and their mix-up with others, including food habits in the name of God. These were related to prevention of infection associated with healthcare system.

However, gradually with the emergence of improved healthcare system with expert medical scientists and other trained personnel traditional system of healthcare based on social culture or traditions is withering away. Gradually, the problem is shifted to other areas of healthcare system. It is a serious challenge to both the service providers and the patients. The World Health Organization is making a global effort to meet this challenge faced by the healthcare system. The most significant one is the Prevention of Infection Associated with Healthcare programme launched by WHO. Fortunately, Gandhi's principles on this is coming back to the modern world with new effort across the world at the initiative of WHO. What the traditional Indian societies practised is reflected in their efforts. Now the problem is to motivate the modern man and woman to extend their cooperation towards the goal of WHO to save the world community.

***Prevention of Infection Associated with Healthcare*:** Prevention of infection associated with healthcare is a significant component of patient safety. In October 2004 World Health Organization launched a patient safety programme in response to a World Health Assembly Resolution of 2002 urging WHO and member states to pay the closest possible attention to the problem of patient safety.

The programme, WHO Patient safety, aims to coordinate, disseminate and accelerate improvements in patient safety worldwide. It also provides a vehicle for international collaboration and action between WHO Member States, WHO's Secretariat, technical experts, and consumers as well as professionals and industrialists.

What is Patient Safety? Patient safety is the absence of preventable harm to a patient during the process of healthcare. The discipline of patient safety is the coordinated efforts to prevent harm, caused by the process of healthcare itself, from occurring to patients.

(http://www.who.int/patientsafety/about/en/accessed on 7/8/2015)

It is said that every year, the treatment and care of hundreds of millions of patients world-wide is complicated by infections acquired during healthcare. As a result, some patients become more seriously ill than they would otherwise have been. Some have prolonged stays in hospital, some experience long-term disability and some die.

To-day perhaps World Health Organization, for the first time in the history of public health is making it possible to launch a powerful global response to tackle the infections that spread in healthcare settings world-wide.

The World Alliance for Patient Safety at the World Health Organization and its technical partners have developed low-cost strategies to address the global challenge. It selected 'Health Care-associated infection' for 2005-2006.

In this context Sir Liam Donaldson, Chairman of World Alliance for Patient Safety says,

> "It is fitting that the World Alliance for Patient Safety has selected healthcare associated infection as the topic for its first Global Patient Safety Challenge. These infections are a major patient safety concern. They affect hundreds of millions of people worldwide every year. Infections take their toll in terms of avoidable patient death and disability. They also waste scarce health-care resources. No country can claim to have solved the problem completely.
>
> Indeed, healthcare associated infection is growing as a problem. Patients are becoming more susceptible to infections because of more serious underlying illness. Poor compliance with hand hygiene by healthcare staff, lack of access to safe water, unclean instruments and environmental surface all contribute to the problem. The environment of patient care is also important. Factors such as understaffing, high levels of bed occupancy and transfer of patients, all create new risks of infection.
>
> The world has the knowledge and resources to dramatically reduce the impact of healthcare associated infection. What is needed is commitment and action at all levels, to ensure that every patient's right to the cleanest and safest care is achieved. We want every country, every hospital and every health clinic around the world to support the Global Patient Safety Challenge."

It is true that healthcare associated infection cannot be entirely eliminated. Nevertheless, several low-cost, simple and effective strategies have proven to be effective in reducing the burden of disease. Many healthcare facilities have succeeded in controlling the problem and decreasing the risks to patients. However, there is gap between the patient safety improvements that are currently possible and the improvements that are actually being made. The gap arises due to non-implementation of tools and interventions.

It also said that risks of infection are high in some parts of the world. In India also the risks are high due to lack of cooperation of the public, negligence and carelessness of service providers both within and outside the hospital system etc.

WHO has, however, addressed four major areas of healthcare associated infection areas:

(a) *Blood products and their use*: as regards the safety measures it has pointed out certain measures—promotion of optimal hand hygiene associated with the procedures for collection, processing and use of blood products;

(b) *Injection practices and immunization*: some significant safety measures are—promotion of optimal hand hygiene practices at time of injection and immunization, strengthening of high-level commitment within countries to use auto-disable syringes for immunization services, actions to ensure safe disposal of sharps as part of integrated management of waste within healthcare facilities;

(c) *Safe water, basic sanitation and waste management*: two significant safety measures are—ensuring access and water quality to support hygiene and hand hygiene in particular, at the level of healthcare facilities.

(d) *Clinical procedures, particularly in first-level emergency care*: significant safety measures are, specific education programmes for promoting safety in surgical procedures, tailored to the needs of healthcare facilities, surgical hand preparation using either antimicrobial soap and water or alcohol-based hand rum to reduce infections associated with surgical procedures, access to safe emergency and essential surgical care, including the availability and use of best practice protocols on clinical procedures and equipment.

(http://www.who.int/patientsafety/events/05GPSClawnchEnglish Final.pdf

To-day World Alliance for Patient Safety is making an effort to save lives with simple and cheap measures which were repeatedly asserted by any attempt to study the social behaviour, attitude and belief of the individuals within and outside the administrative world is not an easy task. Man is conscious of his behaviour and is expert in changing his behaviour depending on the situation. Further every man has at least the minimum capacity to judge what is good and what is bad in the context of the social situation. The behaviour of the people and their social relationship both are very complex problems. The most interesting point is that the different individuals express different views on the same behaviour and attitude and adopt subjective views on them. Experience says that the attitude, behaviour and belief of an individual are generally the products of the past experience which he acquired from his own life and the values and belief transmitted from his ancestors. At the same time, it must be said that an educated man and a member of cosmopolitan society of urban or industrial area and a man who is exposed to outside world due to high mobility from place to place may view the same situation differently from a man who is illiterate, a resident of village and less mobile. What is required is to make the people aware of this problem of infection associated with healthcare and encourage them to take active part to the programme successful in the greater interest of humanity.

Man has the capacity to adjust in the changing situation. Interestingly, while moving from traditional way of life to modern urban life he is compelled to modify his lifestyle. To-day people are giving priority to good health. If in his judgment the modification of behaviour is more beneficial to him and the family then he modifies it accordingly. (Denhradt: 1988)

Changes of Social Culture and Man's Adaptability: Fred W. Riggs is also well known for his contribution to the administrative philosophy. He made an effort to analyze the administrative culture with the help of ecological approach. He borrowed the term 'ecology' from biology, which means the study of life in its surroundings. Riggs had the strong belief that to study the behaviour of a particular administrative system one should have deep knowledge of the environment in which it operates, because the environment has a direct effect on its component system. The medical services cannot be an exception to it. (Maheswari: 1991)

The society changes adopting new behaviour or modifying old one as the environment demands. Here it may be noted that in the process of changes the members may not carry with them the social values needed for survival and promotion of the human society itself. All changes cannot be considered as reforms or direct the changes towards upward trend. In India experience shows that in the process of changes old well established ethical values are withering away. In the administration also ethical vacuity is taking place. The medical service providers, like other persons are also influenced by the changing socio-economic scenario of the country and abroad. To-day the standards, responsibilities of these services have become a core subject of discussion in the perspective of social changes brought by the progress of science and technology and dominance of economics on changes of the society. In India, however, serious effort has yet to be made for an in-depth study of the interrelationship between the society and the service system. It is very essential in the case of medical services as these have direct and immediate effect on human security. Since the medicine is both science and art and has commitment to service to humanity it cannot afford to have ethical vacuity in its functioning.

Under these circumstances if we make an attempt to analyze the ethical issues in the field of healthcare we will certainly be trapped by the multifaceted dilemmas facing serious irresolvable problems or issues.

Dr. Delon Human, Secretary General of World Medical Association, in his foreword to Medical Ethics Manual expressed that healthcare has given rise to extremely complex and multifaceted ethical dilemmas. All too often physicians are unprepared to manage these competently.

It is also stated in the Manual that since ethics deal with all aspects of human behaviour and decision-making, it is a very large and complex field of study with many branches and sub-divisions. Further with the efforts of the United Nations of Organization to make the nations aware of the need of human rights for full development of human personalities, involvement of nation states in the international agreements as signatories and the entrustment of responsibility to the nation state for the safeguard of these rights of their citizens, healthcare services are constrained by various kinds of ethical dilemmas. India occupies a unique position for the diversity in religion, language and culture. Different communities practice different moral or ethical principles. Naturally, healthcare service providers are facing serious challenges, confronting very often with the public or attendants of the patients on ethical issues or violation of human rights.

Again the advances in medical science and technology are pausing several questions about the relevance or utility of traditional medical ethics in India. The World Medical Association's Medical Ethics Manual is clear that the new issues arising out of progress of science and technology cannot be answered by traditional medical ethics. Examples are also cited here—assisted reproduction, genetics, health informatics and life-extending and enhancing technologies, all require the participation of physicians, have great potential for benefitting patients but also potential for harm depending on how they are put into practice.

Another problem referred in the manual is the Dual Loyalty. It says when physicians have responsibilities and are accountable both to patients and third party and when these responsibilities and accountabilities are incompatible, they find themselves in a situation of Dual Loyalty. Here the ethical challenge is to when and how to protect the patient in the face of pressures from third parties.

In 1995 seven advisers from a wide variety of health related professions met with a group of 30 staff members at WHO to discuss the ethical issues currently arising in health and international cooperation. The observations of the study group are as below:

> "Ethical questions related to health arise within a much wider debate, which concerns the societies we live in, what they are becoming and what we want them to become. Though some fundamental ethical issues are unique to the field of health, much of the current debate involves the application to health of basic questions raised by world trends such as—
>
> - Interdependence, action on a global scale, and respect for diversity;
> - Rising individualism and social disintegration;
> - Predominance of economic thinking;
> - Headlong pursuit of technological development;
> - Domination of science by technology and technology by money; and
> - Cultural domination globally by a small number of powerful peoples or groups.

Classical reference points such as the Hippocratic Oath no longer provide a sufficient rationale for specific medical practice, powers and responsibilities, because these have changed in virtually every aspect. In addition, most of the current problems of healthcare go beyond the realm of medicine. The "cosmetic" use of ethical language—to improve appearance rather than to guide decision-making—is a further source of difficulty, and sometimes genuine confusion."

Referring to the emergence of technological influence over the world of health the study group has said that experience has given the scope of increase of suspicion on the ability of technologies to solve all the problems and to satisfy the increased expectations of the people. What is needed to-day is to accept the responsibility by the individuals and the society to direct the development and use of technologies instead of submitting themselves to their expanded world. The gulf between expensive care for the few and the care affordable for all cause serious constraints on ethical issues, which demands cooperation of the non-medical persons to be extended to the medical authorities for resolving conflicting areas of ethics. To them quality of care must be evaluated on the basis of the human and therapeutic needs of the patient rather than, as is too often the case, on the novelty and sophistication of the technology. While doing so various economic, professional and personal interests have to be clearly identified and then prevented as far as possible from influencing the evaluation.

Distribution of society's resources and the promotion of access to healthcare for all are very complex and sensitive issues. Ethically, or even just logically, it is easy to say that healthcare for all is the better choice, but in practice it is constrained by market and other forces. In addition, the development of technologies has radical effects on attitudes, lifestyle and behaviour of men.

As regards the dominance of economics it is stated that the health status of populations is to a great extent determined by economic and social processes outside the medical sector, such as, standard of living, nutrition, education, water supply and sanitation. A number of related factors need to be analyzed and openly discussed, such as, the pressure of macroeconomic policies on health policies, the increasing intervention of financial agencies in the health field, the links between health services, technology and money, the need to rethink the organization and financing of health services in terms of societal choices etc. Here the first ethical demand is to avoid getting trapped, whether defensively or aggressively, within the confines of narrowly economic thinking.

Neither economic thinking nor medical thinking can encompass all of life, though they often claim to. This mutual questioning should offer, as the study team say, good opportunities for renewing the dialogue between WHO and organizations such as the World Trade Organization, UNDP and the World Bank.

It says, "in such a dialogue it will be important to get beyond simplistic concepts, both in the health field and in economics, such as 'public or private' health functioning. Traditional medicine, for instance, makes no such dichotomy, and approaches issues of sickness and health as an inextricable part of individual and social life. The same applies to criteria put forward by funding agencies when they get involved in health: "health costs", for example, cannot usefully be reduced to all-purpose principles such as, "user pays", as recent experience has shown. (World Health Forum: 1996)

In the contemporary Indian society the old ascriptive values have been replaced by achievement oriented values. The modern man has started thinking of personal benefit, convenience and comfort while valuing old tradition or culture transmitted to him by his forefathers. This act of a modern man is situational. The old traditional culture was highly honoured by a traditional man and the cultural unification was possible in the traditional society. Several reasons may be forwarded for it, such as, small size of the village society, simplicity of village life, professional integration, low mobility of the people, aspirations and needs of the villagers were few, lack of exposure to the outside world etc. But in the modern industrialized society with the impact of science and technology and exposure to the outside world cultural unification has been distorted. Diversity of educational and professional background and high mobility compel men to adjust with the professional demands and educational background has given them scope to have fresh look to the old tradition and social values. As a result in the same community or society change of values has become inevitable. For example the nature of family in India changes from joint family to nuclear family system. Both the systems have strengths and weaknesses. But modern Indians give more value to nuclear family system. This system causes great inconvenience to the working parents, children are deprived of due parental care and the socialization process is dominated by e-media. The adverse effect of it is also experienced by the existing society. Various kinds of social ailment like mutual suspicion, adoption of unwelcome behaviour by the youths, heavy influence of peer groups leading to drug addiction and alcoholism, cheating, exploitation etc. are coming to surface. Human culture of traditional Indian society enters into conflicting situation. Imitation of superficial habits, domination of money and muscle power, hypocrisy, multi-standard of life etc. are the major factors which are compelling the modern society to move clumsily. Here, however, one cannot deny that the human culture is dynamic and changeable, but these must sustain their upward trend. It is the man's responsibility to guard the sustainable development of human society. His eyes should not be confined to the nature of the problem only they must move beyond it. Here begins the complexity of identification of ideal way of living in the changing world. In a developing country like India generally people get confused to judge what is good and what is bad.

The progress of science and technology, influencing the lives of the people in India, has made the traditional or agricultural society to move from this stage towards modernized or industrialized society. It invites the State to be dynamic and to undertake developmental programmes in addition to welfare measures. Further India was under the British rule for a long time and the administration of the country adopted British administrative culture. Mahatma Gandhi with active participation of leading personalities of India could make the country free from British rule after a long struggle. The sacrifice of general masses during movement and the efforts of social reformers to eradicate social ailments are also noteworthy. The framers of the Constitution of India made an effort to formulate a Constitution to make India strong within the framework of democracy. Gandhi expressed clearly that democracy was not merely a political concept, it was a way of life. He reaffirmed the deep faith of ancient India on human culture prevalent during that time, which underlined human dignity and human strength. In independent India old values change in the face of transformation of the society. While studying the ethical and moral values in the changing Indian society differences in opinion, attitude and behaviour of the scholars are visible creating confusion in the minds of the people.

The administrative culture (authoritarian, democratic) is a sub-culture derived mostly from society. This may be a major factor for absence of ethical theory of administration. In India, with cultural diversity it is appearing as a herculean task, though not impossible one. Because administrative culture consists of values, orientations, beliefs, dispositions etc. which are, again, rooted in the social culture. Culture is manmade and it is culture which helps an environment for social and individual security. This can be traced from the dawn of human civilization. It is the continuity of culture which helps progress of mankind. It is a social network to unite different groups of people together both vertically and horizontally. Lack of transmission of the social tradition from the old generation to new generation would have compelled the new generation to start the process establishing tradition and culture from zero and in such a situation one cannot expect human progress. Device of family life, discovery of fire, invention of wheel, practice of cultivation etc. though in the rudimentary form were the gifts of old generations or our ancestors. The ethical principles can be traced from the religion which helped development of human personality in the ancient time itself. A modern man while searching for his relevance in the days of science and technology, naturally faces conflicting situation. Human culture always gives weightage to human security and it is a normative science which reflects values. The values are abstract while norms are nothing but principles or guidelines for social life. Here is the significance of ethical principles in each and every social organization. These do not stand on the way of expertise in any service rather help bringing it close to the people who are in need of the expert service.

***Nature of Medicine*:** Since medicine is both science and art. Science deals with what can be observed and measured and a competent physician recognizes the signs of illness and disease and knows how to restore good health. But the scientific medicine has its limits, particularly in regard to human individuality, culture, religion, freedom, rights and responsibilities. The art of medicine involves the application of medical science and technology to individual patients, families and communities, no two of which are identical. By far the major part of differences among individuals, families and communities is non-physiological and it is in recognizing and dealing with the differences that arts, humanities and social sciences, along with ethics, play a major role. Indeed, ethics itself is enriched by the insights and data of other disciplines.

www.wma.net/en/30th publications/30 ethics manual/pdf/ thics_manual_en.pdf)

The contemporary Indian society, like any other society, is dependent to a great extent on scientific knowledge and its technological applications, such as, aircraft, antibiotics, computers, automobiles, telecommunication etc. Robertson, in his book "Sociology" has stated the distinction between science and technology in a simple way. He points out that very often it is noticed that the terms 'science' and 'technology' are used as synonyms in common talks. But both are distinct phenomena. Science refers to the logical, systematic methods by which knowledge of nature is obtained and to the actual knowledge accumulated by these methods. Technology, on the other hand, refers to the practical applications of knowledge about the nature. The goals of science and technology are also not same. Science is concerned with the pursuit of knowledge about nature; technology is concerned with the application of knowledge of nature to some use. Even the primitive people used techniques of making bows and arrow, fire etc. through the trial-and-error methods without the knowledge of principles or reasons of the simple technology. Scientific knowledge requires a logical, systematic understanding of the principles that underlie natural events. A scientific understanding of the world is, however, necessary for an advanced technology. Both are very closely related.

The object of scientific inquiry is innovation, the discovery of new knowledge. This innovation does not occur on random basis. Science is not just the creation of a few curious and inquiring individuals. It is a social institution that is subject to the influence of social forces, both within and outside the scientific community. These social forces strongly affect both the rate and the direction of scientific innovation.

Robertson refers the norms of science as advocated by Robert Merton, who identified four principal norms that constitute the "moral imperatives" of science—Universalism, communalism, disinterestedness, and organized skepticism.

Universalism: Robert Merton emphasized the universal nature of the scientific enterprise and its findings. The particular characteristics of individual scientists—such as their race, class, or national origin—are irrelevant to the validity of their work. Research findings must be evaluated purely in terms of their scientific worth.

Communalism: Communalism is the principle which means that scientific knowledge should not be the personal property of the discoverer. It should be made available instead to the entire scientific community. All science rests on a shared heritage of past discoveries, and no individual can claim property rights over the outcome of research. However, Merton has said that a few scientists may be fortunate enough to have their discoveries after their names, such as, Salk Vaccine, Einstein's theory of relativity, Darwin's theory of evolution etc.

Disinterestedness: Under this principle the scientists are required to be free from selfish interest in their professional roles. However, the scientists may legitimately hope that their work will be recognized and praised by the scientific community. But the recognition should be sufficient reward, and the scientist's main aim should be to contribute to the sum of scientific knowledge. In the scientific community the dishonest manipulation of data or any other fraudulent practice is intolerable.

Organized Skepticism: It refers to the expectation that scientists will suspend judgment until the facts are at hand. No theory, however ancient and respected or new and revolutionary, can be uncritically accepted. There are no sacred areas in science that should not be critically investigated, even if political or religious dogma forbids it. (Robertson: 1977)

This is expressed clearly by "Medical Ethics Manual" published by World Medical Association, which nobody can deny. In addition to significant role of different non-physiological disciplines in medical sciences it has also been realized that with the emergence of big hospitals entertaining huge number of ailing population of a country, the administrative systems and processes have also become very important part of medical sciences. The administrative ethics may flow from three sources—first, the profession itself articulates and upholds certain norms; second, norms laid down by the civil service rules and regulations; and third, personal beliefs and values which are highly individualized but which are reflected in the behaviour, decisions and actions of the public servants.

Human beings unlike other animals, are not born with complex, 'wired-in' behaviour patterns that enable them to survive in specific environments. Instead they must learn and invent ways of adapting to many different environments, ranging from arctic snows to desert wastelands and teeming cities. These learned ways of life, which are modified and passed on from one generation to the next, what sociologists call "culture". An understanding of culture is basic to the understanding of human social life, which again is a very difficult task. (Robertson: 1980)

Medical service constitutes a significant component of administration. Further this service is unique in nature and relationship with the ailing or suffering population of a country. Its activism has direct and immediate impact on life and death of the patient. It has to be within the framework of ethical code in order to be committed to human values and human dignity. Here also one has to admit the existence of diversity of beliefs, attitude and behaviour of the physicians and other medical service providers. The issue of expertise vs. moral principles is still a subject of debate in some cases. It is true that both are different from one another but one cannot replace the other. They must go together by clearing the clouds of discomfort arising on the way to destination.

Religion: Religion is a major component of the culture of a human society. In this context India occupies a unique position due to existence of diversity of religion and culture. With the changes in Gandhi's concept of religion is different from that of common masses. To him religion was not a dogma; not a doctrinal faith like Hinduism, Islam or Christianity. His concept of God was not in terms of Shiva, Brahma or Christ or Allah. It was mysterious power that pervades everything. To him God and religion are manifested ultimately in Truth and Non-violence. His religion is a religion of service and a practical idealism. Through applicability of religion in terms of truth and non-violence Gandhi indicated the significance of *means*. To thinkers like Machiavelli, Kautilya and others *ends* justified the *means*. To Gandhi *means* and *ends* were convertible terms, both are equally important.

It is a unique way of resisting all that is evil, unjust, impure and untrue and resolving all maladjustment in human relations by love and voluntary suffering and by an appeal to, "divine spark in the opponent soul." It is an expression of purest *ahimsa* and it precludes hatred, anger, deception and untruth. To Gandhi *Satyagraha* is a love force or soul force. (Chandra Sekhar Buggi: 1978)

When the insights into truth is gained, passions are subdued, ill-will subdues and inward conflict ceases, it becomes a fire which cleanses the earth. It can be released only if we end our narrow egoism, greed, anger, hatred, all the restricting appetites and passions which keep the individual locked up inside his mortal self. But experience in the contemporary society reveals that most people (even educated men) are failing to safeguard their human personalities from the grab of greed, egoism, revengeful attitude etc. Very often it is experienced that the people while visiting religious temples or offering prayer to God or Goddesses regularly lead their lives with untruth, unethical code, *himsa* and inhumanity instead of allowing their lives to be led by core components of religion—truth, *ahimsa* and humanity. The concept of religion is degenerated to that of rituals. Further on the basis of religions conflicts between two groups of people, politicization of religious activities/faith, divorce of ethical codes from the religious faith etc. are taking place in the contemporary society.

Radhakrishnan said, "Recent developments have given rise to the erroneous impression that while the West is scientific in outlook, the East is spiritually minded. The one is rational while the other is religious. The one is dynamic and perpetually changing while the other is static and unchanging. If we take a long view we find that China and India made fundamental contributions to science and technology till three or four hundred years ago and that there have been illustrious examples or religious idealism and sanctity in the West. The more we understand each other the more we feel that we are like one another. East and West do not represent two different types of consciousness or modes of thought.

Science and religion are aspects of every culture. The rational and spiritual are, two strands inextricably woven in human nature, though in varied patterns. One or the other may be more prominent in different periods of human history."

The purpose of religion is to help us to discipline our whole being, body, mind and will. By prayer, meditation and self-control we integrate our personality.

Progress is not inevitable, raising human generation to new heights of wisdom and virtue. Man is capable of evil as he is capable of good.

The test of true faith is the extent to which it transforms the individual and social order. It must illuminate the dark places of our social life and religious practices. The *Rg Veda* says that the human race is one. All men are brothers. All religions teach that human being is of infinite worth and deserves respect and loving kindness, especially the unfortunate ones. Those who bear the deepest wounds require our greatest sympathy.

The Code of Conduct is called *Dharma*. The institutions and practices that lead to the disintegration of society require scrapped, however venerable their antiquity may be. The spiritual legacy of the past should be distinguished from dead encumbrance. (Radhakrishnan: 1970)

In the similar language Dan Brown, American author said, " all world religions have at their core the same human truth: creation is better than destruction. Love is better than hate."

(http://timesofindia.indiatimes.com/india/Science-and-religion-are-partners-Dan-Brown/articleshow/45103428.cmc)

Gradually, man has failed to make a distinction between greed and need, between human power and money and muscle power, service and exploitation. Religion fails to make a modern man religious or in the true sense by practicing *dharma*.

In this context I am tempted to refer what I am experiencing in Assam, my home state. In Assam a traditional village worked essentially as a democratic institution based on social customs and traditions. It had the authority over every aspect of village life in Assam. It was the privilege of the village elder to occupy the position of leadership and importance. The village was the unit by itself, self-contained, self-regulated and self-reliant in the socio-economic functions. The whole village administration was monitored by the village headman and the religious leader. There are even to-day *Sattras* in the biggest river island, viz., Majuli, such as *Auniati, Dakhipat*, *Garamur*, *Kamalabari* and *Bengenaati*. These *Sattras* worked as very strong federations of villages of Assam commanding mainly religious loyalty and played an important role in the social life of the people. They could maintain unity and integrity among the people of their fold living in different parts of the state of Assam.

The *Namghar*, the prayer house provided the villagers with common platform for free and frank discussions, covering their socio-economic life along with the religious life. A village assembly meeting at the *Namghar* delivered inviolable judgments. There existed a code of morality, humanism and selflessness. It was common among the villagers to help the helpless people, and to extend cooperation to anybody during distress. They observed army like discipline even in the normal situation. They used to work like one man in all walks of life, they move together for cultivation, for fishing, for feast and funeral. Thus among the villagers, the enviable spirit of unity, discipline and social consciousness was practiced. But now the very spirit of democratic society has been destroyed in the process of transformation of social life from traditional to modernity. (Hazarika: 2005)

History of Healthcare System in India: The beginning of healthcare system is accompanied by confusions and controversies. These are reflected in the indigenous *vs.* western systems of medicine, languages used by different Indian communities and foreign language used by the British rulers, western and eastern systems of administration, roles played by Sanskrit college and Madrassas. These are noticed in the origin and evolution of healthcare facilities in the country itself. Let us have look to the evolution of medical services during the British rule in India.

The spread of epidemic in India in the middle of nineteenth century induced the Government to take the trouble of making investigation into the causes of epidemics in the country. The instructions issued by the International Sanitary Congress held at Constantinople in 1867 might provide the scope for it. The Congress pointed out three basic factors for the spread of epidemics as below:

- India was the birthplace of cholera and its permanent home.
- Since 1817 India had been the focus from which the disease had radiated in every direction.
- Indian pilgrims were the most powerful of all the causes which tended to the propagation of epidemics.

Man tainted with cholera was himself the principal agent in propagating the disease. The Bengal Sanitary Commission issued detailed rules for checking cholera epidemic and stressed that without people's cooperation generally it was difficult to check its ravages. It said, "It is only by arousing the people to a sense of preventable nature of great part of the sickness and mortality which prevailed amongst them, and by enlisting their active cooperation that we can ever hope to make such impression on the vast extent of the country concerned." In course of time, the Sanitary Commissions and Boards of Health could secure the support of a sympathetic and instructed public opinion. The sanitary measures in the cantonments were improved. Dr. Macnamara issued reports on water analysis in Delhi and the Bengal Presidency and on the basis of it the Government emphasized the importance of water analysis at different cantonments. It was stated, "the importance of unremitting watchfulness and care to preserve the drinking water in a state of purity, in a country in which the wells are so exposed to contamination owing to the habits of the people, can scarcely be overrated."

The Government then proceeded to organize sanitary supervision in the towns and districts under the jurisdiction of the civil authorities. On 5th September, 1864, Strachey, the President of the Cholera Commission proposed a scheme of sanitary supervision in towns and districts. The important features of the scheme are:

- The appointment of Health Officer for each district.

- The appointment of District Board of Health consisting of the principal civil, military and medical officers of the district.
- A Principal Officer of Health for the Province.
- Establishment of Municipal Committees in civil stations for carrying out the municipal and sanitary services of the locality.

The Government of India suggested that the Sanitary Commissions should devote their attention exclusively to the sanitation of cantonments, while for the civil population in general, new Sanitary Inspector Generals should be appointed who should supervise the sanitary work of the Civil Surgeons, who should act as District Health Officers. The suggestion of the Government of India was accepted by the Secretary of State for India on 29th November, 1878. Accordingly, Malleson, the Bengal Sanitary Commissioner prepared rules for the guidance of local governments in application of measures of sanitation." (Dharm Pal: 1952)

In early 1920s, people of India realized the need of the development of medical sciences. The Hindu physicians made an attempt to find ways and means to improve the science of medicine and to mobilize public opinion in its favour. With this aim in view the All India Ayurvedic Conference was held which was attended by the physicians from different parts of India and Ceylon. The conference was successful in attracting the attention of the Government regarding the need of improvement of medical science.

In Bengal an Ayurvedic Committee was constituted in August 1921 and submitted its report in 1925. It resulted establishment of three Ayurvedic colleges in Bengal and one Ayurvedic Medical college with hospital at Jaffna in Ceylon. The Bengal Government studied the issue of development of medical sciences in a comprehensive way through the committee. Dr. M.N. Banerji, B.A., M.R.C.S. (Eng), I.S.A. (London), was its President. R.N. Chopra, Major, I.M.S., was the Secretary, of the Ayurvedic Committee. They prepared a questionnaire and circulated it amongst the physicians and others to know their views on the matter.

In a reply to the letter with R.N. Chopra, Major, I.M.S., Secretary, the Ayurvedic Committee was Constituted by the Government of Bengal in 1923. Dr. Girindra Nath Mukherjee, B.A., M.D., F.A.S.B. stated many reform proposals for the development of Ayurvedic treatment in India indicating the state of the science of medicine in the country.

Mukherjee referred a statement of Dr. Buchanan, as quoted by Montgomery in his work, "The History, Antiquities, Topography and Statistics of Eastern India, 1807" as regards the province of Behar:

"Medicine is taught by several of Pandits, some of whom also, although they are grammarians, practice the art". Besides the Professors of Medicine, about 700 families of Brahmins, almost all of Sakadwipa, practice the art, and are the only Hindu physicians who possess anything like science, except three of the medical tribes from Bengal, who have settled at Patna. "The traditional system of training of Kabirajes which has lasted for many centuries in Bengal, has always been exclusively literary in character. The Vaidyas learn their medical science mainly from books and from oral tradition from the *Gurus*—the learned physicians of the time, who generally taught a number of students without fees. Similar practice still exists in the Tols".

In 1811 Lord Minto recommended the establishment of Colleges at Nadia and Trihut with a view to the restoration of indigenous learning in Bengal under the management and control of the Government. The East India Act of 1813 authorized the Governor General in Council to set apart a sum of not less than one lac of rupees from the public revenue and spend it for the revival and improvement of Sanskrit literature and to the introduction and promotion of knowledge of European sciences amongst the people of the country. The Court of Directors pointed out that the Sanskrit language contained many excellent treatises on ethics, medicinal plants and drugs, astronomy and mathematics; and they ordered that steps should be taken to induce the people to adopt modern improvements in sciences. The Court directed the Governor General to submit proposals to give effect to the principles laid down. The Sanskrit college was opened on the first day of January 1824. This year may be considered as a landmark in the history of education in India. The Calcutta Madrassa (1781) and the Hindu College (1817) had already been founded but at the personal expenses of Warren Hastings and by public subscriptions respectively. The establishment of this College marked the first definite recognition of the East India Company of its responsibility for the education of the people. The purpose of the Institution was laid down in the famous Resolution of Government dated 21st August, 1821: "The Committee will bear in mind that the immediate object of the institution is the cultivation of Hindu literature. Yet it is in the judgment of his Lordship in Council a purpose of deeper interest to seek every practicable means of effecting the gradual diffusion of European knowledge." In this college, the "General Committee" decided to impart knowledge of medical science—European and Indian—to the student of Sanskrit College. In 1826, Dr. Tytler started educating the students on Medicine according to Western method, and Professors were appointed to teach Caraka, Susruta,

Bhava Prakasa, etc. Classes for the Ayurvedic students were opened in 1827. The classes were well attended. Pandit Madhusudan Gupta was a student of this class and learned the science according to both systems. He became one of the Professors in the college. His students handled bones and dissected animals. We quote the words of Professor Wilson, the Oriental scholar, who examined the students of the medical class: "The triumph gained over native prejudices is nowhere more remarkable than in the class, in which not only are the bones of the human skeleton handled without reluctance but in some instances dissection of the soft parts of the animals performed by the students themselves." In 1831, Dr. J. Grant began his lecture on Anatomy and Physiology, Diagnosis and Surgery.

In 1833, Lord William Bentinck, the then Governor General of India, appointed a committee for the revision of the whole question of medical education in Bengal.

The committee comprised the following gentlemen:

Surgeon J. Grant, Apothecary General.
J.C.C. Sutherland, Esq., Secretary of the Education Committee.
C.G. Trevelyan, Esq., Deputy Secretary, Political Department.
Assistant Spens, Body Guard.
Assistant Surgeon Bramley, Marine Surgeon.
Baboo Ramcomal Sen.

In 1834, the Secretary of the General Committee requested Dr. Tytler about his opinion as to the advisability of adopting English as the medium of instruction, of teaching the students books on European medical science only, and of abolishing the Ayurvedic classes, as many doctors were of opinion that the students should be taught according to a definite system of medical study. Dr. Tytler was for the continuance of the system in vogue, i.e., European and Ayurvedic systems. The Committee worked for twelve months. Rev. Dr. Grant was its President. It was decided that English should be the medium of instruction, and medical classes in Sanskrit College and the Madrassa should be abolished. The final decision of the committee was submitted to the Government in an elaborate Report on the 20th October, 1834.

Dr. Tytler was better known to the public for his correspondence with Raja Ram Mohun Roy, occasioned by a passage in a letter of the Doctor, published in the *Bengal Hurkara* of the 30th May, 1823, regarding the doctrine of Divine Incarnation. It appears that the Doctor was completely silenced by the renowned Raja, under the pseudonym of Ram Dass.

By the famous Minute of the 2nd February, 1835, Lord Macaulay won the definite victory of the Western School over Orientalists. Rev. Dr. Duff and his Anglicist party decided that English should be medium of instruction, against Dr. Tytler, the Superintendent of the "Native Medical Institution", which was founded by Government in 1832, and in which it was found practicable to teach Bengali students the modern science of medicine through the medium of the Bengali language.

Medical College of Bengal was established on the 20th February, 1835, with Dr. Bramley as the Superintendent and H. Goodeve as his assistant. The Government ordered on the 28th January, 1835 abolition of the Native Medical Institution and the medical classes in the Sanskrit College and the Madrassa. Pandit Madhusudan was transferred to the new college and had two assistants assigned to him. The question of dissection of the human body was found to be a stumbling block to the progress of the students in Anatomy, and Pandit showed his manly courage in defying the time-honoured prejudices of the countrymen by his dissection of the cadaver on the 30th January, 1836. This date marks a new era in the history of Western education in India. However, it may be mentioned that opinions differ on this date.

The study of the Ayurveda gradually came to an end with the establishment of the Medical College, where European medicine began to be studied with enthusiasm. No attempt has been made by the Government since then to revive the study of the Indian medical sciences. The torch of teaching Indian medical sciences had been kept burning by the zeal and the scientific spirit of the poor physicians without any help from the State. The scientific men in the Indian Medical Service, trained in the most up-to-date methods of the West, naturally thought the study of the medical sciences of the Hindus was mere waste of time, and the *Kabirajes*, confident of getting no encouragement from a foreign Government, kept themselves aloof from the modern scientific world; even they looked with a suspicious eye towards any interference by the State in the shape of improvement in the various branches of the science.

As regards the importance of Ayurveda it is found that the methods of treatment according to the Ayurveda were called empirical. But the so-called empirical methods of treatment were founded on experiments, observations and treatment which extended over many centuries. Even some of these observations have been declared by competent authorities to be reliable. Here mention may be made of our indebtedness to the indigenous system: the use of the salt-free diet in the treatment of cholera, liquid food in typhoid fever, in which even milk is withheld, cooling regimen in small-pox and measles as advocated by Sydenham, the importance of bael and kurchi in dysentery, the use of preparations of mercury, iron and arsenic internally, use of neem and chalmugra oil in leprosy, musk and makaradhwaja as stimulant, and other medicaments too numerous to mention. In the fields of surgery, obstetrics, pathology, and hygiene, we come across observations, which if known earlier, would have saved the labour of scientific men to an appreciable extent. The use of various cooling oils in the treatment of nervous disorders should be scientifically investigated, as there is a deep rooted belief in the Indian minds that we scarcely posses any curative agents which are equally efficacious.

It may be mentioned that all sections of the Hindu community take advantage of the Ayurvedic system of treatment. The Hindu widows, as a rule, prefer the indigenous medicines and object to taking medicines imported from the West. The old men and patients suffering from chronic diseases show a decided bias towards the medicines prepared by the *Vaids*. The Bengali Muslims also use medicines prescribed by the *Kabirajes*. The educated Indians firmly believe that the indigenous medicines which are generally freshly prepared act better on the constitution of the native population than the medicaments of the British Pharmacopoeia from Europe (Mukhopadhyaya: 1978).

The term "traditional medicine" refers to ways of protecting and restoring health that existed before the arrival of modern medicine. As the term implies, these approaches to health belong to the traditions of each country, and have been handed over down from generation to generation. Traditional systems generally have had to meet the needs of the local communities for many centuries. China and India, for example, have developed very sophisticated systems such as acupuncture and Ayurvedic medicine. In practice, the term "traditional medicine" refers to the following components: acupuncture, traditional birth attendants, mental healers and herbal medicine.

Over the years, the World Health Assembly has adopted a number of resolutions drawing attention to the fact that the most of the populations in various developing countries around the world depends on traditional medicine for primary healthcare, that the workforce represented by practitioners of traditional medicine is a potentially important resource for the healthcare and that medicinal plants are of importance to the health of individual communities (www.who.int/inf-fs/en/fact 134.html).

Through the Traditional Medicine Programme, the World Health Organization supports Member States in their efforts to formulate national policies on traditional medicine including evaluation of practices and examination of the safety and efficacy of remedies, to upgrade the knowledge of traditional and modern health practitioners, as well as to educate and inform the general public about proven traditional health practices.

WHO is working closely with 19 collaborating Centers in ten countries (Belgium, China, Democratic Republic of Korea, Italy, Japan, Republic of Korea, Romania, Sudan, United States of America and Vietnam).

A genuine interest in various traditional practices now exists among practitioners of modern medicine and growing numbers of practitioners of traditional, indigenous or alternative systems are beginning to accept and use some of the modern technology. This will foster teamwork among all categories of health workers within the framework of primary healthcare. The reasons for inclusion of traditional healers in primary healthcare are manifold: the healers know the socio-cultural background of the people; they are highly respected and experienced in work; economic considerations; distances to be covered in some countries; the strength of traditional beliefs; the shortage of health professionals, particularly in rural areas, to name just a few.

A large proportion of the population in a number of developing countries still herbalists and bone-setters and on local medicinal plants to satisfy their primary healthcare needs. WHO estimates the traditional birth attendants assist in up to 95 per cent of all rural births and 70 per cent of urban births in developing countries.

Traditional medicine has maintained its popularity in a number of countries of Asian countries, such as China, India, Japan and Pakistan. In China, for example, traditional medicines (herbal preparations) account for 30 per cent to 50 per cent of the total medicinal consumption. In 1993, the total sales of herbal medicines amounted to more than US$ 2.5 billion. In Japan, from 1974 to 1989, there was a 15-fold increase in Kampoh ("Chinese method") medicinal preparations in comparison with only 2.6 fold increase in the sales of mainstream pharmaceutical products. The Japanese per capita consumption of herbal medicine appears to be the highest in the world.

Recently, there has also been a growing interest in traditional and alternative systems of medicine in many developed countries. One-third of American adults have used alternative treatment and 60 per cent of the public in the Netherlands and Belgium, and 74 per cent in the United Kingdom are in favour of complementary medicine being available within the framework of the National Health Service. A survey among Member States of the European Union in 1991, identified about 1400 herbal drugs used in the European Economic Community.

Medicinal plants are the oldest known healthcare products. Their importance is still growing although it varies depending on the ethnological, medical and historical background of each country. Medicinal plants are also important for pharmacological research and drug development, not only when plant constituents are used directly as therapeutic agents, but also when they are used as basic materials for the synthesis of drugs or as models for pharmacologically active compounds.

Legislative controls in respect of medicinal plants have not evolved around a structured control model. There are different ways in which countries define medicinal plants or herbs. As a result, different approaches have been adopted with regard to licensing, dispensing, manufacturing and trading in order to ensure the safety, quality, and efficacy of medicinal plant preparations.

Herbal medicines are assuming greater importance in the primary healthcare of individuals and communities in many developing countries and there has been an increase in international trade in herbal medicines market is not adequately regulated, and the products are therefore unregistered and often not controlled by regulatory bodies. The establishment of regulation and registration procedures has become a major concern in both developed and developing countries.

WHO has compiled a list of medicinal plants which are widely used in primary healthcare. In July 1996, a WHO scientific group involving 100 experts from various countries around the world adopted the list which includes 28 monographs of 28 medicinal plants originally prepared by the WHO Collaborating Center for Traditional Medicine in Chicago, Illinois, United States of America. www.who.int/inf-fs/en/fact 134.html

There are several areas of conflict between the modern system of medicine and the traditional or indigenous system which are yet to be resolved to command confidence of the people.

Change of Values: The change of values can be understood from the process of transformation of the Indian society from traditional to modernization. The values which prevailed in the traditional society or agricultural society were different from those of modern or contemporary Indian society. Similar is the case with regard to the services provided to the society in both the public and private sectors. Several factors contribute to the change of values—laws of the country, developmental programmes undertaken by the governments, spread of education, progress of science and technology etc. are worth mentioning. In the process of transformation new values are learned and adopted, old ones are abandoned or changed.

The Organizations themselves are potent social and cultural systems. The impact of an organization on its members cannot be rooted out. Because it itself is a human society. The members may change their old values or ideals through exchange of ideas, interchange of opinions and clash of personalities with colleagues and other organizational personnel. (Nigro and Nigro: 1989).

A man from the childhood to adulthood and also during the span of service life gets enough scope to change or modify or replace old values by new ones. Average people go on changing the values they adopted at the childhood or prescriptive values and move towards achievement oriented values. While doing so they may fail to judge what is to be continued and what is to be abandoned. In a developing country it is noticed that average people change the way of living, behaviour etc. through imitation and in some cases due to marketers' motivating compulsion through skillful advertisement for new products. In the process of social transformation many new elements are absorbed by the Indian culture. All changes or entry of new elements into the culture may not contribute to the advancement of human culture in the country. Further, it is experienced that there are contradictions in the values adhered by different individuals or families and communities. In addition, same individual may change his values as he grows up or exposes himself to different situations. So, it is found that though the family plays a pivotal role in socializing the children, the role of school and the profession and the organization in which an individual works is not at all negligible. Family is not the only organization to learn ethical values, the school, service organizations etc. also provide significant platforms to learn ethical values. However, it cannot be denied that the family is a very strong institution where individuals learn ethical values and parents are the chief inculcators of these values in the minds of their children. The codification of ethical behaviour does not necessarily mean that all public servants invariably conduct themselves according to the rules and regulations. The practice of ethics, by any group necessarily depends upon several variables. The civil service is a sub-system and if there is no reinforcing or supportive structure of values in other sub-systems its own articulation would be discovered to be wanting. It would be too naïve to believe that only civil servants are to be cast in the heroic mold while other groups in the society remain under no restrictions whatever.

Ethical behaviour is indivisible, and it may be too much to expect high standards of conduct on the part of the civil servants when the political leadership itself lacks commitment to integrity in public life and public opinion is tolerant of assaults on integrity. The ethical behaviour codified in the rules and manuals are themselves too austere and have become largely inoperable in a society torn as it is by a revolution of rising expectations based on consumeristic culture. (Maheswari: 1994)

The sources of administrative ethics are also very close to the non-rational approach to medical ethics. World Medical Association has made it clear that non-rational approach does not mean irrational approach. Unlike rational approach it is not systematic and no reflective use of reason in favour of a decision. Following are the significant features of non-rational approach to medical ethics:

- **Obedience:** Obedience is a common way of making ethical decisions, especially by children and those working within authoritarian structures. Morality consists in following the rules or instructions of those authority, whether or not one agrees with them.
- **Imitation:** Morality consists in following the example of the role model. This is perhaps the most common way of learning medical ethics by aspiring physicians, with the role models being the senior consultants and the mode of moral learning being observation and assimilation of the values portrayed.
- **Feeling or Desire:** It is a subjective approach to moral decision-making and behaviour. What is right is what feels right and satisfies one's desire; what is wrong is what feels wrong and frustrates one's desire. The measure of morality is to be found within each individual and however, may vary from one individual to another, and even within the same individual over time.
- **Intuition:** Intuition is an immediate perception of the right way to act in a situation. It is similar to desire in that it is entirely subjective, however, it differs because of its location in the mind rather than the will. To that extent it comes closer to the rational forms of decision-making than do obedience, imitation, feeling and desire. However, it is neither systematic nor reflexive but directs moral decisions through a simple flash of insight. Like

feeling and desire it can vary greatly from one individual to another, and even within the same individual over time.

- **Habit:** Habit is a very efficient method of moral-decision-making since there is no need to repeat a systematic decision-making process each time a moral issue arises similar to one that has been dealt with previously. However, there may be bad habits (e.g. lying) as well as good ones (e.g. truth telling). Moreover, the situation that appears similar may require significantly different decisions.

www.wma.net/en/30th publications/30 ethics manual/pdf/ ethics_manual_en.pdf)

Values and Ethics: The values held by persons or groups can be most accurately determined through the careful observation of their behaviour over time. Adherence of certain values by a person can be known by observing his or her behaviour, activities and the style of living. Ethics are statements, written or oral, that prescribe certain behaviours under specified conditions. One cannot deny the differences that exist between generally accepted ethical premises and the day-to-day behaviours of service providers in different sectors which reveal their operating values influencing the ethical principles to be observed by the service providers. (Nigro: 1989)

Medical ethics is a system of moral principles that apply values and judgments to the practice of medicine. Generally, it addresses four principles—*Respect for autonomy*—the patient has the right to refuse or choose for treatment; *Beneficence*—a practitioner should act in the best interest of the patient; *Non-maleficence*—do no harm; *Justice*—the distribution of scarce health resources and the decision of who gets what treatment (fair and equality). In addition to this respect for human dignity, truthfulness and honesty have to be observed. (en.wikipedia.org/wiki/ medical_ethics. 19.11.2014) Ethical principles are rooted in the social culture and religion. Diversity in religion and social culture among the communities spreading over the world and even in the same country creates confusion and contradictions of opinion. The laws of different countries also regulate certain ethical or moral principles directly. The laws relating to domestic violence, care of elderly members including parents etc. may be referred in the case of India. Further, the moral base of the Constitution of India contributes significantly towards values and ethics of social life. Laws differ from country to country and within a country customs, traditions and social values differ from community to community. However, it may be admitted that all religions and social relations are based on human values with the end of service to humanity. Though differences in behaviour, culture, custom and tradition of different communities exist, ultimate goal of all the communities is common, welfare, progress and survival with human dignity.

While admitting that a man learns behaviour, values and other norms of social life at the early age through family environment and these are reflected in his future life whether he is in service or otherwise it is noticed that it is not true in all the cases. Because not all values are acquired early in life and they remain unchanged throughout one's lifetime. The social and psychological environments within which service providers or others function at any given time are strong influences on the pattern of values they apply to the situations. Here again I like to look back to the questions raised by Joan Robinson about group life, he said, "Why does the group exist? Why does the animal not live alone, if not all the year at least for much of it? There are many reasons but the principal one is learning. The group is the locus of knowledge and experience far exceeding that of the individual member. It is in the group that experience is pooled and generations linked. The adaptive functions of prolonged biological youth is that it gives the animal time to learn. During this period, while the animal learns from other members of the group, it is protected by them. Slow development in isolation would simply mean disaster for the individual and extinction for the species." To live in a group and learn correct behaviour requires social discipline. This is how a young physician or any service provider may learn about the ethical principles for survival as human being. The personnel in an organization form a human family in which members belong to different age groups, different expertness, different families and different localities but they meet regularly in this family of organization with well defined goals of service and the medical organizations meet directly the ailing population of a country and thus indirectly render service to the well-being of the whole nation as well as to the world community. Naturally conflict arises in the mind of a member of the service group when there is contradiction in values and ethical principles learned in the family with those in the service group (Robinson: 1989).

***Globalization and Cultural Choice*:** Gandhi said, "I do not want my house to be walled on all sides and my windows to be staffed. I want the cultures of all lands to be blown around my house as freely as possible. But I refuse to be blown off my feet by any of these." This statement of

Gandhi is very much relevant today, especially with the emergence of the process of globalization.

Globalization is a contentious issue. It has both strengths and weaknesses. Generally, controversies rage over the environmental, economic and social consequences of globalization. In addition to it, the impact of globalization on culture and identity is emerging as a strong source of division among the common people belonging to different communities. The negative impact of it has already come to the surface which are experienced by the common masses or the poor people leading to acute financial crisis in the families resulting commitment of theft, trafficking of children and unemployed youths and involvement of people in various unethical activities. The service holders, businessmen and moneyed people are also influenced to a great extent by the negative impact of globalization. The emergence of improved satellite channels, especially foreign channels has brought many changes in the tradition bound Indian society. The socio-cultural pattern of the society is very heavily influenced by these channels.

For many people this new diversity is exciting, even empowering, but for some it is disempowering. Global flows of goods, ideas, people and capital tempted people to change their living styles to adjust with that of a modern man. They started abandonment of traditional values and practices and the dismantling of the economic basis on which the survival of indigenous cultures depends. When such global flows lead to cultural exclusion, multicultural policies are needed to manage trade, cultural differences and identities. The aim of multicultural policies is not to preserve tradition, however, but to protect cultural liberty and expand people's choices—in the ways people live and identify themselves —not to penalize them for these choices. However, these may also go other way round developing the sense of being neglected, exploitation, suspicion in the honesty of the service providers, emergence of protest movements etc.

There is much to cherish in traditional values and practices and much that is consonant with universal values of human rights. But there is also much that is challenged by universal ethics, such as inheritance laws that are biased against women or decision-making processes that are not participatory and democratic.

In no society are lifestyles or values static. As globalization proceeds, this means not only recognizing local and national identities but also strengthening commitments to being citizens of the world.

Today intensified global interactions can function well only if governed by bonds of shared values, communication and commitment.

Corporation among people and nations with different interests is more likely when all are bound and motivated by shared values and commitment. Global culture is not about the English language or brand name sneakers —it is about universal ethics based on universal human rights and respect for the freedom, equality and dignity of all individuals.

Indigenous people see globalization as a threat to their cultural identities, their control over territory and their centuries old traditions of knowledge and artistic expression. They fear that the cultural significance of their territories and knowledge will go unrecognized—or that they will receive inadequate compensation for these cultural assets. In these situations globalization is often blamed.

The historical territories of indigenous people are often rich in minerals and oil and gas deposits. That can set up the potential for conflict between promoting national economic growth through extractive industries and protecting the cultural identity and economic livelihood of the indigenous people, developed over several generations and collectively owned by the community, can have practical uses in agriculture, forestry and health. (UNDP: 2004)

The heavy influence of science and technology on the services provided by the modern state demands building up ethical theory or ethical framework of the services. Ethics in public administration suffers from the absence of theoretical framework. In 1980, Dwight Waldo described the state of moral and ethical behaviour in public administration as 'chaotic' (Waldo, 1980:100). In 1983, James Bowman stated that 'in both practice and theory, the ethical implications of administrative and political conduct remain largely unexplored' (Bowman, 1983a:71) John Rohr, in presenting a 'state of the discipline' report at a major conference, states that 'throughout this report I have stressed the diversity in the ethics field, a diversity that comes close to chaos' (Rohr, 1986a:53). While talking about the absence of theoretical framework for public administration ethics Denhardt said that it is not that public administration acted since 1887 (from the time of Woodrow Wilson) without a sense of ethics nor it is true that the ethics of public servants has deteriorated. Rather, the nature of public administration, the role of public administrators, and societal expectations have gradually evolved to a point that makes it necessary for us to turn our attention to administrative ethics. (Denhardt: 1988).

The Indian experience shows that since independence almost all the services are swallowed by corruption, unethical activities, hypocrisy, violation of human rights and lack of commitment to the principles of the Constitution of India. No doubt the role of the public servants has changed and people's aspirations have gone up to the higher levels day by day. The ethical vacuum in most services is felt and this situation demands the study of state of ethics without delay. This study is required to make public servants responsive, responsible and accountable for their activities.

Terry L. Cooper's discussion in his book, *The Responsible Administrator* (1982) said 'ethics involves substantive reasoning about obligations, consequences, and ultimate ends' and doing ethics .... Involves thinking more systematically about values which are embedded in the choices we make'. To him the process of being ethical ultimately requires the individual administrator to apply those values and make a decision, though Cooper did not define those values.

The author of the book also dealt with the philosophical tradition of ethics. It is stated that an administrator to be ethical must have the capacity to view reasonably with an independent outlook the standards by which the decisions are made in the organization. The standards may change in course of time with fresh look to or analysis of the social values and emergence of new social concerns. While making attempt to adapt decision standards to these changes, an administrator has to reflect a commitment to the core values of our society and goals of the organization. The administrator is to be held accountable personally and professionally for his act or decision.

While talking about philosophical tradition of ethics Denhardt indicated three major aspects of it as below:

1. Ethical action involves a process of examining and questioning, accepted standards for making decisions, a process which must at times be carried out independently. (independent critique)
2. The content of the ethical standards should reflect the core values of society and that the understanding of those values can and will, change over time, thus changing the standards by which actions are to be evaluated. (changing standards)
3. Administrators, because they are not only acting as individuals but also as members of an organization, must consider their role within the organization and the goals of the organization as part of a determination of how to act or standards to use in making decisions. (organizational context)

The terms ethics, values and morality are frequently used interchangeably. It is because the terms 'moral' and 'ethical' are in many ways synonymous. Modern usage might distinguish the two in that, 'ethics' has become associated with both philosophical inquiry and professional standards, while 'morals' continue to hold the connotation of right rules of conduct. In public administration ethics, to be ethical often means to follow right rules of moral conduct, but being ethical can also legitimately mean to be engaged in the inquiry into what those right rules of moral conduct are or should be, or how they might be applied when two or more right rules of conduct conflict.

Richard Means in his book, *The Ethical Imperative* distinguishes between values and ethics, terms he says are intimately related but not the same thing. "Ethics are the normative standards of conduct derived from the philosophical and religious traditions of society" (Means, 1969:55). Values, on the other hand, are norms underlie rational social action and which change over time (Denhradt: 1988).

The norms help maintaining smooth social life through regulation of individuals' behaviour. There is social pressure on individuals to behave in conformity to norms.

Autonomy: Autonomy is a concept found in moral, political and bioethical philosophy. Within this context, it is the capacity of a rational individual to make an informed, un-coerced decision, as stated in the free encyclopedia. It is nothing but freedom to determine one's own action or behaviour. It has its root in the Greek word, *Autonomia*—freedom to live by one's own laws.

Edward Weisband and Thomas M. Franck state, "By ethical autonomy we mean the willingness to assert one's principled judgment, even if that entails violating rules, values or perceptions of the organization, peer group or team." (Nigro)

Jukka Varelius, in the article, titled, *The Value of Autonomy in Medical Ethics* stated that autonomy is a central value in Western medicine and medical ethics, but exactly what kind of role medicine ought to give to patient's autonomy seems to be somewhat obscure. It is that autonomous persons are often in the best position to determine what is good and what is bad for them. Therefore, one finds good reason to consider patient's autonomy to have instrumental value in medicine. Some bioethicists maintain that autonomy is so important that there are cases where patients should be allowed to make their choices about their treatment even if it is clear for parties involved that others would be in a better position to make choices that would serve the patient's well-being. Some philosophers maintain that patient's autonomy can be restricted if there is a threat of very severe harm to patient's well-being, while others seem to accept no limits to patient's autonomy when there is no danger of harming others. *(http://www.ncbi.nim.nih.gov/pmc/articles/PMC2780686)*

In a medical context, respect for a patient's personal autonomy is considered one of many fundamental ethical principles in medicine. Autonomy is nothing but the ability of the person to make his or her own decisions. The faith in autonomy is the central premise of the concept of informed consent and decision making. This idea, while considered essential to today's practice of medicine, was developed in the last fifty years. Beuchamp and Childress, in the book titled, *Principles of Biomedical Ethics*, pointed out seven elements of informed consent. These are: competence and voluntariness (threshold elements); disclosure, recommendation and understanding (information elements); decision and authorization (consent elements). This analysis of Beuchamp and Childress is criticized by philosophers like Harry Frankfurt as inadequate. To the critics an action can only be considered autonomous if it involves the exercise of the capacity to form higher-order values about desires when acting intentionally. It means patients must understand their situation and choices but would not be autonomous unless the patient is able to form value judgments about their reasons for choosing treatment options they would not be acting autonomously.

Autonomy is also defined as relational autonomy, which places the individual in a social context and supported autonomy, which suggests that in specific circumstances it may be necessary to temporarily compromise the autonomy of the person in the short term in order to preserve their autonomy in the long run.

(http://en.wikipedia.org/wiki/Autonomy)

Since long the practice of securing signature of patient's attendant in a form is followed while taking treatment by a patient. Average people who participate in the process of treatment of patients as attendants while signing on the form are under the impression that they have to give the physicians freedom to undertake the task without taking the responsibility of harm caused during procedure, i.e. they will not be held responsible if any worse happens to the patients.

It is also stated that a signature on a form is not a real indication that a patient has understood any of the issues involved. The reason for this is that consent is not about protecting those providing the treatment, it is recognition of patient's autonomy.

Autonomy may also mean different things. In western cultures, the principle behind consent is an ethical one; respect for an individual's autonomy as soon as soon as he/she is able to make his or her own decisions. In some other cultures, personal autonomy may have less importance and the roles of the families, or orders of the elders of the family, may have a far greater influence.

Another aspect of the autonomy is its moral stance, which is related to choice of the patient. The patient has the right to make a choice unimpeded by bias. That choice is made according to the patient's own values and codes of conduct. Further, a reasonable choice to one may not be reasonable to another, including the treating practitioner. Because the second person may not hold the same core values as the patient making the choice.

The next feature of autonomy is the need to ensure that any decisions taken are made freely and without coercion. Achieving such free will choices is easier said than done. Coercion may be overt or it may be subtle. Even with the best intentions, we are often influenced by how others act around us.

(http://www.medicalprotection.org/uk/advice-booklets/mps-guide-to-ethis—a-map-for-the-moral-maze/chpter-8—patient-autonomy-and-consent.)

Robert D. Orr, in his article, *Autonomy, Conscience and Professional Obligation* published in the *American Medical Association Journal of Medical Ethics* highlights an interesting discussion on the issue. Healthcare professionals have a fiduciary relationship with their patients. The expert knowledge and authority in the field which they possess cannot be claimed by the patients. At the same time they are obliged to be trustworthy and to serve the patients' best interest. This has been a lesson taught since the time of Hippocrates till date in medicine.

Healthcare professionals are human beings who are equipped with conscience, i.e. the faculty of judging right and wrong. Sometimes, conscience may direct the individual to perform or not to perform a particular action. The right of conscience allows an individual to refuse to do something by another based on his or her own conscience or religious beliefs.

The right of a physician to refuse to provide a requested treatment has ancient roots. Hippocrates, in writing about the goal of medicine 2,500 years ago, defined good medicine as, "doing away with the suffering of the sick, lessening the violence of their diseases, and refusing to treat those who are overmastered by their diseases, realizing that in such cases medicine is powerless." Though physicians who practice modern palliative care would quibble with his assertion that medicine is powerless when a patient is dying.

For centuries physicians took a primarily paternalistic approach to patient care. Since 1960s, a societal consensus supporting individual autonomy emerged in Western culture embracing patients' right along with other rights, such as, women's rights, minority rights, consumer's rights etc. Many felt that patients should have greater say in their own medical care. One may go a step forward and say that the patient cannot only refuse but also demand treatment.

Robert D. Orr says that there is a misconception on this right of the patient to demand as well as refuse treatment. He analyzes it considering two aspects of autonomy—negative autonomy and positive autonomy. Negative autonomy tells that it is not an easy task to force treatment on someone who refuses it. One cannot deny existence of strong justification to override patient's refusal to medical treatment. As regards the positive autonomy, which means patient's demand obliges a physician to provide a treatment, cannot be considered as a compulsion on physician. Orr points out that a physician is not obliged to fulfill the demands of a patient on a legal ground that—a request for a non-approved drugs, a professional standard—a request for non-beneficial treatment such as, hyperbaric oxygen for a completed stroke; clinical judgment—a request for an antibiotic to treat a viral infection etc.

(http://journalofethics.ama-assn.org/2013/misc1-1303.html)

Indian situation may be x-rayed with the help of what Orr has analyzed. In India even there are enough instances of motivating patients to go for treatment under physician or to be admitted in the hospital after emotional pressure by the family members or neighbours or close friends. They offer even the physical and financial assistance to the ailing person according to their capacity. In the traditional society of the state of Assam to which I belong I find that elderly members of the neighbouring families used to give company to the ailing person in their own locality on rotation basis. Sometimes they used to read loudly religious books to provide some mental relief. Under such situation the refusal of treatment by the patient has become almost irrelevant. In India one experiences the delegation of decision making power of the patient to the family members, especially the sons, daughters, wife/husband for choosing the physician or the kind of treatment, i.e. Allopathic/Ayurvedic/Homoeopathic/or traditional treatment which exists in the rural areas. Even in urban areas it is noticed that there are cases of shift of treatment from allopathic to traditional systems. As regards the positive autonomy, its role is not very significant in the society.

Here one may consider autonomy as the gateway to self-rule. Self-rule provides disciplined life and it is possible through self-knowledge, self-analysis and self-confidence. Thus it has a positive connotation. But there is no guarantee that an individual exercises autonomous power reasonably or the scope of misuse of this power cannot be ruled out. In the contemporary public life in India very often it is noticed that the debate/discussion/justification on the issue of decision making the decision makers try to justify or explain their power of decision making without highlighting the other side of it, i.e. responsibility. Autonomy without responsibility cannot be called autonomy at all. Autonomy and responsibility are the two sides of the same coin. Responsibility is the source of autonomy just as the duty is the source of right. Autonomy is not a self-contained concept. Interestingly, autonomy must be earned to be effective. This is more applicable in the case a physician than that of a patient. There is no point in giving autonomy to a patient who is seriously ill and who is mentally very weak and highly emotional or who is financially bankrupt. In these cases, the decision maker is the patient's attendants. How can a patient exercise the autonomous power to take decision regarding treatment. Even with regard to the attendant it is not possible to know the process of treatment and the consequences of a particular type of treatment to be opted. In India it is also not possible for the physician who is to attend a large number of patients, to explain these to every patient decision maker for receiving effective feedback or to do justice due to time constraint.

Melanie Philips and John Dawson have pointed out similar kind of dilemma. To them the underlying principle behind the informed consent is that the patient must be informed about the nature of suffering and the process of treatment required for his or her cure. Here the difficult task is to decide how much information is required to secure consent of the patient in the interest of the phrase '*do no harm to the patient*'. The principle of '*informed consent*' also is not a satisfactory way to maintain patient's autonomy. The patient's autonomy is shown through this '*informed consent*' principle as regards the nature of treatment to be offered to him or her. Excepting very few patients other patients do not have the knowledge about the consequences of the different types of treatment to be accepted. Generally, the responsibility choosing the type of treatment is entrusted to the doctor. There are basically reasons—patient is physically and mentally weak and constrained by tension, emotion etc., the patient does not have the expert knowledge in the field. So there is no point of giving autonomy to patient in this context. However, in India as largest number of patients are not financially well off, their decision depends on the financial condition also.

On the issue of patient's autonomy Melanie Philips and John Dawson referred in their book, **Doctors' Dilemma**, what Lord Denning set out in 1974 the paternalist's case as: ' first, medical notes and records are very difficult for laymen to understand. They may easily misinterpret them. Second, notes and records may include the medical men's fear of worse things to come which may disturb the patient greatly they were known to him—such as giving six months to live; or saying the doctor suspects a malignant cancer. Third, the notes and records may contain records which may be embarrassing or distressing if made known. These notes and records are confidential documents. The medical man should be able to make them with utmost frankness, and without fear they may be disclosed beyond the profession. They should not be disclosed to other persons except when the interests of justice so require.'

The right to know about one's own health is also constrained by the general principle of 'truth telling'. In India at the school itself a child is taught 'Always speak the truth' on the ground that telling lie is sin. However, there are exceptions to it. In the family the children are not told all the happenings in the four walls of their habitation, because the knowledge about it may harm the children. Similar is the case with regard to the doctors. Most doctors may agree that lying to the patient is absolutely wrong and should never occur. At the same time they have to tell lie on occasions in the interest of the survival of the patients. (Phillips and Dawson: 1985)

While talking about the autonomy of the patients question arises about the ability of the patient to enjoy the autonomy granted to him or her. Physical suffering, mental weaknesses, tension, knowledge of medicine etc. are impediments to take right decision. In the case of children, individuals affected by certain psychiatric or neurological conditions, and those who are temporarily unconscious situation is problematic in to-day's society. In traditional Indian society, the patients were not aware of this right, the physicians were the sole authority to take decision. The family members of the patient had faith in the physician's ability. Gradually with the awareness of the rights of the individuals, increase of the number of physicians in the similar field the decision-making power of the physicians is moving to the patients and the family members. Generally it is found that family members of the patient take decision regarding the consent to be given. According to World Medical Association, if the patient is unconscious or otherwise unable to express his/her will, informed consent must be obtained, whenever possible from a legally entitled representative where legally relevant. If a legally entitled representative is not available, but a medical intervention is urgently needed, consent of the patient is presumed, unless it is obvious and beyond any doubt on the basis of the patient's previous firm expression or conviction that he/she would refuse consent to the intervention in that situation. Here also problem arises when those claiming to be the appropriate decision makers and do not agree among themselves or when they agree, their decision is, in the opinion of the physician, not in the patient's best interest. Autonomy may be given to the patient to take decision on his/her treatment, but without the physician's honest and frank guidance there is every possibility of taking wrong decision by the patient and the family members. Or instances are also found in many occasions to entrust this responsibility by the patient to the physician to do whichever is best treatment according to him or her.

End-of-life-issues: The end-of-life-issues are very sensitive and problematic issues. The World Medical Association discusses these issues in its declaration. It says these issues range from attempts to prolong the lives of dying patients through highly experimental technologies, such as the implantation of animal organs to efforts to terminate life prematurely through euthanasia and medically assisted suicide. In between these two extremes lie numerous issues regarding the initiation or withdrawing of potentially life-extending treatments, the care of terminally ill patients and advisability and use of advance directives.

It emphasized two major issues—euthanasia and assistance to suicide. Euthanasia means knowingly and intentionally performing an act of that is clearly intended to end another person's life and that includes the following elements: the subject is competent, informed person with an incurable illness who has voluntarily asked for his or her life to be ended; the agent knows about the person's condition and desire to die; and commits the act with primary intention of ending the life of the person; and the act is undertaken with compassion and without personal gain.

Assistance in suicide means knowingly and intentionally providing a person with the knowledge or means or both required to commit suicide, including counselling about lethal doses of drugs, prescribing such lethal doses or supplying the drugs.

Euthanasia and assisted suicide are often regarded as morally equivalent, although there is a clear practical distinction, and in some jurisdictions a legal distinction, between them.

Euthanasia and assisted suicide, according to these definitions, are to be distinguished from withholding or withdrawal of inappropriate, futile or unwanted medical treatment or the provision of compassionate palliative care, even when these practices shorten life.

Requests for euthanasia or assistance in suicide arise as a result of pain or suffering that is considered by the patient to be intolerable. They would rather die than continue to live in such circumstances. Furthermore, many patients consider that they have a right to die if they so choose, and even a right to assistance in dying. Physicians are regarded as the most appropriate instruments of death since they have the medical knowledge and access to the appropriate drugs for ensuring quick and painless death.

Physicians are understandably reluctant to implement the requests for euthanasia or assistance in suicide because these acts are illegal in most countries and are prohibited in most medical codes of ethics. The prohibition was part of the Hippocratic Oath.

This kind of dilemma was found in the traditional society also which can be deduced from the behaviour of the family members towards the patient suffering from incurable illness. They used to organize group prayer to God for relief of the patient from the suffering without spelling it explicitly in terms of euthanasia. The family members cannot bear the pain of looking at that stage of the patient. What is the implication of the prayer for relief from the pain by the patient who suffer from incurable illness? God must show some miracle to cure the patient or end the life of the patient.

Here let me mention what is highlighted by Kawal Deep Kour about the euthanasia debate in his article, *Right to die with dignity: the euthanasia debate* published on 20th May, 2015 in the daily newspaper, *The Assam Tribune*. The debate on mercy killing or euthanasia is continuing since ancient time across the world. It has not only moral implication but also legal and professional implications. It is related to the human dignity which is honoured in democracy. Can a man has the right to die with dignity? There is no one answer to it. The origin of the word, 'euthanasia' itself is debatable. Most people are of opinion that it is a Greek word, which means 'good death'. Again Seutonius, the Roman historian used the word, '*Orthothanasia*' for the first time in his work, *De Vita Caesarum*, in which he narrated the death of Augustus Caesar. In order to honour the wish to die of the terminally ill Caesar treatment was withheld. There Seutonius called this act as 'passive action to cause death of a person on his request'. Kour has cited an example from ancient Greece where the physicians assisted the death of a person suffering from terminal sickness by offering a poison to drink on the request of the patient. It may be considered as right to die with dignity. However, there are some who call it as suicide or murder and violation of Hippocratic Oath which may cause tension in the doctor-patient relationship.

A patient who suffers from terminal illness may express such a wish to die due to various compulsions, such as, acute suffering, financial crunch of the family, lack of caretakers. This issue of euthanasia pauses challenges to the medical service providers, particularly to doctors, determination of the extent of his autonomy, denial of right to life, i.e. does the right to life confine to healthy persons only, equal distribution of public resources, it may be an excuse to divorce responsibility for an incompetent doctor. Fortunately, today there has been ways to reduce conflict in the minds of doctors as well as family members and well-wishers to have mental peace through palliative care treatment of patients.

The palliative care treatments for relieve pain and suffering and improving quality of life. Palliative care may be appropriate for patients of all ages from a child with cancer to a senior nearing the end of life. One aspect of palliative care is that it requires greater attention for all patients is pain control. The physicians should not abandon dying patients but should continue to provide compassionate care even when cure is no longer possible.

Truth: Knowledge of the truth is a fundamental key to be a successful physician, though truth telling is constrained by his or own '*Dharma*', "Not to Do Harm" to the patient. The search for truth begins with the conversation between the physician and the patient at the Out Patient Department (OPD) itself in the hospital premises. At this initial stage truth telling as a life saving device in the case of a patient and the technique or approach of the physician as seeker of truth to motivate the patient who is his/her respondent or information giver is the fundamental requirement in the field of medical ethics. The role of a physician as a truth teller is a crucial one in to-day's India due to several reasons— awareness of the individuals their rights; the relationship of the physician is no longer confining to the patient only, it is extended to the social level also; emergence of the healthcare as an important component of the human security concept etc. If we take into account the conversation between the physician and the patient, especially at the OPD of a hospital it is noticed that there is a big gap between the knowledge of the physician and that of the patient, unless the patient himself or herself is a doctor. Another aspect of conversation is the inadequacy of information delivered by the patient to the physician at the time of conversation. Several reasons may be forwarded for this act of the patient-fear psychosis, nervousness, ignorance of the consequence of not telling the truth, too much modesty of average female patients from rural areas, heavy tension etc. However, with the help of modern technology, the true nature of the ailment can be detected by the physicians, but the causes of the ailment or the environment in which the ailment developed may remain unknown or partially known to the physician. Another problem is caused by the constraint of time to be invested by the conversant physician on this process due to heavy rush of patients. Then during the process of treatment when error is committed by the service providers the wrong doers have to be careful to tell the truth, though it is very essential in the interest of the patient. The attendants of the victim patient may also react violently creating unpleasant situation. Due to emotional or mental constraints they may not be in a position to realize the real situation. Or even if they realize the situation they cannot correct themselves in most cases. At the same time disclosure of the error is essential for prevention of it or for the safeguard of the other patients in future. There are also situations in which the patient may not have mental strength to know the truth about his or her ailments provided it is of very serious in nature or difficult to be cured. For example, till recently people were scared of tuberculosis, but now people have come to know that it is curable and preventable disease, gradually tension or nervousness caused by it disappears. To tell the truth to a patient that his or her life is ending is not only a difficult task the necessity of speaking the truth to the patient is also a questionable issue. The experience in the traditional family and social life is that there is always encouraging comments, experience of recovery from serious diseases of various patients are discussed in front of a patient whose life is nearing end. Relatives and the neighbours used to give company to the patient and the family members and make effort to give mental strength to the patient. Here they do not speak the truth nor tell lie but remain silent on the issue. Though in the modern time situation changes one cannot deny that when a patient refuses to know the truth at all, one should not force him to learn it. Here ethics is like a two-edged sword.

Reporting Unethical Practices: Medicine has traditionally taken pride in its status as a self-regulating profession. In turn for the privileges accorded to it by society and the trust given to its members by their patients. The medical profession has established high standards of behaviour for its members and disciplinary procedures to investigate accusations of misbehaviour, and if necessary, to punish the wrongdoers. This system of self-regulation has often failed, and in recent years steps have been taken to make the profession more accountable, for example, by appointing lay members to regulatory authorities. The main requirement for self-regulation, however, is wholehearted support by physicians for its principles and their willingness to recognize and deal with unsafe and unethical practices.

This obligation to report incompetence, impairment or misconduct of one's colleagues is emphasized in codes of medical ethics. For example, the WMA International Codes of Medical Ethics states that "A physician shall.... strive to expose those physicians deficient in character or competence, or who engage in fraud or deception". The application of this principle is seldom easy, however. On the one hand, a physician may be tempted to attack the reputation of a colleague for unworthy personal motives, such as jealousy, or in retaliation for a perceived insult by the colleagues. A physician may also be reluctant to report a colleague's misbehaviour because of friendship or sympathy. The consequences of such reporting can be very detrimental to the one who reports, including almost certain hostility on the part of the accused and possibly other colleagues as well.

Despite these drawbacks to reporting wrongdoing, it is a professional duty of physicians. Not only are they responsible for maintaining the good reputation of the profession, but they are often the only ones who recognize incompetence, impairment or misconduct. However, reporting colleagues to the disciplinary authority should normally be a last resort after other alternatives have been tried and found wanting. The first step might be to approach the colleague and say that he considers his or her behaviour unsafe or unethical. If the matter can be resolved at that level, there may be no need to go further, if not, the next step might be to discuss the matter with him and/or offender's supervisor and leave the decision about further action to that person. If this tactic is not practical or does not succeed, then it may be necessary to take the final step of informing the disciplinary authority.

Accountability: The moral aspect of accountability can help to maintain self-discipline more effectively than any other devices adopted by the government. Democracy, whether political or social depends for its survival on human qualities of the individuals. In ultimate analysis of the concept of democracy there remain moral or ethical principles which bind the human beings together for achieving common good. These principles are rooted in the religion and culture of different social groups. The Constitution of India reflects basic moral principles required for effective functioning of the democracy at both political and social fields. The moral imperatives of the public policies cannot be ignored by the policy formulators as well as by the executors. O.P. Dwivedi has pointed out that an ethical and responsible administrator, believes in self-discipline, humility, and above all shows the absence of arrogance while rendering service to the people. Morality is the source of inspiration for rendering service to the people and to safeguard common good of the society.

To Dwivedi ethical problems among public servants range from the apparently very small and insignificant infractions to those having serious bearing upon the nature and the very survival of the government. He classified unethical conduct into three categories—(a) activities which are contrary to the legal norms of the country and therefore punishable under the law; (b) activities which are contrary to the basic principles of morality/ethics held by the society; (c) activities which are undertaken because of the latent, manifest or perceived pressures felt by a person under the obligations of loyalty, ties of kinship, affection, politics, religion, or sheer need of money. Everywhere there is pressure on public servants from political leaders, influential persons, relatives seeking favours and speed in the work. In addition, money power is very strong in motivating the public servants to be involved in unethical activities. The conduct rules, laws of the country and other legal, administrative and judicial devices have failed to prevent unethical conduct of the public servants. In India almost everyday media is focusing unethical activities of the public servants, the role of the Central Bureau of Investigation in making officials, political leaders and common people accountable for their involvement in corrupt and other unethical activities.

Moral dimension invites the governance to serve the society with aim of common good. This dimension always requires moral responsibility and accountability, sacrifice, compassion, justice, and honest effort to achieve the common good. It is the moral dimension which makes the governance good for all. (Dwivedi: 2002)

Secrecy: Several social scientists have attempted to distinguish the concepts of privacy and secrecy. Both support reduction of observability and an increased potential to deny access to others. They, however, differ in the moral content of the behaviour which is concealed. Secrecy implies the concealment of something which is negatively valued by the excluded audience and, in some instances, by the perpetrator as well. Privacy, by contrast, protects behaviour which is either morally neutral or valued by society as well as by the perpetrators. Privacy has a consensual basis in society, while secrecy does not. There is an agreement on 'right to privacy' in many areas of contemporary life; however, there is no equivalent, consensual to 'right to secrecy'. The idea of right to privacy is an essential attribute of personal and psychological freedom in modern democratic society has been hailed as the most exciting and influential legal development of modern American tort law. (Iyengar: 1979)

The right to privacy is one of the basic human rights in a democratic system. However, there is a dilemma as regards to right to privacy and the need for access to information in the public interest. In this context better to refer what R.B. Jain has pointed out about the right to privacy. It is generally believed that privacy implies a normative element. The right to privacy entitles one to exclude others from—(a) watching, (b) utilizing, and (c) invading his personal realm. According to some scholars privacy is a living reality, the nerve center of a whole creative personality. (Jain, 1979)

It is a known fact that governments have been exercising the privilege of keeping certain facts and documents confidential and secret and their contents were not disclosed to the general public. This privilege had been enjoyed on the ground of national security. With the growth of democratic institutions, the concept of secrecy has also undergone a change. The control of the government on secret documents is not very rigid as it used to be. As people became conscious of their rights they demanded to know from the government the reasons and motives behind a governmental decision which affected their lives. They even asserted their rights to see and inspect the important documents of the government. On the other hand, the government could not concede to place all the documents of the government before the general public and exercised its right under a statute to keep certain types of documents secret. The question of production of confidential and secret documents and papers or revelation of their contents before Parliament or a court of law has been a subject matter of controversy amongst jurists, parliamentarians and academicians.

Secrecy in Indian Government has indeed a long history—longer than in many other countries. As early as 30th August, 1843, the Central Government in India issued a notification asking its personnel not to communicate to the outside world any paper or information in their possession. What was happening at the time was that some civil servants were supplying information on matters relating to government to the press, which had caused occasional embarrassment to the Government. The Government issued a notification as:

> "Some misconception appearing to exist with respect to the power which officers of both services (civil and military) have over the documents and papers which come to their possession officially. The Governor General-in-Council considered it necessary to notify that such documents and papers should in no case be made public, or communicated to individuals, without

the previous consent of the government to which alone they belonged".

In July 1875, the Central Government laid down detailed instructions in a bid to regulate the contemporary administrative behaviour in the face of emergence of press in India. In 1889, Britain passed its first Official Secrets Act and a unique feature of this statute was its applicability to any part of Her Majesty's dominions including India.

In India before 1889 there was no comprehensive legislation on official secrets. The only Indian law on the subject was The Indian Official Secrets Act 1889 as amended in 1904. In addition to this, the British rulers had made applicable to India an Act of British Parliament, namely The Official Secrets Act 1911. Section 2 of the Act deals with the main offence which relates to unauthorized communication of official information including documents by a crown servant. Section 1 is concerned with spying. The main offence created by section 1 may be committed by any person who for a purpose prejudicial to the safety or interests of the state obtains or communicates any document or information which is calculated to be or is intended to be directly or indirectly useful to enemy. Section 2 covers a much wider range of information than section 1. Section 7 of the Act makes it an offence for any person knowingly to harbour a person who has committed or is about to commit an offence under this Act. Section 8 makes it mandatory that any person for an offence under this Act can be prosecuted only by or with the consent of Attorney-General. The Canadian Official Secrets Act 1939 is closely based on British Official Secrets Act, while the French penal code protects two classes of information: first, information affecting national defense and second, information entrusted to certain persons by reason of their profession.

The Government of India in 1923 realized the difficulties and unsatisfactory state of affairs arising out of simultaneous application of two sets of legislation in India. It was therefore decided to enact a law which was not only to be comprehensive but which should also incorporate the experience during Second World War, especially in regard to the protection of military secrets. With this view the Official Secrets Act 1923 was enacted which was later on amended by the Central as well as State Legislature. In 1951, certain minor amendments were effected. In 1967, the Union Government amended this Act to widen its scope.

With the above experience if we look into the situation in medical services in the perspective of medical error and negligence it may be realized that the secrecy is basically needed in the interests of the safety of the medical service providers. The patient's safety requires openness or transparency in the process of treatment. But at the same time one cannot deny the role of secrecy in saving or prolonging the life of a patient.

The term secrecy in its lexicon meaning, stands for things or facts unrevealed, hidden, secluded, kept undivulged or admitted to confidence. In common administrative parlance, it is a synonym for 'confident'. Obviously, it does not imply suppression or distortion of facts for mere heck of it. In administrative procedure, secrecy is to be resorted to for the attainment of a higher purpose. It is always a means to an end. When an organization has to institutionalize secrecy through exclusive structures of confidential cells or intelligence wings to preserve absolute secrecy of procedure in announcing or arriving at certain decisions, it has a higher organizational purpose to achieve. Secrecy of procedure or concealment of facts from a certain section of client or the people in general, temporarily or permanently, can be conceptualized as a 'management need' in all organizations, and especially those which are big, complex and functionally prone to public dealings. Carl J. Friedrich believes that addiction to secrecy is one of the most characteristics of modern bureaucracy.

The administrative interest in carrying secrecy beyond the limits of this general acceptability lies in a widely shared bureaucratic consensus. P.D. Sharma while discussing the issue of secrecy as a management need highlighted the following factors inviting secrecy in the administration:

Depersonalization of Power: Administrative decisions are institutional and not personal. This fact of depersonalization gives a quality of tentativeness to administrative action. No administrator, howsoever, efficient or competent, cannot give assurance which may not be overridden later under the exigencies of a changed situation. The depersonalization of power in public bureaucracies provides a source of interest in secrecy and public bureaucrats in large organizations tend to avoid open positions on issues, which, ultimately, get clinched in the light of inevitable and imponderables.

Administrative Feasibility: Administrative feasibility as a universal administrative concern can be identified as another source of interest in secrecy in administration. Administration is a rational quest and a continuous Endeavour for feasibility of public policy, which by its very nature, has to be somewhat doctrinaire. The people who opt or vote for such idealistic public policies do not want to listen to administrative handicaps that threaten to sabotage them. Naturally, when administrative feasibility is a decisive constraint in the realm of public policy, its open publicity may embarrass the policy-makers. To avoid this embarrassment or popular reaction against administrative handicaps, administrators tend to conceal the reason or basis of action, which in their judgment is a valid fact. In other words, administrative secrecy is a condition conducive for formulation and execution of public policy, which otherwise may be too utopian to be hazarded in practice.

***Camouflaging of Power Conflicts in Hierarchy*:** All organizations have their internal political struggles for power and hidden conflicts of positions in the hierarchy. People in general regard personal appropriation of power and position as contrary to rational administrative norms of action. This being immoral, the taint of personal interest, usually to be found somewhat somewhere in all administrative action, need to be carefully concealed. The bureaucrats never wish to wash their dirty linen in public, because once their personal interests and individual quarrels are exposed to public eye, they cease to be public servants in popular estimation.

The Cementing Force: Like internal power struggles of the hierarchy the deviations caused by lateral interests and other autonomous centres have to be concealed from public discussions. If people tend to feel that hierarchical controls are a mere façade and the dominant stereotypes do not exist, the myth of administrative rationality will be shattered. Here secrecy provides the necessary cementing force and people are made to believe that what they actually do not know, does not exist as well. (Mukhopadhyaya: 1983)

Privacy is closely related to autonomy of an individual. Each individual has the right to control his or her own life and therefore he or she has the right to control the disclosure of information about themselves. Professor Alan Westin defined privacy as, "Privacy is the claim of individuals, groups or institutions to determine for themselves when, how and to what extent information about them is to be communicated'. To Professor Arthur Miller, 'It is the individuals' ability to control the circulation of information relating to him". Ian Thompson said the privacy gives meaning to the concept of private individual. However, privacy is not absolute, like all other rights of an individual. In this context reference may be made of Lindop's comment:

> "In the use that is made of personal data, the interests of the individual and the interests of society may conflict and need to be resolved in the same way as in the context of individual liberty. With data protection, the solution must take the same form: a

> balance must be found between the interests of the individual and the interests of the rest of society, which include the efficient conduct of industry, commerce and administration. But as with our liberties, it is not a single point of balance which must be established.... It may also be settled differently in different societies, and may shift within the same society with changes, for example, in its political climate and institutional structure."

The privacy of medical information is no exception to this general rule. Patients do not have an absolute and inviolable right to confidentiality, and so ground rules have to be laid down about the scope and limits of the right of to clinical privacy, the circumstances in which it can be overridden. However, there are particular reasons why privacy is especially important in the doctor-patient relationship. First is the vulnerability of the patient. The patient comes to the doctor in fear, or pain, need they do not meet as equals. And so the doctor is under an obligation to protect and respect the vulnerability of the patient. The second reason is that the doctor is a member of a consulting profession, consultations are by their very nature private and cooperation is based on the acceptance of the doctor's special skills and knowledge. The third reason is reciprocal confidence, without which the relationship cannot get off the ground.

In the past detailed records were not available as the single handed practitioner could not afford to do this. Now a days all these go in notes. As understanding of human development and behaviour has increased, so medical records have become far more detailed. *The British Medical Journal* took a view limiting the right of patient to control information on him which is as below:

> "Information gained by a professional man in the course of a relationship with a client is the property of the client. The ethical rule is clear. Information so gained should not be passed on to others without the owner's consent save in certain defined circumstances. Doctors, for example, have a statutory obligation to notify certain infectious diseases. Here the interests of society outweigh those of the patient. Other instances occur in which medical men must on their own responsibility weigh their ethical duty to their patients against another, but secondary duty as citizens to prevent harm from befalling others."

The second component of confidentiality is confidence. It is essential mainly for two reasons—practical and moral. On practical reason, the practice of medicine is virtually impossible without it. Unless the patient has a confidence that he or she can talk freely to the doctor without fear that such personal, embarrassing or even shameful information will go any further patient might withhold information, so that, the consultation will be severely hampered. It is not only in the patient's interest, but also in the society's interest the patient should talk freely. The moral reason is closely related to the practical reason for confidence. The patient comes and talk freely to the doctor because there is a *prima facie* assumption of confidentiality. He thinks that what he is saying will go no further. There is a position of mutual trust; the doctor trust the patient to tell the truth about his condition, and the patient expects the doctor to keep his confidence. If the doctor nevertheless discloses the information to someone outside the clinical process, he is abusing that trust and behaving in a dishonest way. And honesty in medicine is absolutely crucial, because dishonesty is wrong in itself.

Disclosure of Medical Records: There are occasions demanding disclosure of medical records. Legal cases, Police enquiry regarding criminal cases, health safety measures, medical errors, medical negligence etc. require transparency in the medical services. The Government of India passed the Right to Information Act under which disclosure of information is mandatory. There is also the need of disclosure of information to the higher authorities, Insurance for security.

However, there is no general guidance on the use of medical records. The disclosure of medical records, generally necessary in the interest of the patients as well as public interest. Here, the delicate question is, can the disclosure of medical records to the patients help cure of their diseases? In some cases, when the knowledge of the problem may help the patient to regain mental strength to overcome the fear complex or darkness about the nature of the problem. But, there are also instances about cases of getting nervous or deterioration of mental condition of the patient after coming to know about the seriousness of the problem. Therefore, it is not an easy task for a doctor to decide whether the record is to be disclosed to the patient and if so to what extent it should be done? Further, all patients may not be in a position to listen or may not understand the medical language. In India, may be in other countries also the general practice is to disclose the record the relatives or the attendants of the patients. Once the recorded information are disclosed to the attendants or relatives, the medical authority loses control over the principle of secrecy to be maintained on the medical record. Similarly, the record on a patient which is kept under the custody of medical authority cannot be controlled by the patient. Once the patient is released from the hospital the question of taking consent of the exit patient for disclosing the medical record to others does not arise. Or it has also become irrelevant to the patient after being recovery of his health. Sometimes, the patient himself or herself discloses to others with proud by narrating the difficult time of suffering from serious diseases and the process of treatment by a doctor. In the case of the death of a patient, the relatives do not bother about the maintenance of secrecy of the medical record.

The information about the patient does not remain either under the custody of the doctor nor under his own custody. Further once these are computerized, the computerizers, if they are not honest may disclose them to others. These information may require for undertaking medical research or improvement of medical treatment in future course of action which demand disclosure to researchers and other doctors. This dilemma is arising due to the fact that a doctor, as a professional is bound by the obligation of professional secrecy and on the other hand as a citizen he must take care of the public or nation's interest. He has the responsibility to contribute to the health security of the citizens. (Phillips and Dawson: 1985)

The negative impact of the maintenance of secrecy in administration has been realized by the people and the scholars in India resulting the passing of Right to Information Act by Parliament on 12th October, 2005. As stated above it is found that the information disclosure in India was restricted by the Official Secrets Act 1923 and various other special laws, which the new Right to Information Act relaxes.

The Act provides that the request for government information by the citizens must be responded timely. It is an initiative taken by the Department of Personnel and Training, Ministry of Personnel, Public Grievances and Pension to provide Right to Information Portal Gateway to the citizens for quick search of information on the details of Appellate Authority, PIO etc. amongst others, besides access to RTI related information/disclosure published on the web by various public authorities under Government of India as well as State governments.

The basic object is to empower citizen/promote transparency and accountability in the working of government/contain corruption and make democracy work for the people in real sense. It goes without saying that an informed citizen is better equipped to keep necessary vigil on the instruments of government and make the government more accountable to the governed.

At the same time it cannot be denied that openness is not free from gaps and flows. It may throw a matter to public debate. In this case there is the possibility of having participants with dearth of knowledge about the consequences of a particular decision, it may invite conflicting views leading to creation of such a situation where the matter remains unresolved solution delayed. One has to realize that the application of the concept of political democracy in the administration of any public organization may cause chaos. In other words, it may be said that democratic principles should be applied in administration to the extent it can maintain efficiency and impartiality to establish social justice. One cannot deny that Delegation of power has the risk of creating the problem of segregation, decentralization in administration may have the risk of disintegration. The medical service is not an exception to it. There is the need of reasonable restrictions on the extent of openness and the person/group of persons to whom a particular matter/problem is to be opened so that a right decision may be taken or a problem may be solved in the greater interest of the nation and the humanity as a whole. No quality of human being is found in absolute nature. All ingredients of human personality must be in the balancing position to have mutual dependence of each other to allow human personality to work.

Whenever body or mind suffers from any ailment there is the need of strengthening the body or mind with the help of medicine to get relief of the suffering. Medicine purifies the body and the mind. The physicians use to impose limit on the quantity of medicine, on the span of time to be used while prescribing medicine to a patient. The restrictions thus imposed by the physicians on the application of medicine is necessary because it is not a regular food of an individual. They also work out what is a balanced diet for an individual to be taken everyday so that body can be strong or purified. The physicians also talk about curing ailments by exercises. Similarly, the Psychiatrists use to treat mental diseases through certain kind of medicines of mind.

Let me refer here to the theories of Greek medicine. Pythagoras and his followers believed in harmonious numbers. Pythagoras was a Greek philosopher, mathematician and founder of the religious movement called Pythagoreanism. He and his followers were well known for vegetarianism, which they practiced for religious, ethical and ascetic reasons. Pythagoreans tried to secure release of the soul from the body. They adopted old ceremonial purification. They talked about two kinds of purification—purification of body and the purification of the mind. The body was purified by abstinence from such foods as meat and beans. This was not based on humanitarian grounds as modern vegetarianism is, but on taboo. In India also there are restrictions on food on religious and caste related reasons, which are nothing but health oriented restrictions, particularly, purification of body and mind. The ancient Indian tradition and philosophy are flooded with this kind of restrictions.

Next is the purification of the soul. The quest for knowledge was regarded by the Pythagoreans as the best means of purification of soul. He who devotes disinterested science is philosopher. By philosophy the Pythagoreans meant the study of sciences. Particularly mathematics is the best means of purging the soul. India also provides many instances of reading religious books in the families having old ailing members with the aim of purging the soul of the ailing person and thereby create an environment for achieving mental peace for all the members of the family.

The Pythagoreans discovered the notion of mean by the study of medicine and music. In music the mean is a mixture of extremes, the higher and lower. It is a blend or harmony fitting together two categories. When the opposites meet their relationship becomes intelligible. So, the mean is the natural limit where the opposites meet. The notion of mean, as a balanced and harmonious mixture of opposites, was reinforced by the Pythagorean medical theories. The body is obviously a combination of the opposite qualities, of dry here, of moist there and of heat in another. When these qualities are harmoniously balanced the body is healthy and perfect. If there is no harmony there is disease.

Both Plato and Aristotle were influenced by Pythagoreans. Plato, in his book, 'Republic' adopted the concept of justice and to him justice means that each of the three elements, reason, spirit and appetite should be kept in proper place. The training of the guardians of the Republic by gymnastics and music corresponds to the purification of the body by medicine and music advocated by the Pythagoreans. Both Plato and Pythagoras emphasized the study of mathematics. They consider mathematics as the ladder for getting up from particularism to universalism.

Aristotle was also influenced by Pythagoreanism, particularly by the theory of mean enunciated by Pythagoreans. Aristotle believed not only in the limit of wealth and in the limit of the size of the state, but also in the mixed, mediatory and moderate constitution which is a blend of two opposite constitutions. (Rao:1980)

Not only in ancient India the restrictions were found in the ways of life of a man. The restrictions were supported by valid arguments. Of course those restrictions were in the rudimentary form. In independent India the Constitution itself provides reasonable restrictions on freedom of the individuals: For example one may refer to the Article 19 of the Constitution of India. The limitations imposed on freedoms guaranteed by Article 19 of the Constitution serve two purposes:

1. They specify that these freedoms are not absolute but are subject to regulation;
2. They put a limitation on the power of a legislature to restrict these freedoms.

There is no general standard of reasonableness applicable to all cases. Court has to decide each case on its own merit by examining if both substantive and procedural aspects of the restriction imposed or sought to be imposed are reasonable.

In determining the substantive reasonableness the court has evolved certain norms. The courts have to consider the factors like the nature of the right alleged to be infringed, the underlying purpose of the restrictions imposed, the extent and urgency of the evil sought to be remedied thereby, the disproportion of the imposition and the prevailing conditions at the time.

Guidelines to determine reasonableness have been spelled out in Pathumma *Vs.* State of Kerala case by a Constitutional-Bench of the Supreme Court. It had held the right conferred by the Article 19 is subject to reasonable restrictions to be placed by Parliament or the legislature in public interest. The Court had also laid down the guidelines to determine the question of reasonableness of "restriction" as follows:

1. That, in judging the reasonableness of the restrictions imposed by clause (5) of Article 19, the Court has to bear in mind the Directive Principles of State Policy.
2. That restrictions must not be arbitrary or of an excessive nature so as to go beyond the requirement of the interest of the general public.
3. That in order to judge the quality of reasonableness no abstract or general pattern or a fixed principle can be laid down so as to be universal application and the same will vary from case to case.
4. That a just balance has to be struck between the restriction imposed and social control envisaged by clause (6) of Article 19.
5. That there must be direct and proximate nexus or a reasonable connection between restriction imposed and the object which is

sought to be achieved. In other words, the court has to see whether by virtue of the restriction imposed on the right of the citizen the object of the statute is really fulfilled or frustrated.

6. That the court must see the prevailing social values whose needs are satisfied by restrictions meant to protect social welfare.

That so far as the nature of reasonableness is concerned it has to be viewed not only from the point of view of citizen but the problem before legislature and the object which is sought to be achieved by the statute. (Ibohal Singh: 2001)

Communication: Communication is a process of sending message from one person to another. Two parties are involved in the process—sender and the receiver. Generally, the sender initiates the process and the understanding is sent in the form of feedback by the receiver to the sender. In an organization the channel for the flow of message is very important. To-day in the big organizations vertical, horizontal and also zigzag channels are noticed. As regards the symbols word is used to communicate any message. The sender cannot observe the information or understanding within the receiver. The sender can know the receiver's understanding in the behaviour and explanation or the feedback. It is also exhibited in facial expression or bodily gestures. The sender's communicative efforts may result in one of the three the effects, in terms of the receiver's behaviour A desired change may occur, an undesired change, or no change. Successful communication involves an effect on receiver's behaviour. Miscommunication, too, involves an effect on the receiver's behaviour, but an undesired change. And no communication involves change in the receiver's action from the behavioural point of view.

When the desired effect occurs in the receiver's behaviour, successful communication has taken place; when on the other hand an undesired effect occurs, miscommunication has taken place while the absence of an effect signifies no communication. Several factors have direct bearing on the success of communication. The sender must have clear identification of the objectives so that these are free from ambiguity. Here the problem arises as the sender cannot directly know the understanding of the receiver. It may create tension in the relationship between the sender and receiver of the message. The receiver may be ignorant of the objective of communication of a particular message of the sender. This happens in the case of average patients at the recovery stage after getting treatment of diseases. Very often it is noticed that in the case of average patients once they get partial relief of the suffering they stop continuing medicine to complete the course or the care to be taken for a prescribed period. This happens due to lack of understanding of the objective of the message of the physicians to the exit patients who are the receivers. This kind of incidence also occurs in the case of the message sent by the supervisors or the higher officials to the subordinates. Sometimes in the case of plural headship or supervision there emerge contradictory instructions or advices making the receivers confusing. Further, unless message of the physician to the exit patient is very clear and strong there is every possibility of setting aside the suggestions/advices by the patient receiver at the influence of the visitors at home and the workplace which may cause harm to the patient and the reputation of the physician. In a country like India where the strength of the patient population in the OPD of the government hospitals is very large and come from very interior places it is difficult to sustain contact with them after discharging them from the hospitals, unless the patients themselves take initiative.

Another factor to be remembered is that all patients are not of similar category. Some of them are stereotype or unchangeable and some are changeable in their thinking. This type of receivers is detrimental to the process of communication.

Coming to the symbol of communication most familiar of it is the use of words. Semantics, which is the science of language and meaning, concerns itself with the study of communication symbols and their meaning. It may be noted that the words do not necessarily have commonly understood meaning. Certain types of words are likely to have ambiguous meanings leading to confusion. (Maheswari: 1991)

***Socialization and Ethical Principles*:** The human infant which is a helpless organism starts learning things and becomes social being through the process of socialization. The socialization is a process in which parents and other family members interact with the child and the child learns by participating in the process through trial and error method at the initial stage and gradually the child's personality grows. Man's personality is the result of the process of socialization in which the parents play a very significant role. In the language of Ian Robertson defined personality as, "personality refers to the fairly stable patters of thought, feeling and action that are typical to an individual." Thus, he tried to analyze the concept of personality into three major ingredients—cognitive, emotional and behavioural. The cognitive ingredient reflects thought, belief, perception, memory and other intellectual capacities; the emotional ingredient reflects love, hate, envy, sympathy, anger, pride and other feelings; and behavioural part reflects skill, aptitudes, competence and other abilities.

It is true that the process of socialization is always conditioned by the values and culture which a community adheres. When in a country different social groups exist socialization process also varies from one community to other. This will have impact on the personality of an individual. In India diversity in culture is prominent and this diversity influences the process of socialization very prominently. The inhabitants of hill areas may be distinguished from those of the plain areas, even in the plain areas different communities adopt different social cultures. It provides scope for diversity in thought process, values, beliefs etc. (Robertson: 1980).

Healthcare services in India have their roots in the Indian culture. *Kabirajes*, *Vaidas*, *tols* were significant and inalienable parts of the healthcare systems during the pre-British rule. The British rulers abolished the traditional medical institutions and put an end to the practice of using Sanskrit language. English language occupied its place. The modern system of medical care does not encourage Ayurveda. It appears that the attitude of modern medical scientists is not cooperative but hostile towards this Ayurvedic system. But at the same time government efforts are flowing to develop Ayurvedic system. The country especially Northeast India is very rich in medicinal plants. These can be used with scientific methods for taking care of health of the people. This was system which was familiar with the people of ancient India and even now average people in rural and hill areas are depending on it. The significant point is that through this system the modern hospital system may be relieved of the heavy burden which can be taken care of by this indigenous system without any risk or the minor cases and secondly people's cooperation can also be secured for both prevention and protection of preventable and curative diseases with care in day to day life by the individuals themselves.

This is expressed clearly by "Medical Ethics Manual" published by World Medical Association, which nobody can deny. In addition to significant role of different non-physiological disciplines in medical sciences it has also been realized that with the emergence of big hospitals entertaining huge number of ailing population of a country administrative systems and processes have also become very important part of medical sciences. The administrative ethics may flow from three sources—first, the profession itself articulates and upholds certain norms; second, norms laid down by the civil service rules and regulations; and third, personal beliefs and values which are highly individualized but which are reflected in the behaviour, decisions and actions of the public servants. Thus big hospitals like any other organization has to depend upon the administrative system manned by non-physicians or non-medical personnel. This kind of situation may also create tensions areas in the process of rendering health services. A big organization always invites formal rules and regulations unlike small ones. Further emergence of the practice of application of modern sophisticated equipment brings gaps in human relations.

At the time of Independence, the country inherited a health system devised during the British imperial rule, essentially to provide services to defense forces and colonial administrators including the native gentry. The system suffered largely in terms of both adequacy of health institutions and facilities as well as health manpower.

The present healthcare system has its origin in the recommendations of the Health Survey and Development Committee appointed in 1943 under the Chairmanship of Sir Joseph Bhore. The Committee's recommendations for future development of the health sector were based on the following main principles:

1. That no individual should fail to secure adequate medical care because of the inability to pay for it.
2. The health programme must, from the very beginning lay special emphasis on preventive work with consequential development of environment of environmental hygiene.
3. The health services should be placed as close to the people as possible in order to ensure the maximum benefit to the communities to be served.
4. It is essential to secure the active cooperation of the people in the development of health programme and administrative support of the people to be sought through the establishment of a Health Committee in every village.
5. The doctor, who is the leader of the health team should be a "Social Physician" who should combine remedial and preventive measures to confer maximum benefits on the community.

Community Development Programme and Srivastava Committee Report: With the launching of the Community Development Programme in October 1952 a modest beginning was made to implement a programme of setting up Primary Health Centres. It was the Srivastava Committee which in its report (1975) suggested that primary healthcare should be provided within the community itself through specially trained health workers.

Poor People Poor Justice: Judicial systems often seem more diligent in prosecuting crimes committed by poor people than crimes against them. According to its Pastoral Land Commission, between 1964 to 1992 Brazil experienced 1,730 politically motivated killings of peasants, rural workers, trade and union leaders and religious workers and human rights lawyers. By 1992 only 30 of these cases had been brought to trial, and just 18 resulted in convictions.

Surveys of poor people find that at best, the police and judiciary are considered unresponsive—at worst, as aggressive abuses of judicial rights. A recent World Bank Survey found that around the world, poor people view the police as:

- Unresponsive: absent when needed, coming only when someone has been killed.
- Corrupt: making false arrests, accusations and imprisonment, with release conditioned on large bribes; stealing money from the children; threatening, blackmailing and extorting citizens; using illegal drugs; conniving with criminals.
- Brutal: harassing street vendors; confiscating identification documents; raping women who register complaints; beating up innocent people, torturing and killing of homeless boys. (UNDP: 2002)

Medical Prescription: The free encyclopaedia says that a prescription is a healthcare programme implemented by a physician or other qualified practitioner in the form of instructions that govern the plan of care for an individual patient. A qualified practitioner might be a physician, physician assistant, dentist, nurse, pharmacist, psychologist, or other healthcare providers. Prescription may include orders to be performed by a patient, caretaker, nurse, pharmacist, physician, other therapist, or by automated equipment, such as an intravenous infusion pump. Prescriptions have legal implications, as they may indicate that the prescriber takes responsibility for the clinical care of the patient and in particular for monitoring efficacy and safety. A medical practice has become increasingly complex, the scope of meaning of the term 'prescription' has broadened to also include clinical assessments, laboratory tests, and imaging studies relevant to the safety or efficacy of medical treatment.

The serious problem as regards the hand written medical prescription.

In most cases the handwritings of the service providers are illegible. Neither the patient nor the pharmacists can read the prescription. In such cases errors inevitably arise in the process of treatment. In this context, mention may be made of the report of the National Academies of Science's Institute of Medicine (IOM) of July 2006 which stated that death occurred to 7,000 people annually for it. In India effort has yet to be made to make a survey of such problems. However, electronic system emerged in the process of communication in the healthcare system.

http.//en.wikipediaorg/wiki/Medical_prescription

Social Responsibility: Organizational ethics must reflect social responsibility. It is influenced by personal ethics of the persons working in the organization. Personal ethics is the product of one's education, religion, and family and community values. In India, cultural diversity and social values are changing fast. In the contemporary society experience shows that moneypower is more valued by a modern man. It is degenerating his need to greed and compelling him to be involved in corrupt practices. Corruption is standing as a serious impediment to carry out social responsibility of a public servant. In most cases the service provider, political leaders forget that they are the trustees of public money and the citizens whom they are to serve are the taxpayers. Nobody can deny that democratic administration is needed for establishing good governance and these leaders and administrators are the role models for the common masses. The concept of 'democracy' and 'governance' include both rulers and the ruled. The social responsibility of the service providers is reflected well in John and Johnson's "Our Credo" as quoted by Donald Treadwell and Jill B. Treadwell, in their book, "Public Relations Writing". It goes as below:

"We believe our first responsibility is to the doctors, nurses and patients, to mothers and fathers and all others who use our products and services.

In meeting their needs everything we do must be of high quality.

We must constantly strive to reduce our costs in order to maintain reasonable prices.

Customer's orders must be serviced promptly and accurately.

Our suppliers and distributors must have an opportunity to make a fair profit.

We are responsible to our employees, the men and women who work with us throughout the world.

Everyone must be considered as an individual.

We must respect their dignity and recognize their merit.

They must have a sense of security in their jobs.

Compensation must be fair and adequate, and working conditions clean, orderly and safe.

We must be mindful to ways to help our employees fulfill their family responsibilities. Employees must feel free to make suggestions and complaints.

There must be equal opportunity for employment, development and advancement for those qualified.

We must provide competent management and their actions must be just and ethical.

We are responsible to the communities in which we live and work and to the world community as well.

We must be good citizens—support good works and charities and bear our fair share of taxes. We must encourage civic improvements and better health and education.

We must maintain in good order the property we are privileged to use, protecting the environment and natural resources……"

Generally ethical standards are codified in the organization's mission, values, or vision statements and express the standard under which the organization will relate to its many publics. (Treadwell and Treadwell: 2005)

References

Buggi, Chandra Sekhar, 1978: *Relevance of Gandhian Political Ideas To-day*; *Journal of Gandhian Studies*; Vol. 5, No. 18, January; Institute of Gandhian Thought and Peace Studies, Gandhi Bhawan, University of Allahabad, Allahabad.

Dharm Pal, 1952: *Administration of Sir Lawrence in India* (1864-1869); Minerva Book Shop, Shimla.

Dwivedi, O.P., 2002: "The Challenge of Cultural Diversity for Good Governance", *Indian Journal of Public Administration*; Vol. XLVIII, Jan-March, 2002, No. 1.

Hazarika, Niru 2005: *Ethnic Autonomy Question in NE India*; Spectrum Publisher, Delhi.

Maheswari, S.R. 1991: *The Theories and Practice of Public Administration*, Allied Publishers Ltd., New Delhi, 1991.

Mukhopadhyaya, Girindra Nath 1974: *History of Indian Medicine*, Vol. II; Oriental Books, Reprint copy; pp 1-30, Traditional Medicine.

Nigro, Felix and Lloyd G. Nigro: *Modern Public Administration*, 7th ed. Harper & Row Publishers, New York.

Philips, Melanie and John Dawson, 1985: *Doctors' Dilemmas: Medical Ethics and Contemporary Science*; Harvester Press.

Radhakrishnan, S., 1970: *The Present Crisis of Faith*: Orient Paperbacks: first edition; A Division of Vision Books Pvt. Ltd., New Delhi.

Rao, V.V. 1980: *A History of Political Theories*: S. Chand & Co., Delhi.

Robertson, Ian 1980: *Sociology*, Worth Publishers, Inc. 444 Park Avenue South, New York.

Sethi, J.D. 1980: *Health and Development—A New Focus*, IJPA, July-Sept, 1980, Vol. XXVI, No. 3.

Treadwell, Donald and Jilli B. Treadwell, 2005: *Public Relations Writing*; Second Edition: Response Books; A Division of Sage Publications, New Delhi.

The Times of India, New Delhi, Tuesday, 20th August, 2013.

UNDP Report, 2002: *Deepening Democracy by Tackling Democratic Deficits*: Human Development Report: UNDP.

Ibid: 2004, *Globalization and Cultural Choice.*

World Health Forum. Vol. 17, 1996 (Seven advisers were 1. Professor Dimitri Barreto, 2. Professor Mohamed Larbi Bouguerra; 3. Mrs Barbar Kelly, 4. Dr Rainer Land; 5. Mr. Emmanuel Seyni Ndione; 6. Dr. Hiro Wakasugi and 7. Dr. Sergio Biros and Mr. Pierre Calame).

NINE
Conclusion

Survival and progress of global society demand respect for human values which require existence of ethical principles for safeguarding these values. The modern state and the progress of science and technology cannot do away the need of these values. The state policies and its activities may be considered as the mirror of these human values. Professor Z. Bankowski, who was the Secretary-General of the Council for International Organizations of Medical Sciences (CIOMS) in the article, titled, *Ethics and Human Values in Health Policy* published in the World Health Forum, Volume 17, 1996 also said, "A healthy policy reflects the fundamental beliefs and commitments of the nation or the people. These commitments are its human values... Ethics is itself grounded in socio-cultural, philosophical, or religious convictions. These convictions are the yardsticks for right and wrong, good and evil." These are conditions of man's way of life in a society. Freedom is no doubt man's birth right, his freedom to a certain extent is limited not only by the social norms but also by his connection with the past life.

In India the traditional societies expressed human values, though in the rudimentary form and without scientific interpretation, through the customs and traditions and religion to be observed by the families and the social groups. An analysis of them reveals that most of them had also health orientation to a great extent.

Human civilization is a continuous process and modern civilization cannot be rooted out from the past. Here, one has to remember the contributions of Radhakrishnan and Mahatma Gandhi for their contribution to the Indian culture and civilization. As distinguished Professor of Philosophy, Radhakrishnan has contributed very significantly to the Indian philosophy and religion. K.M. Munshi and R.R. Dwiakar, general editors of the book titled, *Hinduism Through the Ages* mentioned very clearly as, "His (Radhakrishnan's) two volumes of *Indian Philosophy* and his editions of the *Upanishads*, the *Bhagavad Gita*, the *Brahmasutra* and *Dhammapada* are monuments of deep erudition, penetrating insight and lucid exposition"

In order to create new social order Gandhiji introduced *Nai Talim* in the year 1937, which could not be continued for several socio-political reasons, is based on certain values cherished by him. He wanted that these values should be internalized by the younger generation also through new system of education evolved by him. The NCERT and Gandhi Peace Foundation had jointly sponsored studies on Gandhian values which he practiced himself in his personal and public life, experimented with them and suggested that our society should be instructed on the basis of these values if we want to remodel the social set-up through education. These values are as follows:

1. Truth (Honesty),
2. *Sarva Dharma Samabhava* (Composite culture, reverence for other's beliefs, communal unity) Non-violence (Love for mankind, service of humanity, *Satyagraha*, compassion, Universal love),
3. Freedom (Fearlessness),
4. Democracy (Rights, Duties, Responsibilities, National Integration),
5. Equality (Removal of Untouchability, Social Justice, Non-exploitation),
6. Self-Realization (*Swadeshi*, dignity of labour),
7. Purity of ends and means (Integrity between thought and action),
8. Self-discipline (self-control), and
9. Cleanliness (*Suddhi*, simplicity of life, non-consumerism, aesthetic).

To cultivate these virtues a man requires education basically through family and educational institution from his childhood. These two institutions should create a congenial environment by practicing them in the day-to-day activities. A child learns at the initial stage by imitation and out of compulsion or fear. Gradually, he starts developing habit for practicing them.

For the realization of these values in the system of education, a properly planned curriculum, organization of community life based on these values inside the educational institution and a programme of social service integrated to school life are very necessary. Without the development of the inner culture of man all our worldly possessions become the means of his own destruction, science and technology, if recognized as ethic neutral, will surely destroy our great civilization. Without a perception of the morality of the means and ends intellect becomes a self-stultifying instrument.

In modern time due to misconceptual notion of modernity and development the cultural values have deteriorated in India as in other parts of the world. It is a global crisis. A modern man has freedom to develop his personality and it is necessary for full development of the inner qualities or to shape the personality for realization of a healthy human society. But, as Radhakrishnan said, "Perfect freedom is impossible in an imperfect world and so those who have secured a vision of spirit work in the world so long as there is wrong to be set right, error to be corrected and ugliness to be banished from life. The individual who achieves unity within himself sets other men forward in desiring the same good. In a true sense, the ideal individual and the perfect community arise together."

Now, let us look to the changing situation in India. We fought against subjugation, cruelty and exploitation through the struggle for Freedom of India. We demanded our birth rights. Now the question arises, after gaining independence are we free from these in India? The answer is 'No' to a great extent. Even today we are facing rather more starkly the aliments of exploitation, cruelty, violation of human rights in all possible forms. These are multiplied by some fresh problems like strife, rivalry, unhealthy competition, blackmailing, conflicts, hypocrisy, mutual suspicion, revengeful attitude, greediness, maximization of selfish interest, lethargy, indolence, criminalization of profession etc.

The government is making efforts to remove all these ailments from our social life through formulation of new laws covering moral or human aspect of our social as well as personal life. The laws relating to the maintenance of elderly parents by the children, prevention of domestic violence against women, the establishment of Human Rights Commissions and Women Commission etc. are some of the examples. These are in addition to the provision of rights and duties of citizens and the welfare measures embracing downtrodden people or in short the constitutional provisions of the country. However, it cannot be denied that some acts of men are morally bad but legally valid. In this context mention may be made of Raja Ram Mohun Roy (1772-1833), the great Indian political thinker who acquired comprehensive knowledge of ancient religious, secular and philosophical literature, pointed out that in India father had an absolute right to sell or mortgage the ancestral property without consulting his sons even though such act might sometimes cause distress to the family and thus become morally indefensible. (Gupta: 2000-2001) This kind of situation is noticed even today in the relationship of husband and wife, parents and the children, mother-in-law and daughter-in-laws and even in the relationship amongst the neighbours in the existing social scenario.

Raja Ram Mohun Roy had the fear that some sound moral practices like obedience to parents, teacher, showing gratitude to benefactors cannot be given through legal force. Similarly, the laws relating to the maintenance of aged parents by the children, prevention of domestic violence against women as formulated by the government, unless the children have attachment or love for their parents from the core of their heart mere formulation and even its implementation will be a futile exercise.

Looking to the situation in which this kind of moral degradation is taking place it is found that with the transition of the society from the traditional status to modernization we have uprooted most of our old values existed in the traditional society from time immemorial due to impact of science and technology. Today we are in search for the ways of comfort, we have been exposed to outside world and are influenced by the impact of globalization. Certainly these cause change to our life.

The traditional society of the state of Assam maintained its social norms for flourishing human values to live together happily and peacefully, while recognizing the differences on caste, language, religion and culture, it was well known for tolerance, mutual respect for each other, fellow feeling, hospitality. The members of the traditional society could not even imagine the use of the socio-cultural pluralism of the society for personal gain. Nor one group of people considered other group as a threat to its survival and each group enjoyed freedom to preserve its own culture and tradition without any kind of exploitation and fear. In the primitive tribal society provision was made for the dormitory system in which the youths were taught about community life and it helped development of sense of belonging, feeling oneness, mutual respect for each other and commitment to the cause of the community. In the non-tribal society also through the celebration of different social and religious festivals the youths were given platforms for developing their personal qualities in the perspective of the social life. The religious leaders and the heads of the village could administrate the society very effectively. This was possible due to their honesty, sincerity and commitment to the cause of the village. With the adoption of modern democratic political system situation changes. The traditional society has been exposed and involved in the modern democratic process in its degenerated form. Most rural people were simple not only in the way living but also in the thinking process. They have been exploited emotionally just to gain political and economic power section of the people. These people have also been engaged in various illegal and immoral activities by these dishonest people by offering certain amount of money. Thus, the number of immoral activities in the state has increased and the nature of their involvement in the process is so complex and circuitous that it is not possible to most of them to realize the worse consequence of it on their own life.

Here, I may refer to another situation that in the case of India, the economic poverty of the masses was the main concern immediately after gaining independence. These were reflected in the voices of Mahatma Gandhi, Jawaharlal Nehru and several other leaders of the nation who devoted themselves to the movement for the freedom of the country. The government made the right effort to feed the hungry masses, to clothe the naked one and to shelter those who are exposed to all kinds of natural calamities. During that time national situation demanded it. Unfortunately, the human aspect of the process slipped away from their mind due to which its importance was lost in our fundamental programmes. Our planners and the leaders of the nation had overconfidence on the continuation of the human culture of the society without special care as it was the foundation of our country. The unfortunate result is that it has created flaws in our social life affecting the administration very badly. It is natural because the administrative system is a sub-system of the social system. It will certainly be influenced by the values in the society. Due to this situation with the progress of modern civilization various other serious social ailments have encroached upon our social life.

The leaders did not give due care to find space in their thought to enhance the quality of human resource which was the fundamental requirement to climb up in the escalator of the nation's progress. During freedom movement the efforts of the movement leaders provided lessons from different dimensions to realize that a democratic administration was necessary for good governance. In independent India the way in which the leadership moves gives scope to feel that due weightage is not given to the ideals of the constitution of the country. Grassroots level democracy was neglected. The election process, though held periodically, human values are not respected, public opinion is not honoured, shift of goal from the commitment to the cause of the nation to the power struggle of political parties based on money power and muscle power is noticed. As a student of political science, I also realize that politics is basically the struggle for power, but my realization is that this struggle must be rooted in the service to the nation, not in any other consideration. Further democracy at the top levels cannot be strengthened with very weak or withering grassroots democracy. The role of the political parties as socializing agencies has become very insignificant.

While looking at the social life it is noticed that the religion which is an inalienable part of the culture fails to influence the devotees in the right direction. The rituals are the aids religion, but it is felt that rituals are clouding the true spirit or the ethical aspect of religion. The social control over the members of the society has become very fragile.

A democratic country cannot be built by undemocratic leaders. No human society can be built by half human beings or by devils, no mischievous person can be empowered by human power and no money gatherer can claim to be an earner of wealth.

Further the federation cannot be strengthened unless the principle of the democratic decentralization is followed in its true spirit. This is the best device of self-help and to inculcate in the people the sense of belongingness and responsibility through direct involvement at the ground of the nation. The Union Government at the higher level can be empowered with the power of the people. The leaders of the nation try to have power with the people not over the people. Because by throwing out the sovereign nobody can wipe out the sovereign power of the people in a democracy. The leaders of independent India neglected the grassroots level power. Human power cannot be imposed from outside, it has to be generated by the individual itself through self-realization. Just as Plato said until philosophers were kings ideal state could not be achieved, until man cultivates human qualities through education we cannot think of good governance. Krishna Iyer, in his book titled, *Justice and Beyond* has said, the purpose of education is to culture the mind of a man so that he can accomplish all his aims in life. Education to justify itself, should enable a man to use the full potential of his body, mind and spirit. It should also develop in him the ability to make the best use of his personality, surroundings and circumstances so that he may accomplish the maximum in life for himself and for others. Today the education process is deviating from this which may appear as a threat to the nation soon. Iyer has quoted George A. Ellis, "Man is not on this earth merely to be happy, not even to be simply honest. He is there to realize great things for humanity, to attain nobility and to surmount the vulgarity in which the existence of almost all individuals drags on.... Art is not vague production, transitory and isolated, but a power which must be directed to the development and refinement of the human soul... the artist must have something to communicate, since mastery over form is not the end but, instead, the adopting of form to internal significance."

We forgot that it is only the democratic society which can help the individuals to acquire traits like tolerance, mutual help, sharing of feeling and care for the elderly and helpless people. The seeds of these must be sowed in the mind of a man at his early age by the parents in the family itself and environment has to be created for nurturing these qualities at the later stage by him at the instance of the teachers in the educational institutions and at the workplace under the guidance of the moral leadership of the higher authorities.

In to-day's India most people of both sexes are confronted and confused with the existing social values and the problem of adjustment becomes a serious challenge for them. The agencies for regulating the process of socialization like families, educational institutions, even the religious institutions have become very weak having very little impact on the life of a modern youth. Surprisingly, even these socializing institutions are also affected by confrontation and confusion as regards values to be adhered for the service to humanity. It results that the youths in most cases started imitating many things available in e-media as it is easily accessible to them without any constraint. It is a common practice in any developing country. India is not an exception. This process provides enough space to think of being engaged in various other activities accompanied by moral neutrality. The moral vacuum and human society cannot go together. This situation goes long way in destroying the human values in all the institutions in the state inviting all kinds of constraints. The efforts of the modern administration devoid of human orientation are self-defeating efforts. Now, we find that the leaders of the state and the society are struggling for survival.

In earlier times the people lived simpler lives. Their sphere of action was limited. Their intellectual development was low. There needs were few and were easily supplied. So, they had fewer opportunities for vice. Our life is more complex; our needs are many; we have to deal with many more persons; our struggle for existence is very great; our intellectual development is great. So, we are exposed to various kinds of vice. Surprisingly, men recognize broader and nobler ideals. But they do not practice these ideals in their lives and have become more selfish and narrow. Because it is difficult to practice these ideals they are in search of more comforts.

In a country like India it is really a difficult task to respond effectively to the challenges faced by it. The transitional society like ours always pauses confusion, conflicts and indecisiveness in the minds even of university degree holders while talking about the values in life. Ultimately, imitation has its way in their behaviour in this confusing situation.

The progress of science and technology no doubt, makes our life comfortable and fast. It also helps us to have access to all kinds of information about the world. Or in other words we are now living in a global village. At the same time it is also multiplying our wants, expose us to undesirable materials and physical comforts. This is the crux of the problem of transitional society. The desire of a man goes on increasing and desire multiplication is an unending process and can never be fully satisfied as each desire is followed by another and hence we lose control over it. In such a situation human qualities cannot flourish in a man. In order to establish a human society, the value of love, humanness, responsibility, care for civic and national property must be inculcated in the minds of the students or the children. We should not forget the rise and fall of a nation is directly related to the enhancement and deterioration of the quality of thought process of at least the leading personalities of the nation.

In Independent India with the adaptation of the Constitution and spread of education people have become conscious of their rights and other opportunities for their development. It was thought that the education will develop the intellectual horizon. It is essential for self-expression and self-development. More emphasis has been given on women education. Because to educate a woman means to educate a generation. This conclusion was based on the role of the family and again the role of a woman as mother teacher in the family in the traditional society. In the process of modernization and the impact of science and technology, the impact of family on the children has become insignificant. Today family plays a very insignificant role in molding the character of the children. The social control over individual disappears. In the traditional society the economic dependence caused obedience to social customs or elderly members in the family. This tie has become very fragile to keep people together with the assertion on individual right as citizen of an independent country. As citizen of the country everybody can enjoy the rights guaranteed by the Constitution. Thus, there emerged the constitutional protection and control of individualism. It is more specific based on the law of the country. It changes the social environment of man and broken the fabric of the traditional social life. We are still struggling to stabilize our status. We are to make sincere efforts to reactivate our human values along with the process of modernizing our lives.

In the traditional society of India several social customs were followed which indicated the merge of individual in the family. Especially, the prevalence of *Sati-pratha*, Child marriage etc. were some of the examples which did not recognize the individual status of wife or girl child. With the reform of the society and the adoption of the constitution the individual status is recognized. Today they are enjoying the economic independence also now they have been exposed to new challenges of adjustment with the husband and other family members, i.e. role adjustment with their habitation and environment in the workplace. While removing our social ailments like *Sati-pratha* and other we have failed to innovate alternative ways of integrating individuals with the society.

Further, the way of adjustment of the parents with children also changes. With the growth of the child they seek emotional and economic independence from their parents. They try to fulfill their desire in all possible ways. The parents also satisfy their wants without having a critical look to the consequence of it. The socializing agencies have to be strengthened to build up the character and habit of the future generation in the right direction. It is required due to changing situation in independent India.

Govind Ballabh Pant pointed out in his radio talk on 18th August, 1955 rightly as, "The new tasks of Civil Servants are therefore all comprehensive and include planning, control and guidance of the entire economic as well as social activities... the manner in which work is done and is efficiency now directly impinge on the lives of individual citizens. The welfare of the people will to an ever-growing extent depend on the imagination and sympathy and the efficiency with which work is understood and done by the civil servants.

A close analysis of the various components of the vast intricate mechanism that has to handle and grapple with these problems of growing moment and import will be necessary so that proper comprehension of its overall functions and requirements may be possible and automatic checks and control and adjustments may be provided to ensure the speed of work without impairing efficiency.

These are the problems that inhere in the running of any large concern and with them are linked the questions such as those of requirement, training, inter-departmental co-ordination, effective delegation of authority at all levels...rationalization of procedure, elimination of cumbersome apparatus of forms, maintenance of happy personal relations to evoke the best out of colleagues or subordinates, provision of effective punishments and suitable rewards where necessary, proper incentives for efficient work, deduction of time required for taking decisions, prompt attendance to correspondence, even distribution of work load, quick flow of communication vertically and horizontally, constant evolution and appraisal of effort, and continuous scrutiny of methods of working for introducing improvements.

Another very important factor of Public Servants to bear in mind is with regard to proper use of public funds. The tax-prayer's money is hard-earned money and Government servants are trustees of the public fund to ensure that every single pie of it is properly spent and utilized for the fullest benefit of the citizens. Sometimes those who have to spend this money seem to overlook the supreme duty that full worth has to be extracted over the money spent.

It is apt to be forgotten that this money is more sacred than their own and no part of its has to be spent in any waste-full manner. A proper climate of economy has to be produced. Economy never means sacrifice of efficiency or of the objectives. The welfare-state ideal will require the expenditure of huge sums on schemes of public weal, benefit or advantage. These sums must be spent but they must be well spent with care and prudence so that while on the one hand waste is eliminated on the other the purpose underlying the expenditure is completely achieved.

The problem of administration is not mechanical. It is essentially human. Unless, therefore, it is approached in that right spirit with sympathy, solicitude and understanding the desired results become difficult of achievement. The administrators have to serve the people because that is the only purpose for which they can and they ought to exist. Every ounce of their energy, their intellect, their capacity has to be surrendered to the devoted service of their masters, the people. That has to be their all-consuming passion, and their guiding mission. It needs a full missionary approach for results to be abiding and sweet, and to carry succor and service and light and hope to those still living in hamlets and hutments throughout the country and to apply the soothing balm to the sufferers." The expertness of a man must be added with human qualities if we are to contribute to the progress of humanity. Both must move together.

Bibliography

Abadi, Shirin (2003): Nobel Peace Prize Winner, *Human Development Report,* 2002, UNDP.

Abraham, S.J. Prasad, A. Joseph and K.S. Jacob (2000): *Medical Ethics: Confidentiality,* Partner Notification and HIV Infection: Issues related to Community Health Programmes; Int. *Medical Journal of India,* Vol. 13, No. 4.

Acharya, Binoy: *Occupational Health and Safety in India Legislations Inadequate*: Published in *IJPA*; July-September Issue, 1989, Vol. XXXV, No. 3.

Adams, Guy. B. and Danny, L. Balfour (1984): Ethical Failings, Incompetence and Administrative Evil (Lessons from Kartina and Iraq) published in the book, *Ethics and Integrity in Public Administration: Concepts and Cases*; edited by Raymond W. Cox III, published by M.E. Sharpe, New York.

Administrative Reforms Commission: GOVERNMENT OF INDIA constituted the Second Administrative Reforms Commission in August 2005 to prepare a detailed blueprint for revamping the public administration system. It consisted of the following members:

(i) Shri Veerappa Moily—Chairperson
(ii) Shri V. Ramachandran—Member
(iii) Dr. A.P. Mukherjee—Member
(iv) Dr. A.H. Kalro—Member
(v) Dr. Jayaprakash Narayan—Member
(vi) Smt. Vineeta Rai—Member-Secretary.

The Commission was asked to suggest measures to achieve a proactive, responsive, accountable, sustainable and efficient administration for the country at all levels of the Government. The most significant aspect is 'ethics in governance'.

Agarwal, R.C. (1986): *Constitutional Development of India and National Movement,* S. Chand & Co. Ltd., New Delhi.

Anand, Dr. V.K. (2001): Allahabad Law Agency, 16/2/Mathura Road, Plot No. 33, Faridabad.

Annan, Kofi (2002): United Nations Secretary General: *Human Development Report* UNDP Human Development and Human Dignity.

Babu, B. Ramesh: His address on *Legitimate Globalisation: Towards New Universal Norms and Values: Man in India*: 90 (1-2): 309-409.

Bakshi, P.M. (2004): *The Constitution of India*: 5th edition; Universal Law Publishing Co. Pvt. Ltd., New Delhi.

Baeva, L.: Existential and Ethical Values in an Information Era, *Journal of Human Values*, Vol. 20, April 1, 2014.

Baxi, Upendra (1994): *Inhuman Wrongs and Human Rights*: Har-Anand Publications, New Delhi, 1994.

Bharadwaj, H.R. (2007): *Heritage of Unity, Harmony and Peace;* published in the book, *Understanding India*, ed. by Subhash Chandra Kashyap and Abhaya Kashyap, Vitasta Publishing Ltd., New Delhi.

Bhardwaj, Rekha (2000): article, Significance of Scriptures in Highlighting Human Rights, published in the book titled, *Human Rights: Global Perspective* edited by Hemlata Talesa, Nalini Pansholy and Mangi Lal Nagda; Publisher, Rajasthan Council of Educational Administration and Management, Udaipur.

Bhaskara Rao, V.: Frederick Taylor; *Administrative Thinkers*, edited by D. Ravindra Prasad, V. Prasad, P. Satyanarayana and Y. Pardhrasaradhi, Sterling Publishers Pvt. Ltd., New Delhi-22.

Bharatiya, L.K.: *Prospect of Change on Gandhian Lines*; *Journal of Gandhian Studies* in 1987 by Institute of Gandhian Thought and Peace Studies, Gandhi Bhawan, University of Allahabad.

Bharato, K.S. and Mani (1987): *The Foundations of Gandhian Thought,* Bharati.

Bhattacharya, Buddhadeva: Gandhian Socialism and Its Relevance in India Today; *Journal of Gandhian Studies:* Institute of Gandhian Thought and Peace Studies, Gandhi Bhawan, University of Allahabad, Allahabad, Vol. 7, No. 27, Jan-Apl. 1980.

Bhattacharya, Mohit (1987): *Public Administration*, World Press Private Ltd.

Bhattacharya, Mrs. Gauri (1981): Political and Social Ideas of Mahatma Gandhi: A Critique: An unpublished Ph.D. thesis submitted to Gauhati University in 1981.

Boorstin, Daniel J. (1974): *Democracy and Its Discontents*; Random House; New York, 1974.

Bose, N.K. (1957), *Selection from Gandhi*, Navajivan Publishing House, Ahmedabad.

Bowman, James and Donald C. Menzed (ed.) (1998): *Teaching Ethics and Values in Public Administration Prorammes*, State University of New York.

Barnabas, C. Joseph: article, *Religious Freedom and Human Rights*, published in the book Human Rights in India: ed. by Chiranjivi J. Nirmal, Oxford University Press.

Barnett, John H.: Action and Symbolic Viewing (An investigation of the *Gita* and Executive Ethics; *Journal of Gandhian Studies*; Institute of Gandhian Thought and Peace Studies; Gandhi Bhawan, University of Allahabad, Volume 12; No. 46, January, 1985.

Basu, Acharya Dr. Durga Das (2007); *Commentary on the Constitution of India*: eighth edition 2007: Wadha & Company: Agra, Nagpur and New Delhi.

Bharatiya, L.K.: Prospect of Changes on Gandhian Lines; *Journal of Gandhian Studies* in 1987 by Institute of Gandhian Thought and Peace Studies, Gandhi Bhawan, University of Allahabad.

Bhatta, P.C., Compiler: Proceedings of the International Conf. on Health Policy: Ethics and Human Values, held in New Delhi 1986. It was held in collaboration with the Council of International Organization of Medical Sciences (Geneva). Compiled by, Secretariat, IMA House, May, New Delhi.

Bowman, James and Donald C. Menzed (ed.) (1998): *Teachings and Values in Public Administration Programmes*; State University of New York.

Budhachandra Singh, Khundrakpam (2011): Gandhian Approach to Non-Violence and Peace: An unpublished Ph.D. thesis submitted to the Department of Political Science, Manipur University.

Buggi, Chandra Sekhar: articile, Relevance of Gandhian Political Ideas To-day; *Journal of Gandhian Studies*; Vol. 5, No. 18, January 1978; Institute of Gandhian Thought and Peace Studies, Gandhi Bhawan, University of Allahabad.

Canley, Simon and Peter Jones (ed.) (1945): *Human Rights and Global Diversity*, Frank Cass: London, 1945.

Chandra, Bipan (1971): *Modern India*, National Council of Educational Research and Training, New Delhi.

Chatterjee, Aneek (2010): *International Relations Today*: Longman (Pearson), Kolkata.

Chaturvedi, Urmila (2002): *Priority to Duties in Indian Tradition*, published in the book *Governance and Human Rights*, edited by Jhunjhunwala; Kalpaz Publications, Delhi.

Chaturvedi, T.N. ed. (1998): *Fifty Years of Indian Administration*: *Retrospect and Prospects*; Published by IIPA, New Delhi, 1998.

Chowdhary, T.H.: *Relevnce of Hinduism*, National Council of Educational Research and Training, New Delhi.

Chiranjivi, J. Nirmal (ed.) (1999): *Human Rights in India*: Oxford University Press.

Choudhuri, Dr. Keshab: A Limited-frame reference to Gandhian relevance: *Journal of Gandhian Studies*; April-July, 1976, Vol. No. 10-11.

Cox III Raymond W. (2009): *Ethics and Integrity in Public Administration: Concept and Case*; M.E. Sharpe, Armonk, New York.

Deep Dogra, Km. Sandhya, 1980: Mahatma Gandhiji's Social Philosophy: *Journal of Gandhian Studies*: Vol. 7. No. 28, July, 1980; Institute of Gandhian Thought and Peace Studies, University of Allahabad, Allahabad.

Denhardt, Kathryn G. (1988): *The Ethics of Public Service: Resolving Moral Dilemmas in Public Organizations*. Greenwood Press, New York.

Desai, Suresh A.: The Role or Price System in Gandhian Economics: Gandhi Marg, *Journal of the Gandhi Peace Foundation*; No. 24, Vol. 2, Number 12, March, 1981.

Devadoss, Dr. T.S.: Freedom, Equality and Peace—A Gandhian Perspective: *Journal of Gandhian Studies*: Institute of Gandhian Thought and Peace Studies, Gandhi Bhawan, University of Allahabad, Allahabad, Vol. 14, Nos. 54-55, Jan-April, 1987.

Devi, Ksh. Bimola: *Relevance of Gandhian Thought in the Present Day Society*; Manipur Today, Republic Day, Dept. of Information and Public Relations, 26.12.2010, Vol. XXXI, No. I.

Dharm Pal (1952): *Administration of Sir Lawrence in India* (1864-1869); Minerva Book Shop, Shimla.

Dias, R.W.M. (1994): *Jurisprudence*, Aditya Book Pvt. Ltd., New Delhi.

Diwakar, R.R.: Trying to Understand Gandhi: *Journal of Gandhian Studies*: Vol. 14, No. 53, October 1986. Institute of Gandhian Thought and Peace Studies, Gandhi Bhawan, Allahabad University, Allahabad.

Doctor, Adi H. (1997): *Political Thinkers of Modern India*; Mittal Publications, New Delhi.

Dogra, Km. Sandhya Deep: Mahatma Gandhiji's Social Philosophy: *Journal of Gandhian Studies*: Institute of Gandhian Thought and Peace Studies, Gandhi Bhawan, University of Allahabad, Allahabad, Vol. 7, No. 28, July, 1980.

Dubhasi, P.R.: Accountability and Ethics, *Indian Journal of Public Administration*, Vol. XXIX, No. 3, July-Sept. 1983.

Dutta, Sashi Dhar (1990), Chairman, National Integration Committee; National Integration.

Dutta, Keshab Narayan (1956): *Culture and Civilization of Assam*; published by Mahendra Kumar Barua, Shrimanta Sankar Krishi Bikash Samiti; 1st edition.

Dwivedi, O.P.: *Ethics and Accountability*: *IJPA*; July-Sept; 1983, Vol. XXIX, No. 3.

Dwivedi, O.P; The Challenge of Cultural Diversity for Good Governance: *Indian Journal of Public Administration*; Vol. XLVIII, Jan-March, 2002, No. 1.

Dwivedi, O.P.: Ethics and Administrative Accountability, *Indian Journal of Public Administration*, Vol. XXIX, No. 3, July-Sept, 1983.

Dwivedi, O.P.: (Presidential Address of O.P. Dwivedi on "Moral Dimensions of Statecraft: A Plea for an Administrative Theology" delivered in June 1987 to the Canadian Political Science Association, Hamilton, which is being recorded from *Canadian Journal of Political Science*, Vol. XX, No. 4. December 1987 published in *Indian Journal of Public Administration*; October-December 1988; Vol. XXXIV, No. 4.

Ebenstein, W: *Introduction to Political Philosophy.*

Edelstein, L. (1943): *The Hippocratic Oath, Text, Translation and Interpretation; Baltimore*, Johns Hopkins Press.

Elliot, Frederick (1971): *Goals for Quality must be based on Values derived from Changing Society*, Modern Hospital, August.

Emden, S. Cecil (Ed.): *Selected Speeches on the Constitution*, Oxford University Press, London, Humphrey, Milford.

Frankiln, D.: "Relevance of Gandhi for Our Time" *Souvenir*, Gandhi Centenary Celebration Committee for Assam.

Gallaghar Eagene B. (Ed.): "Doctor-Patient Relationship in Changing Health Scene": (Conf. proceedings and papers organized in USA in 1976 by Department of Health Education and Family Welfare, Public Health Service, National Institute of Health), ed. by Eagene B. Gallagher, Professor of Medical Sociology, Professor of Behavioural Science, Kenttucky College, Medicine).

Gandhi: An Autobiography; (1959). Navajivan Publishing House, Ahmedabad, 1959.

Gandhi, M.K. (1985): *From Yeravda Mandir, Ashram Observance in Action*, Sage Publication, New Delhi.

Gandhi, (1948): *Key to Health*, this book was written by M.K. Gandhi in Gujrati language and translated in English by Sushila Nayar, first published in October 1948, Navajivan Publishing House, Ahmedabad-380 014.

Gandhi (1957): *The Story of My Experiments with Truth*, Beacon Press, Boston.

Gandhi (1924): *Young India*; 13th November.

Ghosh, Dr. Raghunath: *The Gandhian Concept of Truth: In the Light of Advaita Vedanta and its Relevance in Modern Society*: *Journal of Gandhian Studies*: Institute of Gandhian Thought and Peace Studies, Gandhi Bhawan, University of Allahabad, Allahabad, Vol. 12, Nos. 47-48, April/July 1985.

Giddens, Anthony (ed.) (1992): *Human Society: An Introductory Reader in Sociology*; Polity Press, 65 Bridge Street; Cambrifge CB21 UR UK.

Gill, Deepak G.: *Limitation upon choice and constraints over decision making in doctor-patient exchanges*: University of Missouri-Columbia Medical Center, Columbia, Missori.

Gopalakrishnan, Dr. R.: Gandhiji's Ashram Vows and their Relevance for the Contemporary Social Situation: *Journal of Gandhian Studies*: Institute of Gandhian Thought and Peace Studies, Gandhi Bhawan, University of Allahabad, Allahabad, Vol. 12, Nos. 47-48, April/July, 1985.

Goyal, O.P. (1984): *Studies in Modern Indian Political Thought*, Kitab Mahal, Allahabad.

Goel, Dr. Aruna and Dr. S.L. Goel (ed.) (2005): *Human Values and Education*; Deep & Deep Publications.

Government of India, Ministry of Information and Broadcasting, New Delhi: *Collected Works of Mahatma Gandhi*, 1969, Vol. 22.

Grover, Dr. D.C. (1977): *Satyagraha: An Answer to International Conflict*; Institute of Gandhian Thought and Peace Studies, Gandhi Bhawan, University of Allahabad, Allahabad, Vol. 4, No. 16, July.

Guha, Ramchandra (2013): *Gandhi Before India*, Penguine Book.

Ibid., Vol. XII, 1969.

Ibid., Vol. XIII, 1964.

Gupta, M.G.: *History of Political Thought*; Chaitanya Publishing House, Allahabad, 1972.

Gupta, N.L. (1995): *Education and Values in the Mahabharata*, Concept Publishing Company.

Gupta, R.C. (1963): *Great Political Thinkers: East and West*, Lakshmi Narain Agarwal, Agra.

Gupta, R.C. (2006): *Great Political Thinkers*: Lakshmi Narain Agarwal, Agra.

Hasan, Nawab Md. Dilwar: The Saint we know as Gandhi: *The Assam Tribune*, 2nd October, 2014.

Hazarika, Niru (2005): *Ethnic Autonomy Question in NE India*; Spectrum Publisher, Delhi.

HRH, the Prince of Wales: Text of Speech at the Royal Albert Hall, London, 1969.

IWCOHR Occasional paper No. 4 on *Human Rights in India: An Overview*; January 1997.

Iyengar, N.K.N.: Personal Privacy in the United States: (review Article) *Indian Journal of Public Administration*, October-December, 1979, Vol. XXV; No. 4.

Iyer, Raghavan (1986): *The Moral and Political Writings of Mahatma Gandhi*, Oxford.

Iyer, V.R. Krishna: *Justice and Beyond*: Deep & Deep Publications; New Delhi, 1988.

International Medical Journal of India, Vol. 13, No. 4, 2000.

Jain, R.B. and Kanchan Sharma: *Implementation Machinery for Environment Protection in India*: *IJPA*; July-September Issue, 1989, Vol. XXXV, No. 3.

Jha, Vidyananda (2002): *Priority given to Human Rights in Ancient Indian Tradition*: *Governance and Human Rights*, edited by Bharat Jhunjhunwala, Kalpaz Publications; Delhi.

Jhunjhunwala, Bharat Ed. (2002): *Governance and Human Rights*, Kalpaz Publications, Delhi-110052.

Kampadoo, Peter Lakhsmanen: *Way Five: The Sarvodaya Way: Journal of Gandhian Studies:* Vol. 14, No. 53, October 1986 Institute of Gandhian Thought and Peace Studies, Gandhi Bhawan, University of Allahabad, Allahabad.

Kapur, Anup Chand (1989): *Indian Political System*: published by S.Chand & Co., New Delhi, 1989, Kempadoo, Sri Peter Kempadoo: *Sarvodaya: Gandhi's Alternative To Development Strategy for Today's World.* Published in Jan. 1983, *Journal of Gandhian Studies*, Vol. 10, No. 37-38, Oct. 82, Institute of Gandhian Thought & Peace Studies, Gandhi Bhawan, University of Allahabad.

Kerridgelan, Michael Lowe and Camerun Stewart (2009): *Ethics and Laws for the Health Professionals*; published by Federation Press, Australia.

Khanna, Dr. B.S: Asstt. Prof., IIPA, New Delhi, Paper: Morale in Public Services presented in the Conference on Morale in Public Services, held on 3-4 January 1959.

Khan, Zia Uddin, Mathur and Iqbal Narain (Ed.) (1969): *Panchayati Raj, Planning and Democracy*, Asia, 1969.

Khatami, Seyyed Md.: President of the Islamic Republic of Iran: Chapter 2: Deepening Democracy by Tackling Democratic deficits: Human Development Report: 2002; UNDP.

Kirpal, Prem: *Culture and Development*: pubished by Har-Ananad Publications, 364-A, Chirag, Delhi-110017.

Kistaia, M. 2007: Article: George Elton Mayo (2007); Published in the book *Administrative Thinkers*: edited by D. Ravindra Prasad, V.S. Prasad and P. Satyanarayana; published by Sterling, New Delhi.

Krishna Iyer, Justice V.R. (1995): *Human Rights—A Judge's Miscellany*: B.R. Publishing Corporation, A Division of D.K. Publishers Distributors, Delhi.

Kurien, K. Mathew and Mythily Sivaraman: *Gandhian Approach to Property and Relations and Class Comflict*: 1986 Institute of Gandhian Thought and Peace Studies, Gandhi Bhawan, University of Allahabad, Allahabad, Vol. 3, Apl.-July, 1976, No. 11-12.

Kumar, Dr. Vipul (2008): *Legal Solutions for Medical Profession*: published St. Matthew's Scientific Research Foundation; 2010; (Here reference is made of the Law of Torts, Ratanlal & Dhirajlal (twenty fourth Edition 2002, edited by Justice G.P. Singh).

Lambert Commission: In March 1979, Royal Commission on Financial Management and Accountability (also known as Lambert Commission) submitted its final report to Government of Canada. Published in *IJPA, Special number on Administrative Accountability,* July-September, 1983, Vol. XXIX, No. 3.

Laski, Harold J. (1960): *A Grammar of Politics,* London, 4th edition, 1960, reprint.

Leighton, Alexander H. (1956): Preventive Psychiatry in Industry; *Management News*, January 28, 1949, as referred in the book titled, "*Public Personnel Administration*" by O.G. Stahl; fifth edition of earlier work of William E. Mosher, J. Donald Kingsley and O. Glenn Stahl, Oxford & IBH Publishing Co., New Delhi.

Madhulika, Smt.: Gandhiji and Contemporary Ideologies Regarding Freedom, Peace and Equality. *Journal of Gandhian Studies: Institute of Gandhian Thought and Peace Studies*, Gandhi Bhawan, University of Allahabad, Allahabad, Vol. 14, Nos. 54-55, Jan-April, 1987.

Mahanty, Jaganath (2000); *Human Rights Education*; Deep & Deep Publications.

Mahatma Gandhi, *Harijan,* 5th May, 1946.

Maheswari, Shriram (2002): *Administrative Theory*: MacMillan India Ltd., Delhi, 2002.

Maheswari, S.R.: Accountability in Public Administration: A Conceptual, *IJPA*; July-Sept., 1983, Vol. XXIX, No. 3.

Maheswari, S.R. (1994): *Theories and Concepts of Public Administration*, Allied Publishers Ltd., New Delhi.

Maheswari, S.R. (1991): *The Theories and Practice of Public Administration*, Allied Publishers Ltd.; New Delhi.

Malhotra, Dr. S.L. and Dr. S.K. Sharma (1977): *Towards Village Swaraj, Research Monograph*; Department of Gandhian Studies, Punjab University, January, Chandigarh.

Mallay, N.N., *Public Enterprises in India (1971): The Control and Accountability*, Delhi, National.

Melanie Phillips and John Dawson (1985); *Doctors' Dilemmas: Medical Ethics and Contemporary Science*; Harvester Press, 1985.

Merriam, Charles A. (1939): *The New Democracy and the New Despotism*, McGraw-Hill Book Company, New York.

Minocha, O.P.: Article, "*Accountability in Public Sector Enterprises*", *IJPA*; July-Sept., 1983, Vol. XXIX, No. 3.

Misra, Sridhar (2002): The Social Good in Indian Tradition: published in the book titled, *Good Governance and Human Rights*, edited by Bharat Jhunjhunwala, Kalpaz Publications, Delhi-110052.

M.K. Gandhi (1989): *An Autobiograhy Or The Story of My Experiments with Truth*, Navajeevan.

Monhot, S.R. (2007): *Relevance of Hindu Philosophy to Understand India* published in the book, *Understanding India*, ed. by Subhash Chandra Kashyap and Abhaya Kashyap, Vitasta Publishing Ltd., New Delhi.

Mukhopadhyaya, Girindra Nath (1974): *History of Indian Medicine*, Vol. II; Oriental Books, Reprint copy; pp. 1-30, *Traditional Medicine*.

Mukherjee, Subrata and Sushila Ramswamy: *A History of Political Thought (Plato to Marx)*: Prentice Hall of India; New Delhi.

Mukhopadhyaya, Ashok; Article: *Administrative Accountability: A Conceptual Analysis*; *IJPA*; July-Sept 1983, Vol. XXIX, No. 3.

Mukhopadhyaya, Lipi: Social Conditioning and Deviant Behaviour, *IJPA*, *Spl. Number on Social Tensions: Administration and Political Responses*; July-Sept. 2002, Vol, XLVIII, No. 3.

Nagarjan, Rema: *The Times of India*, 15th December, 2013: Article: Clean Slate for Doctors on Medical Negligence?

Narayan, Shriman (2005): *Gandhi: The Man and His Thought*: Publication Division, Government of India, New Delhi.

Naseema, C. (2002): *Human Rights Education: Conceptual and Pedagological Aspects*; Kanishka Publisher Distributors, New Delhi.

Nathan, Lord (1957): in collaboration of Anthony R. Barrowclough: *Medical Negligence*; Butterworth & Co. Ltd. (Lord Nathan: 1957).

Nayar, Sushila (1948): Translator of the Book, *Key to Health authored by Mahatma Gandhi*, Navajivan Publishing House, Ahmedabad.

N.D. Palmer (1973), *The Indian Political System*, Houghton Mifflin Co. Boston.

Nehru, Jawaharlal: A Word to the Services; speech made by Nehru as Prime Minister, at Kurnool, in Andhra, on 9th December, 1955 to an audience of Public Servant, *Indian Journal of Public Administration*, Vol. 1, Oct-Dec., 1955, No. 4.

Nehru, Jawaharlal (1946): *The Discovery of India*; New Delhi, 1946, 12th impression 1992, Delhi referred in IWCOHR Occasional Paper No. 4 on *Human Rights in India: An Overview*; January 1997.

Nirmal, C.J. (1999): *Human Rights in India*; Oxford University Press.

Nigro, Felix and Lloyd G. Nigro: *Modern Public Administration:* 7th ed. Harper & Row Publishers, New York.

Mani, V.S.: *Human Rights in India: An Overview*, IWCOHR Occupational paper No. 4.

Pal, Dharm (1952): *Administration of Sir John Lawrence in India* (1864-1969). Published by Minerva Book Shop.

Palkhiwala, Nani A. (1997): *We The People*; UBS Publisher' Distributors Ltd., New Delhi, 11th print.

Pandya, V.D. (1987): *Gandhian Perspective to Democracy and Socialism*: Institute of Gandhian Thought and Peace Studies, Gandhi Bhawan, University of Allahabad, Allahabad, Vol. 14. Nos. 54-55, Jan.-April.

Philips, Melanie and John Dawson (1985): *Doctor's Dilemmas: Medical Ethics and Contemporary Science*; Harvest Press.

Prabhu, R.K. and U.R. Rau (1945): *The Mind of Mahatma Gandhi*, Oxford University Press, London.

Prakash, Dr. Jagadish and Nageswar Rao (1980): *Gandhian Perspectve to Socialism*: Institute of Gandhian Thought and Peace Studies, Gandhi Bhawan, University of Allahabad, Allahabad, Vol. 7, No. 27, November.

Prasad, Prof. Kali: Paper: Morale in the Public Services: A Social Psychological Analysis; *Ibid.*

Prasad, D. Ravindra: Abraham Maslow published in the book titled, *Administrative Thinkers*, edited by D. Ravindra Prasad, V.S. Prasad, P. Satyanarayana and Y. Pardhasaradhi, Sterling Publisher, New Delhi, 2011.

Pushparanjan, A.: Are Religions One? *Journal of Gandhian Studies*: Institute of Gandhian Thought and Peace Studies, Gandhi Bhawan, University of Allahabad, Allahabad, Vol. 7, No. 27, November, 1980.

Pushparajan, A.: *Environmental Challenges of Today and Gandhi—The Only Hope of the Twenty First Century*; published in Gandhi-Jyoti, *Journal of Gandhian Thought*, 1st January, 1992—6th April, 1992.

Pyasi, Mala (2002): *Duties Before Rights*; published in the book, *Governance and Human Rights*, edited by Bharat Jhunjhunwala; Kalpaz Publications, Delhi.

Quartey, Francis Ofosu: Gandhian Concept of Non-violence: Published in *Journal of Gandhian Studies*, Vol. 7, No. 28 July, 1980. Gandhi Bhawan, University of Allahabad, Allahabad.

Rader, Melvin (1964): "*Ethics and Human Community*" Hott Rinehart and Winston, USA.

Radhakrishnan, S. (1961): *Recovery of Faith*; George Allen & Unwin Ltd., References, Radhakrishnan: *The Present Crisis of Faith*: published by Orient Paperbacks, first edition, A Division of Vision Books Pvt. Ltd., New Delhi, 1970.

Radhakrishnan, S. (1992): *The Present Crisis of Faith*: Orient Paperbacks, New Delhi, 11th Edition.

Radhakrishnan, S. (2013): *Indian Philosophy*, Vol. 2, Oxford University Press, Ninth Impression.

Raj, Dr. Hans (2001): *Principles of Public Administration*, Surjeet Publication, Delhi.

Rajkhowa, J.P.: *Sankardeva: His Life Preachings and Practices*, published by Rupsmita, Rajkhowa, Guwahati, Assam.

Ramesh, Babu (1990): *Address on Legitimate Globalization Towards New Norms and Values*, published in Man in India.

Rao, B. Shiva (1967): *The Framing of India's Constitution*; Vol. II, The Indian Institute of Public Administration, New Delhi.

Rao, V. Venkata (1980): *A History of Political Theories*: S. Chand & Company, New Delhi.

Robertson, Ian (1980): *Sociology*; Worth Publishers, Inc., 444 Park Avenue South, New York.

Robinson, Joan (1970): *Freedom & Necessity; An Introduction to the Study of Society*: George Allen & Unwin Ltd.

Rolland, R. (1969): *Mahatma Gandhi: The man who become one with the Universal being*. Translated by Catherine D. Groth, New Delhi, Publication Division, Government of India, (referred in Budhachandra's unpublished Ph.D. thesis, titled Gandhian Approach to Non-Violence and Peace).

Rowatt, D.C. (1964): Ombudsman.

Roy, A.C.: *International Relations Since 1919*, World Press, Calcutta, 9th edition.

Ruthnaswamy, M. (1972): *Principles and Practice of Public Administration*: Fifth edition; Central Book Depot, Allahabad.

Sabine, G.H., (1949): *A History of Political Theory*; 3rd edition.

Sadana, B.L. and M.P. Sharma (2004): *Public Administration in Theory and Practice*, Kitab Mahal, Allahabad.

Sapru, Dr. R.P.: *The Conflict of Ethics and Social Justice in Developing Countries*; Dr. R.P. Sapru was an Associate Professor, Dept. of Cardiology, Postgraduate Institute of Medical Education and Research, Chandigarh. Published under the auspices of Indian Council of Medical Research the Conference papers. The International Conf. was held in New Delhi 1986. The topic was *Health Policy: Ethics and Human Values*. It was held in collaboration with the Council of International Organization of Medical Sciences (Geneva). Compiled by Dr. P.C. Bhatta, Secretariat, IMA House, May, New Delhi.

Sarma, D.S. (1967): *Hindustan: Through Ages*, Bharatiya Vidya Bhawan, Chowpatty, Bombay.

Seshachalam, P., Rensis Likert (2007): Published in the book *Administrative Thinkers*: edited by D. Ravindra Prasad, V.S. Prasad and P. Satyanarayana; Sterling Publishers (P) Ltd., New Delhi, 2007.

Sethi, J.D.: *Bureaucracy and Accountability: Indian Journal of Public Administration*, Vol. XXIX, No. 3, July-Sept., 1983.

Sethi, J.D. 1978: *Gandhi Today*: Vikash Publishing House; Delhi, 1978.

Sethi, J.D.: *Health and Development—A New Focus*, *IJPA*, July-Sept, 1980, Vol. XXVI, No. 3.

Sinari, Dr. Ramakant: *The Culture of Peace and Gandhi's Commitment*, *Journal of Gandhian Studies*, Vol. 5, No. 21, Oct. 1978.

Singh, Dr. Deepa, (2002): *Human Rights and Police Predicament*; the Bright Law House, Delhi-110006.

Singh, M. Ibohal (2001): *Human Rights in India*, Vibhav Law Publications.

Singh, Nagendra (1981): *Human Rights and The Future of Mankind*: Varsity Books.

Singh, S. (1966): *A History of Political Thought*; Rastogi & Company, Meerut, 1966, pp. 280-320.

Sinha, Anil Kumar (2002): *Human Rights in Mahabharata,* Governance and Human Rights, edited by Bharat Jhunjhunwala, Kalpaz Publications; Delhi.

Sinha, Jadunath: *A Manual of Ethics*, New Central Book Agency, 8/1 Chintamoni Das Lane, Kolkata-700009.

Sharma, Gakulesh (2000): *Human Rights and Legal Remedies*; Deep & Deep Publication Pvt. Limited, New Delhi.

Sharma, P.D. article, Doughlas McGregor (2011): *Administrative Thinkers*, edited by D. Ravindra Prasad, V.S. Prasad, P. Satyanarayana and Y. Pardhasaradhi, Sterling Publisher, Delhi.

Sharma, P.D. (1979): *Secrecy Needs in Public Administration*: *Indian Journal of Public Administration*, October-December 1979, Vol. XXV; No. 4.

Sharma, Dr. S.K (1979): *Gandhi's Objectives and Development Styles*; Institute of Gandhian Thought and Peace Studies, Gandhi Bhawan, University of Allahabad, Allahabad, Vol. 7, October, No. 25.

Sharma, S.R. (1965): *The Soul of Indian History*: Bharatiya Vidya Bhawan, Sharma, M.L.: *Gandhi as a Socialist*, Deep & Deep Publications, New Delhi, 1980.

Srivastava, V.P. and R.S. Narayan (2002): *United Nations on Human Rights*; Vol. 1, 1st Edition 2002.

Stahl, O.G.: *Administrative Accountability*: *Indian Journal of Public Administration*, Vol. XXIX, No. 3, July-Sept., 1983.

Staub, E.: *Roots of Evil* (1993): *The Origin of Genocide and Other Group Violence*., New York, Cambridge University Press, Katz F., 1993.

Stimson, Gerry V.: *Interaction Between Patients and General Practitioners in the United Kingdom*: Institute of Psychiatry, London, England.

Study Report: A Study Report on Voluntary Efforts: Their Contribution and the Methodologies of People's Participation, sponsored by the Department of Rural Reconstruction, Ministry of Agriculture, Government of India in 1978. Referred in Gandhi Marg, *Journal of the Gandhi Peace Foundation,* 24 March, Sunanda Raj 1999; article, Awakening of Human Rights; published in the Book, "Human Rights in India" ed. By C.J. Nirmal, published by Institute of Indian and International Studies, Oxford University Press.

Tewari, A.P. (1976): *Gandhian Approach to Class Conflict and Property Relations*: Institute of Gandhian Thought and Peace Studies, Gandhi Bhawan, University of Allahabad, Allahabad, Vol. 3, April-July No. 11-12.

Tewari, A.P. (1983): *Gandhiji's Concept of an Ideal State*; Institute of Gandhian Thought and Peace Studies, Gandhi Bhawan, University of Allahabad, Allahabad, Vol. IV, July, No. 40.

Tripathi, Amrit Kumar: Intergenerational Differences in the Preferences for Family Values: An Indian Perspective, *Journal of Human Values*, Vol. 20, April 1, 2014.

Tiwari, Kedar Nath: *Comparative Religion*, Motilal Banarasi Dass, Delhi.

Urbano, Ryan C.: Public Administration Ethics: James Svara's Model, *Journal of Human Values*, Vol. 20, April 1, 2014.

The Assam Tribune, 8th October, 2014: Note (Eating white meat, fish may lower liver cancer risk: Washington: 7th Oct - eating lots of white meat such as poultry or fish may reduce the risk of developing liver cancer, scientists say.

Ibid., 8th Apr., 2014.

Ibid., 7th Nov., 2014.

Ibid., 28th Nov., 2013.

Researchers studied the relationship between meat intake and the risk of hepatocellular carcinoma (HCC).

They analyzed studies published between 1956 and 2013 and found that eating white meat or fish may reduce the risk of developing liver cancer by 31 per cent and 22 per cent respectively. Consuming red meat, processed meat, or total meat was not associated with the liver cancer risk.

"The present mega-analysis indicates that a high level of white meat or fish consumption can reduce the risk of HCC significantly, while intake of red meat, processed meat or total meat is not associated with HCC risk," researchers wrote in the study published in the *Journal of Alimentary Pharmacology and Therapeuticsgest* that dietary intervention may be a promising approach for prevention of HCC, which still need to be confirmed by further well-designed prospective studies and experimental research." *PTI.*

The Government of India: Swachchh Bharat Mission; Ministry of Urban Development, Ministry of Drinking Water & Sanitation, Ministry of Panchayati Raj; appeared in *The Assam Tribune*, 2nd October, 2014.

The Times of India, New Delhi, Tuesday, 20th August, 2013.

Treadwell, Donald and Jill B. Treadwell (2005): *Public Relations Writing*; Second edition, Response Books, A Division of Sage Publications, New Delhi, pp. 57-59.

Tripathi, Anil: *Gandhiji's Social Philosophy*: *Journal of Gandhian Studies*, Vol. 7, No. 28, July 1980, Gandhi Bhawan, University of Allahabad, Allahabad.

Tripathi, B.K.: *Gandhian Approach to Economic Development*: Institute of Gandhian Thought and Peace Studies, Gandhi Bhawan, University of Allahabad, Allahabad, Vol. 7, No. 25, October 1979.

Tyagi, A.R. (1989): *Public Administration*; Atma Ram & Sons.

Umapathy, N.: Herbert Simon, *Administrative Thinkers.*

Umarani, R.I. *Gandhiji's Asharam Vows and their Relevance for Contemporary Social Situation*: *Journal of Gandhian Studies:* Institute of Gandhian Thought and Peace Studies, Gandhi Bhawan, University of Allahabad, Allahabad, Vol. 12, Nos. 47-48, April-July, 1985.

UNDP Report, 2002: Deepening Democracy by Tackling Democratic Deficits: Human Development Report: 2002, UNDP.

Ibid., 2004, *Globalization and Cultural Choice.*

Veeranghavan, J., *Dharma: The Values that Sustain* (2007): ed. *Understanding India*, ed. by Subhash Chandra Kashyap and Abhaya Kashyap, Vitasta Publishing Ltd., New Delhi.

Verma, Dr. Surendra: *Modern Search for Peace*: *Journal of Gandhian Studies*, Vol. 5, No. 21, Oct., 1978.

Vij, D.R. 2000: article, United Nations Decade (1995-2004) For Human Rights Education: A Challenge and Opportunity for the Educators; *Human Rights: Global Perspective* edited by Hemlata Talesa, Nalini Pansholy and Mangi Lal Nagda; Rajasthan Council of Educational Administration and Management, Udaipur.

Wilson, Harold: *Text of Speech by the British Prime Minister*, the Rt. Hon. Harold Wilson, M.P.

World Health Forum. Vol. 17, 1996 (Seven advisers were 1. Professor Dimitri Barreto, 2. Professor Mohamed Larbi Bouguerra; 3. Mrs Barbar Kelly, 4. Dr Rainer Land; 5, Mr. Emmanuel Seyni Ndione; 6. Dr. Hiro Wakasugi and 7. Dr. Sergio Biros and Mr. Pierre Calame).

Index